THE MULTIPLE SCLEROSIS DIET BOOK

The Multiple Sclerosis Diet Book

A Low-Fat Diet for the Treatment of M.S.

ROY LAVER SWANK, M.D., Ph.D.
and
BARBARA BREWER DUGAN

DOUBLEDAY
NEW YORK LONDON TORONTO SYDNEY AUCKLAND

PUBLISHED BY DOUBLEDAY
a division of Bantam Doubleday Dell Publishing Group, Inc.
1540 Broadway, New York, New York 10036

THE MULTIPLE SCLEROSIS DIET BOOK is an extensively revised
edition of *The Swank Low-Fat Diet,* published in 1972
by Willamette Publishers, Beaverton, Oregon.

Library of Congress Cataloging-in-Publication Data
Swank, Roy L. (Roy Laver), 1909–
The multiple sclerosis diet book.
Bibliography: p. 365.
Includes index.
1. Multiple sclerosis—Diet therapy—Recipes.
2. Low-fat diet—Recipes. I. Dugan, Barbara Brewer.
II. Title. [DNLM: 1. Cookery. 2. Dietary Fats—
administration & dosage. 3. Multiple Sclerosis—diet
therapy. WL 360 S972m]
RC377.S94 1987 616.8'340654 86-16819

ISBN 0-385-23279-9

PRINTED IN THE UNITED STATES OF AMERICA

27 26 25 24

To Eulalia Swank, my wife

To Patricia Brewer, my sister

CONTENTS

SECTION V: RECIPES

INTRODUCTION

It has been thirty-six years since our investigations of multiple sclerosis (M.S.) were undertaken. The early history of the development of the low-fat diet therapy was described in the Introduction to the 1977 edition, which is included in this book following this introduction.

During this period, Dr. Roy Laver Swank has interrogated and examined about thirty-five hundred M.S. patients and maintained contact with approximately two thousand of them for ten to thirty-six years. Since his retirement as head of neurology in 1974 and the publication of the 1977 edition, research has continued. Studies of cerebral blood flow, a series of papers on the red-cell mobility test for diagnosis of M.S., papers describing abnormality of blood plasma in M.S., and a paper concerning the benefits derived by patients from infusion of normal blood plasma have been published. In addition, the statistical analysis of the Montreal patients who have been on the Swank low-fat diet for up to thirty-six years was completed. This new material has been integrated with the older material and is presented here in a manner we hope will be of help to both patients and their physicians.

This book describes methods by which patients with multiple sclerosis can take the best possible care of themselves. By following the precepts developed over the years, the great majority of patients can expect to remain free of disability for up to thirty-six years if these methods are initiated before disability has developed and are faithfully adhered to. If the treatment is started late, marked reduction in the frequency of exacerbations, increased stability, and slowing of deterioration can be expected.

It has been said that patients on the Swank low-fat diet prosper because it is basically a healthy diet. It is the opinion of the authors, however, that the very close relationship of the progress of the disease to the amount of fat intake, and the marked intolerance of the disease to animal and butterfat, argue for a direct relationship of the fat intake not only to the clinical course but also to the basic mechanism of the disease.

In this edition, we explore the early symptomatology of the disease, and we examine additional factors that influence the course of the disease and advise the treatment for them. The diet instructions have been made easier to master, new recipes have been added, and others have been removed. We offer suggestions for adhering to the diet while traveling abroad, as well as while eating in restaurants or at other peoples' houses. There are new sections on condiments and helpful cooking aids for disabled patients. And we explore the relationship of traumatic and psychological stress to multiple sclerosis and recommend treatment for this.

A chapter on the use of the Swank low-fat diet in the treatment of heart disease and stroke was included in the 1977 edition. Although it has been deleted from this edition to focus attention on our main interest, M.S., we still advise the diet for treatment of these vascular diseases. The diet is easy to learn and is well tolerated. In addition, it reduces blood cholesterol concentrations, in most patients to very low levels (133),* and by reducing both blood viscosity (134) and aggregation of blood cells (see Chapter 9) it increases circulation.

Roy Laver Swank, M.D., Ph.D.
Barbara Brewer Dugan

* Numbers in parentheses throughout this book, both in the text and in the figure captions, refer to the Bibliography.

INTRODUCTION TO THE 1977 EDITION

To immerse oneself completely in research of a single disease is unusual, but in August 1948 Dr. Wilder Penfield, then director of the Montreal Neurological Institute, invited me to Montreal to undertake studies of multiple sclerosis. My knowledge of multiple sclerosis changed rapidly as I interviewed and examined many patients at the clinic and spent hours in the library. Three useful clues to the disease came to light. First, in many cases relapses occurred quite suddenly, suggesting a vascular cause. Second, the neurological literature suggested that the frequency of the condition varied geographically. Third, post–World War II nutritional studies revealed a marked variation in fat consumption in different parts of the world, suggesting a possible correlation between high-fat intake and a high frequency of multiple sclerosis.

We began to place patients with multiple sclerosis at the institute on the low-fat diet in December 1948. The diet was closely supervised until 1954, when I moved to the University of Oregon Medical School in Portland. The Montreal patients were then checked frequently by mail and by a yearly visit to Canada until October 1974. Communications continued to remain open, but the patients did so well that only occasionally did one need help. This was taken care of by telephone or letter. Since moving to Portland, I have seen and treated many new patients, but they have not been added to the original study group in Montreal, now under observation for twenty-nine years.*

* Thirty-five years as of November 1984.

In addition to following closely the progress of our multiple sclerosis patients, we pursued other related studies over the years. At first these were epidemiological, to determine if wartime deprivations of food in Europe had altered the frequency of multiple sclerosis (9), and if the natural geographic variations of the disease that we had observed in Norway could be explained by difference in food intakes (10). Other studies of nutrition and blood viscosity were carried out later in Tokyo, Japan; Mesina, Italy; and Israel; as well as in Portland, Oregon.

In the laboratory it was shown that high-fat meals caused the blood cells to aggregate or clump (97), seeming thus to obstruct the circulation (98), reduce the oxygen supply to tissues (102), and alter the function of the brain, heart, and other organs (103, 104). This led to the observation that paraffin particles (emboli), about the size of aggregates, introduced into the bloodstream produced demyelinated lesions in the brain not unlike those seen in multiple sclerosis, and also scattered focal breakdown of the blood-brain barrier (75, 78, 79). Larger particles caused lesions of a more destructive type in the gray matter. Meanwhile we studied the blood protein changes in patients with multiple sclerosis and the effects of fat meals on blood plasma proteins (121, 122, 123).

Because of the observation that fat meals lead to the clumping of red cells in animals and man, and that similar clumping occurs in patients with multiple sclerosis, an instrument known as the screen filtration pressure machine was developed for measuring the presence in the blood of aggregated blood elements. By accident, this led to the discovery of aggregated platelets and leukocytes in blood that had been stored for transfusion, and to aggregates composed of the same blood elements during very low blood pressure that resulted from rapid bleeding (135, 136). These studies were done first on animals but were later confirmed elsewhere on humans at the time of the Vietnam war. These aggregates were sufficiently large and numerous to obstruct the smaller blood vessels and cause pathological and physiological abnormalities.

By chance, it was found that these aggregates could be removed by passing blood through a layer of polyester wool (135). In 1961 during a sabbatical leave to the University of Cologne in Germany, we were able to show that removal of these aggregates from the blood by filtration improved the circulation, the metabolism, and the function of perfused isolated organs. A polyester wool filter for the heart-lung machine used during cardiovascular surgery was the next step, followed by the transfusion filter. Both filters have been very extensively tested on both animals and humans; the results of these tests indicate that removal of the aggregates from circulating blood tends to normalize the blood flow, allow maintenance of normal oxygen and carbon dioxide contents in blood, and minimize tissue damage. Needless to say, many patients have benefited.

In recent years we have concentrated on the nature of the destruction of small blood vessels and surrounding tissues that is produced by these platelet-leukocyte emboli. The emboli not only block blood vessels, but they also erode away the blood vessel inner lining (endothelium) and destroy the surrounding tissues, primarily in the lung, and also in the kidney, liver, and brain (110, 111). When the emboli are removed by filtration, these deleterious changes do not occur.

Present studies of the amount of blood circulation in the brain of patients with multiple sclerosis and stroke in comparison to normal subjects will soon be finished.* Our next interest will center on the nature of the surface membranes of the cellular elements in the circulating blood.

These efforts have been directed to explaining the lesions of multiple sclerosis, as well as heart disease and stroke, on a vascular basis due to embolic occlusion of blood vessels by aggregated blood cells. These studies are reviewed in this book along with the work of many other researchers to give the reader an opportunity to view the results and possible progress in this field. Our patients wanted not only to participate in our studies, but understandably also to know what was happening in our research. One of the aims of this book is to make this knowledge available to many more patients, their friends, and their relatives.

Obviously, many scientists have helped in the individual studies, as shown by the co-authors listed in the Bibliography. The final form of the diet and the many recipes have been developed over the years with the able help of a number of research assistants as well as by interested patients and their families. Among the former were Miss Eddy, a dietitian from the Royal Victoria Hospital, who helped to work out the mechanics of the diet in 1948 and 1949. She was followed by Aagot Grimsgaard, who accumulated the recipes for the first publication in 1958, which she co-authored. Aagot's dogged determination kept many patients on the diet early in the experimental period before its benefits had become known. She and Kathleen H. Prichard, who started with us in 1962, worked in the laboratory and were valuable contributors to our research efforts. Kathleen Prichard

* This material has been published. See the Bibliography (81).

with Mary-Helen Pullen co-authored the 1972 edition of the diet book. The 1977 edition was co-authored by Mary-Helen, who has been associated with our work since 1969.

It has been our intent through the years to give the patient a more complete understanding of multiple sclerosis, its history, nature, and possible causes as well as therapy. In addition, we would like to bring into stronger focus the rationale for the use of low-fat diets, and especially the Swank low-fat diet, in heart disease and stroke.

It will seem to many people accustomed to a high-protein and high-fat diet that the very low fat allowance in this book demands considerable self-discipline and ingenuity. However, the diet has proven easy to learn and follow after an original adjustment period of several months. Approximately two thousand patients have done just that for up to twenty-nine years with very good results. Although the diet was experimental for the first years, during which time patients had to be urged to stay on it and closely checked to see that they did, in recent years the patients have been very receptive to dietary management. Those on the diet for many years know its value. Those seen more recently, most of whom come from all over the United States and Canada, have been encouraged by the success reported to them by other patients, and they consequently are easily started and maintained on the diet.

We offer the low-fat diet to those with multiple sclerosis, heart disease, or stroke with the belief that it will benefit them. For others we suggest it as a means of enriching their lives through increased energy and quite possibly increased longevity.

Roy Laver Swank, M.D., Ph.D.

Portland, Oregon
May 1976

THE MULTIPLE SCLEROSIS DIET BOOK

Section I

PERSPECTIVE

CHAPTER 1

A Legacy of Fats and Oils

The diagnosis of a disabling disease necessitates a considerable reassessment of one's life and goals, as well as an adjustment of everyday patterns of living. If the diagnosis is made shortly after onset of the disease, as it usually is with heart disease and stroke, the patient soon develops a sense of security in the knowledge that he or she will at least have some positive guidance, and that all known therapeutic agents will be made available. On the other hand, if several years elapse between the onset of the disease and the formulation of a diagnosis, as frequently happens in multiple sclerosis, the patient usually experiences severe frustrations and anxieties. As the symptoms wax and wane, he or she comes to believe that the physicians (and there may be many) are either incompetent or are withholding the diagnosis. It is only natural that the patient imagines all sorts of horrible things and that anxiety and even agitation may result. When the diagnosis of multiple sclerosis is finally made, the patient experiences a sense of relief. He or she can now make plans for the future and is able to seek more expert guidance.

To obtain maximum benefit from treatment, we advocate its application as early as possible. In multiple sclerosis this is while the symptoms are transient, in heart disease and stroke before a major disabling attack. A change of life style from a diet of high-fat foods to one with low-saturated fats and an increase in polyunsaturated oils is strongly recommended. This should be accompanied by adequate rest, a reduction of stress, and the adoption of a mental attitude that fosters optimism and a determination to live a satisfying life within the limitations of the disease. The goal of the multiple sclerosis patient is to reduce the attacks and promote a state of remission that will add years of fruitful activity to his or her life. It is our belief that the Swank low-fat diet plays a major role in accomplishing this.

During the past thirty-six years, we have collected a wide variety of recipes to assist the dieters in decreasing the saturated fats and increasing the unsaturated oils in their diets. These recipes have been home-tested so that patients and their families may enjoy nutritious and diversified food. These recipes, along with everyday menus and additional chapters covering different aspects of life, including suggestions for eating out and traveling, make up a large portion of this book.

The Swank diet is not a new treatment. Our ancestors ate much less fat than we do, both for economic reasons and because it simply was not available. Today many have returned to this more natural diet for reasons of health. Another aspect of the Swank low-fat diet is the elimination of various types of canned, frozen, or processed foods unknown to previous generations. These foods are too often the mainstay of teenage diets and snack foods for everyone. They are aptly termed junk foods. It is impossible to gauge accurately the amount of fat or oil contained in these foods, and eating them adds unwanted fats to a measured diet while adding calories of questionable nutritional value.

For the average person, accustomed since childhood to a high-fat intake involving large quantities of whole milk, butter, and meat, this diet will constitute not only a new way of eating but a new way of living—more healthfully, happily, and energetically.

CHAPTER 2

Dietary Fat—Past, Present, and Future:

Its Relationship to Multiple Sclerosis and to Heart Disease and Stroke

One result of our rising prosperity and higher standard of living has been an increased consumption of animal fat and butterfat. Until about two hundred years ago, the fat intake of our Western ancestors was probably about 60 grams (two ounces) daily, and much of this fat was contained in vegetable and fish oils (1). The development of pasteurization, refrigeration, and rapid transportation; the improvement of dairy herds (with a corresponding increase in the butterfat content of milk); and the fattening of beef cattle in feeding pens have all contributed to a steady increase in the amount of our daily animal and butterfat intake. Vegetable oils, formerly used in their natural state, have been processed into margarine and shortening and consequently have taken on the character of animal fat.

In 1909, when the average amount of fat available for consumption in the United States was first recorded, the amount per person was 125 grams (four ounces) daily. As a result of technological advances, it had risen to 141 grams by 1948, 13 percent for the thirty-nine-year period (2), or an increase of about 0.33 percent each year. Other technologically advanced nations had shown similar increases by that time (3). Canada had a daily fat supply per person of 132 grams; Denmark, 129 grams; and England, 97 grams. On the other hand, Italy had 50 grams; Cuba, 60 grams; China, 38 grams; India, 27 grams; and Japan, 14 grams. Further increases in fat availability have occurred since 1948 in the high-fat-consuming areas and among the low-fat-consuming urban dwellers in Japan. In the United States, fat consumption had increased to 150 grams by about 1972, a rate increase since 1948 of about 0.26 percent per year. Available evidence would suggest a faster rate of increase in the high-fat-consuming countries of Western Europe.

It should be kept in mind, however, that the actual consumption of food is less than the amount purchased at the retail market. This is particularly true of those countries, such as the United States and Canada, with an abundant nutrition. Since much of the purchased food, in particular bacon and meat fat, is discarded during food preparation, it is therefore possible to speak only of the prepreparation product. The estimate of lost or wasted food varies from 10 to 30 percent, the greatest loss being in the fats.

One probably can speak of relative changes in food intakes in the United States with greater accuracy (5). In the past sixty years, the daily total caloric intake per person has decreased, primarily because of a substantial decrease in carbohydrate intake. The calories available from fat, however, have steadily increased from 32 to 42, or to 44 percent of the total. The total protein intake has remained essentially unchanged, but the proteins of animal origin have increased from about one half to two thirds of the total with a corresponding decrease in the intake of proteins of vegetable origin to one third of the total. This shift in proteins from plant to animal origin has been partly responsible for the large and steady increase in fat intake. Furthermore, it has resulted in a shift from the relatively unsaturated vegetable oils to the more saturated fats. If this recent change is a continuation of a trend that began 150 to 200 years ago, a fat increase of two to three times is understandable.

Fat intake or consumption also can be expressed as a percentage of total caloric intake. The estimated 60 grams of fat consumed two hundred years ago produced 540 calories (9 calories per gram of fat). If we assume that the total caloric intake then was 3,500, about the same as that consumed per person in the United States in 1911, then fat furnished 15 to 16 percent of the daily calories. This is about the same percentage or slightly more than is consumed by most Orientals today. By 1911 fat consumption in the United States accounted for 32 percent of the total calorie intake; since then the figure has risen to about 42 to 44 percent.

Despite the decreased daily caloric intake, life insurance tables between 1941 and 1967 indicate a significant *increase* in weight of males of all heights and ages. This trend toward obesity was confirmed by studies of the general public in a National Health Examination Survey and in similar surveys by Selective Service examinations.

The explanation for this appears to be a reliance by man on power-driven substitutes for physical labor, high-fat foods consumed in fast-food restaurants, and the ever available food-dispensing coin machines.

From the standpoint of fat intake, the world can be divided into two areas (3): high-fat (the United States, Canada, northern Europe, and the British Isles), and low-fat (the Mediterranean area, Latin America and Caribbean countries, India, and the Middle and Far East). Israel is an exception in the Middle East. There the European Jews consume a relatively high-fat diet; the Yemenite Jews, a very low-fat diet. The fat intake of the remaining Oriental Jews is probably also low or moderate. People in the areas of high-fat intake have been consuming an ever-increasing amount of animal fat and butterfat.

This diversity in eating habits has not escaped the notice of anthropologists. They have observed that in Europe two parallel and little-mixed cultures based upon food have evolved. These are the "beer-butter" and "wine-oil" cultures. The first extends across northern Europe (Scandinavia, Germany, Holland, Belgium, northern France, northern Switzerland, and the British Isles) and has come to be the mode of life in the United States and Canada. The second predominates in the Mediterranean area (Spain, Italy, southern France, southern Switzerland, and Greece) and stretches to the Middle East and North Africa. The beer-butter culture corresponds geographically to the area of high incidence of multiple sclerosis and vascular disease; the wine-oil culture corresponds to the area where these conditions have a low incidence.

Until very recent times almost all peoples consumed only a small amount of fat, much of this in the form of vegetable and fish oils. Today approximately three fourths of the world population follows a similar diet, with ample evidence that this practice has not weakened human resolve or strength. Many great feats of physical endurance in history were accomplished by men who from infancy consumed a diet containing very little fat. The Egyptian and Mayan pyramids were constructed by laborers consuming a basic grain and vegetable diet. The great conquests of antiquity by Alexander and his Macedonians, who frequently marched fifty miles a day before going into battle, and the conquest of the Mediterranean countries by the Romans, were accomplished by men who ate chiefly grains, fruits, and vegetables washed down with wine. Caesar's legions complained when they had too much meat, preferring to do their fighting on a basic diet of corn and other grains (7). They walked to battle, marching from one end of the known world to the other.

In our own times, a number of champion distance runners have followed a basic vegetable-cereal diet supplemented by milk and a few eggs. We also read about the Hunzas, who remain physically very active until 80 or 90 years of age (and many live to be 120) (6). These people are locked in an isolated valley of the Himalayan mountains and depend entirely upon their valley for food. Their diet consists of vegetables and cereals, very little meat, no fish, some goat milk, and goat cheese. For a beverage they drink wine in moderate amounts. They have unexcelled energy and endurance and experience very good health. Of further support for our developing thesis, scientists have shown that the energy to be derived from carbohydrates is significantly greater and more easily available than from fats or proteins (see Chapter 10).

Today in the predominantly high-fat-consuming Western world, the story is different. While much of the world's population exists on a near-starvation diet, nutritionists estimate that more than 50 percent of Americans are overweight, many of them suffering the health hazards and discomforts of obesity.

As peoples' intake of fat increased, at least two diseases increased in frequency. One of these, multiple sclerosis, is a relatively uncommon disorder, but it produces a degree of disability and socioeconomic havoc out of proportion to its frequency because of the time of onset and its long duration. The geographic distribution of multiple sclerosis has been of interest to neurologists since before the beginning of this century. The early hypotheses on the possible connection between the prevalence of multiple sclerosis and geographic location were based on the relative numbers of multiple sclerosis patients admitted to hospitals and clinics in different parts of the world. The first formal geographic distribution study, and incidentally one of the more valuable to date, was done in Switzerland between 1918 and 1922 (8). It showed a high prevalence of multiple sclerosis in the northern, German-speaking part of Switzerland (up to 1/1,000 of the population). In the southern, Italian-speaking area, there were very few cases (0 to 0.1/1,000 of the population). In the western, French-speaking area, the prevalence of multiple sclerosis fell between that in the German- and Italian-speaking areas. Available evidence pointed toward a correlation of these differences in frequency of multiple sclerosis with the fat intake. The German-speaking, northern Swiss were known to consume a large amount of fat of animal origin; the southern, Italian-speaking Swiss followed a low-fat diet much like that of the Italians. The French-speaking Swiss were believed to consume a diet somewhat intermediate between the two (9, 50).

A similar study of Norway in 1949 recorded all new cases that developed between 1935 and 1948 (10). Not only the prevalence

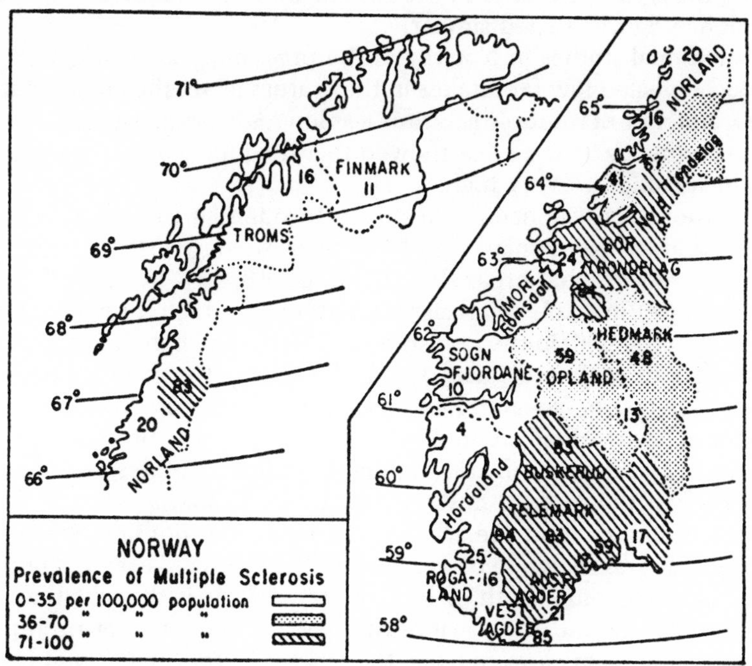

Figure 1. The prevalence of multiple sclerosis in Norway in 1948. The numbers indicate cases per 100,000 population. Note the low prevalence (0–35/100,000) along the coast, the high prevalence (71–100/100,000) in the inland mountainous areas, and intermediate rate (36–70/100,000) in the more level inland farming areas. Rates listed were for rural populations, but in the cities the rates were similar to the surrounding rural areas (10). From Roy L. Swank, *A Biochemical Basis of Multiple Sclerosis.* Charles C. Thomas, Publisher, 1961, p. 33, Springfield, Ill.

(number of cases) but also the incidence (number of new cases each year) were determined (see Figure 1). Along the entire Norwegian coast from 71° north latitude near the Arctic zone, south to the 58° latitude well inside the temperate zone, the prevalence of multiple sclerosis was low along the coast (0 to 35/100,000). The incidence was also very low. In inland farming areas the prevalence was high; especially so in the isolated mountainous areas where the population was relatively sparse (71–100/100,000), and moderately high in the more accessible farming areas (36–70/100,000). The ratio of the number of cases in central farming areas to those in coastal fishing areas was nearly 4 to 1. If one considered only mountainous farming areas, the numerical ratio to the coastal areas was about 8 to 1. The incidence figures varied similarly.

Nutritional studies in Norway in the pre– and post–World War II period revealed low-fat intakes in those areas along the coast where the frequency of multiple sclerosis was low. Additional studies in the high-frequency inland areas showed that the intake of fats of animal origin was high to very high.

Additional prevalence studies done throughout the world established that the frequency of multiple sclerosis varied significantly in different geographic areas (9, 10, 11, 12, 13, 14). In general, the frequency of multiple sclerosis was high to very high (prevalence of 50 to 200/100,000) in the industrialized West, which included northern and central United States, Canada, England, Germany, northern France, Belgium, Holland, Denmark, central Norway, Sweden, and northern Switzerland. A somewhat lower rate was present in the northern Mediterranean area and southern United States, and a very low rate in the Middle East, Africa, India, China, southeast Asia, Japan, Indonesia, and Mexico (11). In Japan the multiple sclerosis prevalence was shown to be very low both in the cold extreme north and warm extreme south of the country (17). It is thought that in South America and the Caribbean area the frequency of multiple sclerosis also is very low. In Israel the rate for European migrant Jews is high; for African-Asian migrants, low (12).

From studies by the Food and Agriculture Organization of the United Nations in 1948 (3), the fat available for consumption in those areas with a high frequency of multiple sclerosis was high—in general more than 100 grams per person daily. In those areas of low frequency of multiple sclerosis, the daily fat consumption per person was low to very low—in general fewer than 50 grams (see the table on the relationship between daily fat intake and multiple sclerosis). Based on these observations, in 1950 we suggested (9) that the frequency of multiple sclerosis was related to the amount of the daily consumption of animal fat and butterfat. Our studies in Norway (10) not only confirmed the possibility of this correlation, but also singled out animal fat and butterfat (saturated or hard fats) as the more harmful. The oils seemed to play much less of a role. This was borne out by the low frequency of multiple sclerosis among Eskimos and Laplanders in the north, who consume large amounts of highly unsaturated oil in the form of blubber and cod-liver oil, and among the Italians, who consume large quantities of olive oil.

In another survey, this time in Montreal, Canada (14), we found that the prevalence of multiple sclerosis was highest in the areas of best housing, and lowest where the housing was poor. This was true in both French- and English-speaking sections of the city. This did not seem to be a reflection of differences in medical care and diagnosis, since free clinics were readily available to people of lesser means. We knew, however, that poorer families generally consumed a high-cereal and low-fat and low-protein diet for reasons of economy. This survey also appeared to be consistent with the basic thesis that the frequency and severity of multiple sclerosis was related to the amount of the animal fat and butterfat intake.

A recent, more detailed study of the relations of nutrition to frequency of multiple sclerosis (15) confirmed that a strong correlation exists between fats of animal origin and the frequency of multiple sclerosis. Where much animal fat was consumed, the frequency of multiple sclerosis was high; where little animal fat was part of the diet, the frequency of this disease was low. Other studies in England (16, 18) showed that when an emulsion of sunflower seed oil containing 30 milliliters of the oil was taken daily in two equal doses, the exacerbation rate in multiple sclerosis patients was lower (.54 relapses/year) than when an equal amount of an emulsion of olive oil containing 9 milliliters of the oil was taken by another group of patients (.76 relapses/year). The investigators concluded that the slight drop in relapse rate in the sunflower-oil-treated patients was due to its high content of essential fatty acid (linoleic acid). Other similar studies were grouped and analyzed statistically. They confirmed that the addition of linoleic acid to the diet did reduce the frequency of relapses of the disease (18). Unfortunately, no record was kept of other foodstuffs, including animal fats and butterfats consumed by the patients. We have observed that when oil is added to the diet of patients with multiple sclerosis they automatically choose to reduce their intake of saturated animal fat. The amount of reduction varies directly with the amount of added oil, as is shown in Figure 8. The sunflower-oil group would be expected to reduce their fat intake 30 to 60 grams; the olive-oil group, by perhaps 10 to 20 grams. The reduction in exacerbation rates would be substantially greater in those patients receiving the greater amount of oil.

Based on our Norwegian studies and the observations in Switzerland and elsewhere, we have illustrated what we consider the probable relationship of the prevalence rate of multiple sclerosis to the

RELATIONSHIP OF DAILY FAT INTAKE
TO PREVALENCE OF MULTIPLE SCLEROSIS

High Prevalence Countries	Daily Fat Intake	Low Prevalence Countries	Daily Fat Intake
U.S.A.	120.9	Cuba	48.6
Canada	118.3	Italy	60.0
British Isles	122.5	South Africa	49.9
Norway	118.0	China	40.1
Denmark	150.8	Japan	24.5
Sweden	116.0	Mexico	42.9
Netherlands	114.7	Turkey	46.8
Germany	111.4	Brazil	51.7
Switzerland	104.7	Romania	52.7

grams of animal fat and butterfat eaten daily (see Figure 2). The highest rate recorded to date is 2/1,000 population in several northern areas of the United States and in northern Switzerland where the fat intake is very high. These rates apply only to readily diagnosed cases.

A graph for frequency of death from heart disease related to fat intake is also shown in Figure 2.

* * *

In contrast to multiple sclerosis, which has a relatively low prevalence, vascular disease (heart disease and stroke) has become highly prevalent, and in recent years has been the cause of approximately 50 percent of deaths in the United States. Heart disease and stroke are due to hardening of the arteries (arteriosclerosis), a normal accompaniment of old age. But the degree to which arteriosclerosis is present in our Western civilization, due to the superimposition of atherosclerosis, is unique and worrisome. It is generally believed the condition is increasing in severity and prevalence. Fortunately, the public is increasingly aware of and concerned with the problem—no one can ignore a disease that will kill approximately one of every two Americans living today!

Several observations during World War II helped to focus the attention of American investigators on the relationship of various diets to atherosclerosis and heart disease. A large number of young Ameri-

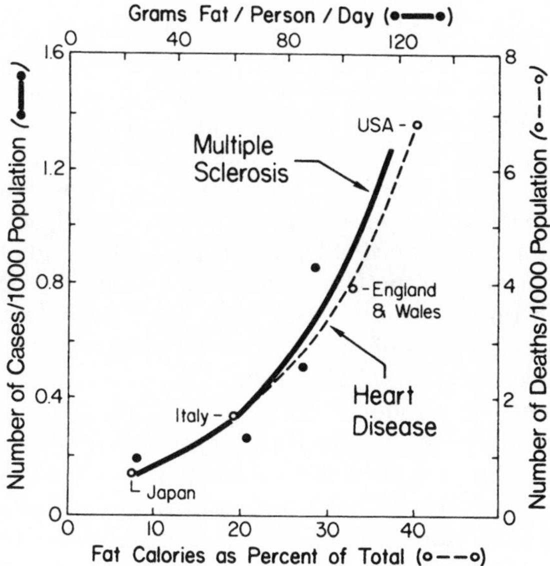

Figure 2. An increase in the grams of fat consumed (milk and animal fat) accompanied by an increase in the prevalence of multiple sclerosis (solid line). Also, the percentage of calories from fat directly correlates with the number of deaths per 1,000 population from heart disease in different geographic areas (broken line). The relationship of heart deaths to animal fat consumption is taken from Ancel Keys and Joseph Anderson (23, 24).

can servicemen died of heart attacks (myocardial infarctions) under the stress of military training and combat. At the same time, in contrast with marked vascular changes that were observed in young American troops, pathologists were finding very little atherosclerosis at postmortem examinations in the arteries of Okinawans and other Orientals of all ages killed during the war (19). These observations were confirmed in Korea (20) and still later in Vietnam. Whereas the Orientals' diet had contained very little fat (20 to 30 grams daily) and consisted mainly of vegetables and cereals, by cultural tradition the American troops had grown up on a high-fat diet (approximately 140 grams daily), the result of a liberal supply of meat, butter, eggs, and so on.

During the World War II period, the fat consumption in Norway was reduced about 50 percent due to food shortages (21, 22). Concurrently, there were significant reductions in the death rates from heart diseases and other occlusive vascular diseases. After the war both the fat intake and death rate from vascular disease returned to the prewar level. The rate of multiple sclerosis was similarly affected (10).

Because of these war-related observations, an intensive international effort began to relate differences in geographic distribution of heart disease to diet (23, 24). The studies over several years revealed that as the fat intake increased in different geographic areas there was a corresponding increase in the mortality rates from heart disease (see Figure 2). Somewhat later, a collaborative study by investigators in England and the United States also showed a significantly higher death rate from heart attacks in ulcer patients whose diet included large amounts of milk and cream compared to those who did not receive this kind of treatment (25).

More recently a number of controlled clinical studies have suggested substantial benefits to heart patients as a result of a low-fat diet (26). Some results have been judged inconclusive, but nowhere has the diet been detrimental. Although the experiments have varied considerably as to composition of the diet, duration of the test, and criteria of improvement, a general consensus is developing that a diet with reduced saturated fats and the addition of unsaturated oils benefits patients with heart disease. The composition of the diet that will render maximum benefit to patients and the stage or point in the disease that diet must be started still needs clarification.

* * *

The apparent similarities of the relationship of prevalence of both multiple sclerosis and heart disease to the consumption of fat (see Figure 2) would suggest basic similarities in the two conditions. However, this is obviously not the case, since the clinical histories and findings at examination, ages of onset of the diseases, and neuropathological findings are so different.

* * *

What is the future of dietary fat? There are reasons to suspect that its consumption is at or near its zenith and will decrease in the not too distant future. At present in most of the Western world we are able to raise enough food to supply our needs. This will continue until our population growth is such that the demand for food exceeds the supply. At that point, the fat in our diet will begin to decrease because less fat will be produced. This has already started. The sale of red meat has decreased and many ranchers have been hurt by this. Still, the extent of this trend has yet to be determined.

The production of animal proteins and fats requires several times the acreage needed to produce the same number of calories from carbohydrates. When cattle are fattened in feeding pens, an even greater amount of acreage is necessary to grow the needed cereal grains and corn. When the population pressure becomes great, the increasingly valuable land will be devoted to the production of economical foods such as cereals; less and less land will be used for grazing of beef cattle and dairy herds. Economics will force the substitution of vegetables and cereals for fats and animal proteins in our daily diet.

In the overcrowded Orient, this shift to a predominantly vegetable and cereal diet probably occurred many centuries ago as the forest disappeared, population density increased, and available good farmland became scarce. Although it will be slow, a similar change undoubtedly will occur in our country. Technological advances can delay this trend for only a few years.

There have been various estimates of the time when the population of the United States will exceed the ability of the soil to satisfy the demands of our present diet. The recent trend toward zero-population growth in this country suggests that shortages of foodstuffs by themselves will not dictate our eating habits in the foreseeable future. Weather changes, however, could alter this prediction. A shift to a vegetable-cereal economy probably will occur for health and international economic reasons. This transition has already begun, precipitated in part by the recent energy crisis and because we have chosen to supply food to the "have-nots" of the world. We can continue to produce agricultural products in excess; they are resources like trees, which by careful nurturing will never be depleted. These resources are in short supply in most of the world and can be exchanged to advantage for other diminishing necessities such as oil. To get the most from our forests and farmlands, changing to a vegetable-cereal-based diet now would be advantageous; in time, it may be necessary.

It should be remembered that history, both ancient and recent, bears out the fact that people are generally healthier on a low-fat diet. Gluttony and chronic degenerative disease have been linked in the minds of both laymen and scientists for many years. The saying "You dig your own grave with your teeth" has been around for a long time. In the prosperous areas of the Western world during the past few decades, the maxim applies to a majority of the population, not to just a few as it did in former years. It is only in modern times that our bodies have harbored so many degenerative diseases—and the physician has become so important.

If our theories concerning the importance of fat in the causation of degenerative diseases are correct, we can expect that these ailments will become less prevalent as we change to a cereal diet. But this does not mean that economics and population growth will solve all multiple sclerosis, heart disease, and stroke problems. Possibly, as we change to a vegetable-cereal diet, stresses will develop in other metabolic weak spots in the human body and new dietary difficulties will replace the old. This will depend to a large extent upon the ways in which we grow and process our food in the future, a worthwhile challenge to the American farmer and to the food-processing and energy industries (see Chapter 10).

Section II

MULTIPLE SCLEROSIS

CHAPTER 3

Multiple Sclerosis: History's Latecomer

The clinical features and pathology of multiple sclerosis appear not to have been recognized or described by ancient or medieval physicians. The earliest case history is found in the diary of Augustus d'Este, written in the beginning of the nineteenth century. At the age of twenty-eight, d'Este suffered his first attack, followed by a complete remission. The subsequent periodic relapses with varying disabilities were so characteristic of multiple sclerosis that the modern physician could not avoid this diagnosis. Yet physicians at that time, and they were the best from England and the Continent, were apparently not familiar with the disease.

The recognition of multiple sclerosis as a medical entity dates from a series of pathological and clinical studies by French, English, and German scientists between 1835 and 1872 (14), which was followed by widespread familiarity with the disease in Europe around the turn of the century.

Comparable familiarity with the clinical and pathological features of multiple sclerosis appears to have been delayed in North America, probably until after World War I. This increased awareness led to recognition of the socioeconomic gravity of the disease and to a realization of the depth of our ignorance regarding its cause.

In the 1930s a surge of interest in multiple sclerosis was followed by the organization of national and local societies dedicated to its research and treatment. One natural, but not planned, by-product of raising funds by these societies was a dissemination of information about the disease. Known to a large segment of the medical profession by name alone, multiple sclerosis very rapidly became familiar to a surprisingly large number of the lay public, as evidenced by the frequent diagnosis of the disease by the patient or by family, friends, and neighbors in the process of referral to the physician. This familiarity has not contributed materially to a solution of the mystery of the grave malady, but it has stimulated interest into many of its facets.

One wonders if multiple sclerosis is actually, or only apparently, a disease of very recent times. Did it occur before the nineteenth century or was its occurrence so infrequent that it failed to be recognized? These questions have yet to be answered satisfactorily. It is difficult to believe that intelligent observers would fail to recognize a condition so striking in its clinical manifestations if it occurred in anything like its present form and high incidence. If multiple sclerosis is a disease of modern times, then it is important to ask if the disease has been and is continuing to increase in frequency. Certainly we are becoming more aware of its frequency because of familiarity with its clinical features. As we diagnose the disease in milder forms, the number of cases known to us, and the diseases' statistical prevalence in the population increases. This could mislead us to assume that the incidence of the disease is increasing.

A review in 1922 (27), including data from many sources, concluded that the average incidence of multiple sclerosis in the United States had increased in the previous twenty years. It could not be determined whether this was due to an increased occurrence of the disease, or to more accurate diagnosis or extension of the disease concept. In 1952 it was stated that the incidence of multiple sclerosis in Europe had doubled early in the twentieth century (28). Using mortality statistics, a report in 1950 (29) stated that deaths due to multiple sclerosis had steadily increased in Australia, Canada, and the United States during recent years. Hospital admission figures taken from the Montreal Neurological Institute annual reports showed a nearly 50 percent increase in the admission rate for multiple sclerosis from 1935 to 1958. These data are probably as reliable as any available for this period. The personnel of the Montreal Neurological Institute changed relatively little and it seems unlikely that diagnostic criteria changed significantly during this period (14).

These combined data indicate an increasing incidence of multiple sclerosis, but whether the increase is real, or it is our awareness of the disease and improved diagnosis, continues to be the question. We believe that until modern times multiple sclerosis did not occur or was very rare. In all probability some element or influence in the environment changed, or new elements emerged 150 to 200 years ago, that so altered the metabolism of man that the complex of symptoms that we have come to recognize as multiple sclerosis appeared, particularly in the Western world. It is our opinion, based on clinical observations and impressions, and upon meager objective data, that the incidence of the disease had increased remarkably by about 1950. Subsequent events are difficult to evaluate, but we feel that the incidence of the disease is still increasing. The nature of the causative factors and how the disease is established remain in large part unknown, but they are being extensively investigated at present. Some facts, however, are known, some of which we will discuss in subsequent chapters.

CHAPTER 4

Multiple Sclerosis: General Information

Personal Characteristics

With few exceptions multiple sclerosis patients before becoming disabled are active, energetic, and highly productive. Generally they are intelligent and vital individuals. Physically they are of average height and weight, and athletic in build and inclination. They are usually attractive. They are nervous (tense) and perceptive. As the disease progresses, the "inbuilt" nervous tension increases and they become irritable. They rarely lose their inclination to work and produce unless severely disabled. In general, they become very well informed about their disease through reading and discussions with one another. It is, therefore, very difficult if not impossible to keep information concerning their disease from them. These characteristics are so frequently observed in the multiple sclerosis patient that their absence in the early phase of the disease should cause one to reexamine the history for clues to another diagnosis.

Most patients have cold feet and hands, and they are often cold in a warm room. Some may also have spells of being overheated and many experience night sweats. They bruise easily and often suffer from multiple subcutaneous hemorrhages for no known reason.

Effects of Stress

Patients with established multiple sclerosis withstand both psychological and physical stress poorly. In the face of anxiety or nervous tension, whatever the cause, patients note fatigue and a reduced ability to perform. The news of a death in the family, continuing domestic and marital difficulties, loss or threatened loss of the means of financial support, and accidents of a frightening nature are frequently followed by increased disability. Totally new symptoms are not produced by these stimuli as a rule, but exacerbation of existing systems is common. Such aggravations may last a short time and pass completely. Sometimes the additional disability is prolonged or permanent. Physical stress and/or fatigue, particularly when deep and prolonged, whether from work or exercise, are equally deleterious to patients. Probably a combination of the above stresses explains the high frequency of deep fatigue, particularly in mothers of children, following Christmas each year and extending well into January.

Intolerance to Heat

Patients with multiple sclerosis also have a very low tolerance for heat (30, 31). The onset of warm, humid weather, or a hot bath, leaves many patients with marked fatigue and increased disability that is usually temporary but can be permanent. Total immersion of the patient or immersion of an extremity in hot water is followed by an elevation of skin temperature of nonimmersed as well as immersed parts of the body, and subsequently by fatigue and increased neurological disability. A tourniquet on the immersed extremity to prevent blood from circulating to and from the immersed part of the body is said to prevent this. Immersion of subjects in cold water while they are still suffering the effects of earlier immersion in hot water may quickly remove the disability. We have patients who report marked, though temporary, improvement after a cold bath or a swim in cold water. Recent studies have shown that the temporary improvement of the patient upon cooling occurs if there is a drop in body temperature of at least 0.6° F to 1.2° F. We feel this degree of temperature change is not always necessary since we often observe improvement in patients who have had *only* their hands in cold water for a few minutes.

Intolerance to Weather Changes

Our studies have shown that about 5 percent of attacks occurred several days after a weather temperature change of more than 20° F upward or downward in a single day (32). These attacks were usually not severe. The absolute temperature, wind velocity or direction, precipitation, amount of sunshine, barometric pressure, and other factors seemed not to influence the disease. Temperature fluctuations (commonplace in the north temperate zone) are probably the reason for the seasonal variation in the well-being of multiple sclerosis patients twice a year, usually during October and November, and again in April and May. At these times of changing weather, patients experience more than the expected number of exacerbations, fluctuations, or fatigue spells.

Seizures

Grand mal seizures are rarely seen in multiple sclerosis. In our own cases they have occurred in about 3/1,000 patients. However, mild focal seizures of short duration and short confusional or "absence"-type seizures have occurred in well over 5 percent of our patients. These seizures keep recurring, sometimes frequently, for three to six months, then disappear. In most cases they are completely controlled by therapy with Dilantin. In some cases phenobarbital has been effective. Antiseizure therapy usually can be discontinued slowly after six months without recurrence of the seizures. Electroencephalograms have not been helpful in recognizing these brief seizures.

Headaches/Migraines

Scintillating scotoma (focal impaired vision), with or without migraine headaches, nausea, and vomiting have been observed frequently. These symptoms were recorded in eight (10 percent) of eighty consecutive new patients seen during the first half of 1975. On treatment of multiple sclerosis with the low-fat diet, these headaches usually become much less frequent and less severe, and they often disappear after one or two years. Headaches from tension, starting usually in the back of the head and neck and radiating to the back of one or both eyes, also occur and are usually relieved by mild sedation and the reassurance that comes as the patient improves.

Blood Pressure/Hypertension/Diabetes/ Hypo- and Hyperthyroidism

Hypertension is rare, most patients having decidedly low blood pressure. Diabetes has been a rare complication, although it is common for multiple sclerosis patients to have a slightly elevated blood sugar curve (but not abnormally elevated). There seems to be a tendency for a family history of diabetes. Both hypo- and hyperthyroidism are rare. Because of the patient's weakness, a clinical diagnosis of hypothyroidism is often made early but is not supported by laboratory evidence.

Sexual Problems

Partial or complete loss of potency in males, which cannot be alleviated by hormones, and a loss of sexual interest (drive) in females occurs, sometimes early, but usually later during disability. Irregular or absent menses in females is a frequent complication of multiple sclerosis. These symptoms may develop early or late and are usually accompanied by fatigue. In many cases, potency, sex drive, and normal menstruation return after recovering from the fatigue—usually after a long rest.

Genetic Considerations

Familial cases (presence of multiple sclerosis in one or more brothers or sisters of a patient) were not considered seriously until the early 1930s. It was then noted that a sibling of a multiple sclerosis patient was twenty times more likely to have the disease than someone not related to a patient. Subsequent studies in the late 1940s and 1950s (33, 34, 35, 36) and again in 1981 (37) found the familial incidence of multiple sclerosis to be about eighteen times greater than the occurrence of multiple sclerosis in the general population, and to involve second and third degree relatives (two and three generations removed) as well as first. Four to 6 percent of the patients' blood relatives were found to have the disease. The incidence in children of patients with multiple sclerosis may be slightly lower than that observed among brothers and sisters. From these observations it seems likely that genetic factors exert their influence on patients with multiple sclerosis. One should not forget, however, that members of families are subject to similar diets and other environmental influences. It is therefore possible that the suspected genetic factors are less important than they appear.

Extensive studies of multiple sclerosis patients with identical twins have revealed that in about 80 percent of them only one member of each pair developed multiple sclerosis. We have observed five such pairs of identical twins for up to twenty-six years, and only one of each pair has developed multiple sclerosis.

Wives and husbands of patients with multiple sclerosis have rarely developed the disease. In our own thirty-six-year experience with continued observation of more than two thousand cases for ten to thirty-six years, and a total experience of about thirty-five hundred cases, no husband or wife of a patient with multiple sclerosis has developed the disease, nor has any of their children. Keep in mind that we insist that the entire family be placed on the same low-fat diet whenever possible.

Racial Considerations

It is still not understood how or why racial differences influence the frequency of multiple sclerosis. The prevalence of the disease in greater New York City has been shown to be about the same for all racial groups (about 6/10,000) (38). One exception was a very low prevalence in poor blacks (1.4/10,000). This could be due to their tendency to consume more cereals and less meat and other fat foods than do more affluent segments of our population. However, one cannot dismiss a possible racial difference. Recently it was shown that Japanese Americans have a higher rate of multiple sclerosis than is known to occur in Japan (39). Even so, the frequency of cases among Japanese Americans is still well below that of Caucasians living in the same areas. Our observation of Japanese Americans in the Pacific Northwest is that they tend to consume a diet not totally different from the diet of their Japanese ancestors.

Latitudinal Influence

For many years it has been postulated that the frequency of multiple sclerosis was determined by latitude. The farther one lived from the equator, the nearer to the colder areas of the world, the greater the risk of acquiring the disease. A casual survey of the prevalence data would appear to bear this out. However, when analyzed carefully, several studies indicate that such a relationship is misleading.

The first of these in Switzerland (8) showed a change from very high to very low frequency of multiple sclerosis in the very short distance from northern to southern Switzerland (less than 1° latitude change). The second, in Norway (10), showed a very low frequency of multiple sclerosis along the entire coast from near the Arctic Circle south through 13° of latitude to well inside the temperate zone (see Figure 1). Another study in Japan (17) revealed the frequency of multiple sclerosis to be very low in two areas, one in the far northern part of the country and another in the near southernmost area. The northern area is relatively cold; the southern, warm. They are separated by 10° of latitude.

These particular observations indicate that latitude plays little if any part in the causation of multiple sclerosis or in its frequency of occurrence. This conclusion is supported by a recent statistical study of geography and nutrition in relation to multiple sclerosis (15).

Frequency of Multiple Sclerosis in Males and Females

In our Norwegian study (10), the new cases of multiple sclerosis that developed each year were split evenly between males and females 1:1. However, this ratio could have been altered by the long duration of the disease (approximately twenty-five years), and because the disease usually treats males less kindly than females. As a result there are present in the multiple sclerosis population more females than males in the ratio of about 3:2. This is probably related to the greater stress to which males are subjected, plus less opportunity to rest when fatigued. This difference in prevalence (number of cases present in the population) of multiple sclerosis is reflected in our thirty-six-year study of the disease.

Intolerance of Alcohol

Patients have a greatly reduced tolerance to alcohol. Many seem to be less tolerant of wine than of beer, whiskey, and other similar spirits. In general, our patients tolerated about 50 percent as much alcohol as they did before the onset of the disease. Thus, if a patient could readily drink and tolerate about four cocktails before, his tolerance after onset of the disease would be two cocktails.

This intolerance to alcohol could be related in part to the low-fat diet. The diet increases the motility of the gastrointestinal tract so that the alcohol would be absorbed more rapidly than normal. Although this may be a factor, we find other reasons to suspect a general intolerance to alcohol. For example, many patients are markedly affected by small doses of sedatives and antidepressants. Perhaps the increased porosity of the blood-brain barrier permits a rapid passage of sedatives, including alcohol, to the brain.

The basic fact remains that patients are intolerant of alcohol, and many suffer unusually severe hangovers after consuming relatively small amounts of it.

Nicotine/Marijuana/Caffeine

Some of our early studies suggested that smokers tended to deteriorate faster than nonsmokers. The differences were not great and lacked satisfactory statistical significance. However, both temporal vision and balance were found to be almost immediately depressed by smoking, the effect lasting for about one hour. The flicker-fusion scores in ten of twelve subjects and balance scores in four of ten subjects deteriorated within ten minutes of starting to smoke (42, 43). Repeating the test after recovery, one hour later, resulted in similar results. Although recovery did occur, it seems likely that repeated insults of this type would cause additional damage to the nervous system.

Marijuana has been hailed in the press as beneficial to multiple sclerosis patients. Our experience confirms the general opinion that the drug serves to calm the patient and puts aside his or her anxieties, but in the long run it appears to cause a breakdown or perversion of the personality. The few patients we have followed become irresponsible and shiftless, which could be due in part to the underlying M.S.

Also, vision may have been harmed, since after discontinuing the use of the drug temporal vision (flicker-fusion) improved.

The use of caffeine in coffee, tea, and soft drinks has been discouraged because it often causes or increases nervousness and anxiety in patients. This tends to intensify symptoms and signs of the disease and in some patients, causes greater difficulty in personal relationships and in the ability to perform physical and mental tasks. This is an opinion based on many cases. When it is recognized, deleting or reducing caffeine in the diet relaxes and improves the patient's performance.

Memory and Mentally Related Functions

Impairment of memory, primarily for recent events, develops in many patients slowly and insidiously. The degree of loss usually parallels the general neurological involvement, but may be more or less severe. Later in the disease memory loss may interfere with function and judgment in some patients. Stress, anxiety, fatigue, fever, and overheating usually intensify the memory loss and often lead to mild to severe confusion that is temporary but may be sufficient to interfere with work or schooling. Patients may experience temporary confusion of varying degrees during an exacerbation, even if they have not experienced stress or fatigue.

Age of Onset of Multiple Sclerosis

Multiple Sclerosis is considered a disease of young adults. About 85 percent of cases have their first neurological symptoms between the ages of twenty and thirty-five, although a diagnosis may be delayed for years. Most of the remaining cases develop before the age of fifty, but an onset in the fifties or even the sixties is not outside our experience. Less than 1 percent of our cases have had onset between the ages of fifteen and twenty, and we have rarely seen cases with earlier onsets.

CHAPTER 5

Multiple Sclerosis: The Clinical Picture

The diagnosis of multiple sclerosis should be made as early as possible and the low-fat diet started immediately. If the diet is continued, it will prevent disability in a majority of patients. Once permanent disability has developed, one can expect to do no more than "hold the line," or more likely to slow down the rate of progress of the disease. For these reasons this chapter is devoted to a description of *the unfolding of the clinical picture. Particular attention will be paid to the early symptoms.* We will consider three periods: the prodromal, early, and late phases of the disease.

The Prodromal Symptoms

The prodromal period is characterized by vague symptoms without clear-cut neurological signs. It is during this period that patients first consult their family physicians and for the first time are referred to a neurologist. Neither physician as a rule recognizes the significance of the symptoms and, judging from our experience, more than half of the patients with multiple sclerosis are at first considered to have a nonorganic psychiatric disease. At some point they may be referred to psychiatrists, who usually agree with the referring physicians' diagnosis. The patients are usually unhappy because their complaints are not taken seriously. Consequently, the advice of other physicians is sought. Repetition of this series of events results in frustration, anger, and resentment.

These very early symptoms are not specific for multiple sclerosis and develop as follows: an individual who formerly was very energetic and productive begins to suffer for no obvious reason from *periodic fatigue, difficulty sleeping,* and *nervousness.* Gradually this becomes accompanied by a general loss of strength and endurance, and occasionally by depression. The fatigue is precipitated by physical and even mental effort, and finally becomes continuous. It can only be partially relieved by prolonged rest, much of it in bed.

Many then notice sensitivity to the *heat* and *burn* of the *sun,* to *marked changes in ambient temperature,* to *hot baths,* to *fevers* from intercurrent infections, and to both physical and psychological *stress.*

Muscle aching and cramping, joint pains, and *diffuse slight weakness* of the extremities often develop during long walks, or after standing for long periods, in patients who formerly were energetic and athletic. These symptoms are usually most severe in cold or damp weather and are relieved as the weather moderates. The usual laboratory tests and X rays for arthritis are negative, yet the patients are considered to have, and many are treated for, arthritis.

Peculiar visual symptoms described by the patients as unclear or blurred vision, and periodic foggy vision, also occur in patients with normal full visual fields and normal visual acuity.

Sensory complaints that the patient describes as "peculiar feelings" lack objectivity and are not taken seriously by the examiner.

Finally, some patients complain of *deteriorating memory, cloudy mentation,* and occasionally of *confusion.*

All of these symptoms are usually periodic at first; only later do they become continuous. They are brought on by physical or psychological stress, hot weather, hot baths, exposure to sun, and intercurrent infections both with and without fever. They are not specific for multiple sclerosis since they may occur in other diseases, for example, hypoglycemia, hypothyroidism, hyperventilation, and middle ear disease.

Cold, pale hands and feet, periodic subcutaneous hemorrhages without obvious cause, and *often a pale, drawn face* during the periods of fatigue complete the picture.

These prodromal symptoms have come to light in the last ten years as we have interrogated and examined increasing numbers of patients in early phases of the disease. These symptoms do not lead to a diagnosis of multiple sclerosis and are often confusing. They finally merge with the more definite neurological symptoms in the early phase of the disease. It is of interest that in this stage of the disease the red-cell mobility test (see p. 39) often confirms the possible presence of multiple sclerosis.

Early Phase Symptoms

Fatigue is still the most persistent symptom. It may continue to be periodic. Following physical or psychological stress, it often becomes so severe that the patient is unable to do more than rest: the patient is exhausted. Generalized weakness and varying degrees of instability appear from time to time. Often *double vision* and *foggy vision* occur, both of which are transient. Lack of *mental clarity, memory loss,* and slight *confusion* may soon become obvious to the patient and to the family and friends. These symptoms usually clear in a few days and are usually missed by the examining physician. Tendon reflexes are apt to be slightly hyperactive, but *pathological reflexes* will usually be absent. The patient will describe areas of altered *sensations,* which the physician will not be able to confirm.

The patient frequently becomes *exhausted,* has a drawn, pale face, and/or may become increasingly *nervous and irritable,* unable to work for days, weeks, or months. He or she usually recovers slowly but on occasion will suddenly feel much better and soon return to normal activities. Objective findings of significance begin to appear, but they may not satisfy the criteria for diagnosis of multiple sclerosis.

These symptoms are usually sufficiently severe to alarm the family and friends of the patient. The patient feels relieved that his or her complaints of several years' duration are finally taken seriously. The family physician is also alarmed and again refers the patient to an internist and finally again to a neurologist. Since objective neurological signs are either absent or not impressive, there is another delay while routine testing is undertaken. The usual tests of the spinal fluid; and the visual-, auditory-, sensory-evoked potentials may still be normal; and the CT scan with enhancement and Nuclear Magnetic Imaging (NMI) are also apt to be normal. Medical people recognize, though, that the patient is ill, and in some cases one or more laboratory tests will support this opinion.

During this phase the basic character of the disease unfolds.

Exacerbations (attacks or relapses) begin to occur. They can have a sudden onset with full development of a symptom (or symptoms) in a few minutes or hours, a slower onset during a period of several days before maximum disability is reached, or a gradual development during a period of weeks or months. The characteristic feature is that the attack, after a variable period of time, recedes (remission occurs), sometimes quickly and seemingly completely; at other times, slowly and incompletely.

Early in the disease, remissions tend to be quite complete and often develop soon after the exacerbation or attack. As the disease progresses, remissions are slower to develop and less complete. Later, remissions fail or nearly fail to occur. For this reason, patients respond well to almost any treatment (or merely observation) in the early phase of the disease (see the insert in upper right corner of Figure 6).

If the diagnosis is made in the early stage of the disease, the patient will probably avoid serious disability if he or she follows the low-fat diet carefully and minimizes physical and psychic stress.

Late Symptoms and Signs

The later symptoms are more severe and are accompanied by clear-cut objective signs. At this point the diagnosis by clinical means is usually possible, and there is additional support for the diagnosis from the laboratory, which we will discuss in the next chapter.

These are the major symptoms and objective findings that appear and continue to develop to total disability:

The more important visual symptoms are double vision and loss of vision in one or both eyes. The double vision is often accompanied by nystagmus (rhythmic oscillation of eyes when gazing off center) or by incoordinant or simply jerky movements of the eyes. Visual loss can be confirmed by careful examination of visual fields or by measuring reduction in visual acuity. It may be accompanied by paleness of one or both optic discs.

The important motor symptoms are weakness, and rarely paralysis, of one or more extremities, the face, or trunk. This weakness may, in time, develop into a state of marked stiffness (spasticity).

The usual sensory symptoms are alteration or loss of sensitivity to pinprick, light touch, position sense, and/or vibration sense. This usually occurs in the extremities and lower trunk and in the face.

Coordination and stability may be impaired, leading to loss of coordination of the extremities and occasionally the trunk. Other manifestations of this are vertigo, with or without double vision, nystagmus, nausea, and vomiting.

Added to these symptoms are urgency and frequency with occasional loss of control of the bladder and less often of the bowels. Impairment of memory and occasional confusion may occur, especially when under stress.

Neurological signs such as hyperactive reflexes, extensor plantar responses, reduced sensitivities and incoordination, and ataxia are the common findings upon examination.

From this point the disease becomes progressive with or without occasional relapses. We are not going to go into a description of advanced permanent disability here; it can be found in dictionaries and textbooks of neurology.

CHAPTER 6

Multiple Sclerosis: Diagnosis

In the early phases of multiple sclerosis, when the diagnostic laboratory procedures are of limited help, the neurologist must depend almost entirely on the patient's history and examination, and upon his own clinical acumen. Familiarity with the early symptomatology of the disease is necessary if a correct judgment is to be made at that time. Later the laboratory may add confirmation and even identify lesions in the "silent areas"* of the brain that produce no signs or symptoms. Even then the laboratory can be misleading. Application of the low-fat diet plus reduction in physical and psychological stress at an early stage results in remarkable recoveries and prevents disabilities for up to thirty-five years in a majority of patients. The same treatment applied after disability has become established can do no more than arrest the disease, or slow down its progress (see Figures 6, 7, 9, and 10).

Clinical Diagnosis

The clinical diagnosis of multiple sclerosis is based upon two main characteristics that are found rarely in other diseases. The first is that the lesions causing the symptoms and signs are multiple and usually

* "Silent areas" refers to lesions exhibited by magnetic imaging or CT scanning not reflected by clinical symptoms or examination.

randomly disseminated in the brain and spinal cord. Consequently, the symptoms and signs are unpredictable and vary a great deal. The lesions are also scattered with respect to time—not all lesions occur at the same time.

The second unique feature of multiple sclerosis is that all but a few cases are exacerbating-remitting in character. The exacerbations (attacks or relapses) may develop abruptly, in some instances resembling stroke. Also, they may develop slowly during several days or weeks, or still more slowly during several months.

After a variable period, which may be as short as one day or as long as several months, the symptoms abate, sometimes rapidly but usually more slowly. The improvement may be slight, but early in the disease the remissions are usually remarkably complete, so complete that the patient considers that recovery has occurred. These improved states constitute a remission (see the insert in Figure 6).

Exacerbation-remission cycles vary with the individual case. The usual rate is about one cycle per year, but the frequency may be as high as 5 per year and as low as 0.1 per year. In either event, it can be assumed that complete recovery from a cycle is rare: some residue of the neurological lesions is usually retained (40). This is indicated by the return of symptoms years after apparent complete recovery when the patient is exposed to stress: for example, bright sunlight will cause temporary foggy vision; and nervousness and physical stress will cause weakness, incoordination, reduced vision, and sensory changes, all of which are temporary.

To satisfy these two criteria and arrive at a clinical diagnosis, it is necessary for a minimum of two exacerbation-remission cycles (relapses) or their equivalent to have occurred. Unusual cases occur in which the first exacerbation is accompanied or followed by a CT scan or other diagnostic test indicating the presence of a second lesion in a silent area. In such cases the diagnosis is accepted by an increasing number of neurologists, but not by all (41).

In the prodromal phase of the disease, the symptoms are usually transient and in a sense are exacerbating-remitting. They may or may not suggest involvement of the central nervous system (CNS) and as a consequence multiple sclerosis is rarely considered and the laboratory tests at that time are of limited help.

In the early phase of disease the patient begins to experience relapses with involvement of the CNS. By the time the patient is examined by his or her physician, the symptoms may have cleared, and the neurological findings are no longer present or are not convincing. At this time the physician has the choice of relying on, or ignoring, the patient's history, or of dismissing the episode as functional. The diagnostic methods could be of help at this point, but are often overlooked.

Later in the early phase and extending into the late phase of the disease, symptoms begin to be supported by positive neurological findings, at which time a clinical diagnosis can usually be made. Support by the laboratory is often available then, but it may not be needed.

Our experience indicates that about 97 percent of cases are exacerbating-remitting from the beginning. As disability develops, the remissions are less complete and eventually do not follow an exacerbation. Then exacerbations no longer occur and the disease becomes progressively disabling. No more than 3 percent of our cases have been progressive from onset.

Laboratory Diagnostic Methods

In general, it can be stated that when the diagnosis is already obvious on clinical grounds alone, and laboratory confirmation is not needed, most laboratory procedures will confirm the diagnosis in a relatively high percentage of cases. However, in early cases when laboratory confirmation would be welcomed, this support dwindles to unsatisfactory levels.

For example, *oligoclonal bands* can be demonstrated in samples of spinal fluid in a very high percentage (up to 97 percent) in clinically certain (advanced) multiple sclerosis cases. Confirmation then drops sharply in early, often questionable cases, to 50 percent and lower. Furthermore, the spinal fluid from other neurologic diseases such as neurosyphilis, stroke, amyotrophic lateral sclerosis, and so forth sometimes exhibits the same bands. We feel, therefore, that the withdrawal of spinal fluid by spinal puncture is not warranted except in unusual cases, or unless other diseases are seriously in contention. An added objection is raised by the frequency of postpuncture headaches and general discomfort, and by the *frequent worsening of the disease following the puncture.*

Evoked potentials (EP) of vision, sensations, and the brain stem measure alternations and slowing of nerve transmission within the central nervous system after appropriate stimulation. These tests normally confirm information obtained from history and examination and, on occasion, are useful in bringing to light lesions in silent areas, which would otherwise be missed. In these cases, a positive result would often be equivalent to a second relapse and add a degree of certainty to the diagnosis. These methods are confirmatory in a high percentage of advanced cases, but they fail to help in many early cases when the diagnosis is in dispute. In addition, they are not specific for multiple sclerosis, being abnormal in other neurological diseases that cause damage to the nervous system and are difficult to discern from multiple sclerosis in the early stages.

The *flicker-fusion and enhanced flicker-fusion tests* (42) have been used in our clinic for six years. These psychophysical methods test the patient's ability to discern the rapid flickering of a small red light. In multiple sclerosis, the flicker fuses and appears as a solid glow at slower than normal flicker rates. These tests are abnormal in about 75 percent of multiple sclerosis cases, and often in early cases as well as in late cases. The mechanism of the test is unknown. There is no definite relationship between flicker-fusion scores and visual acuity. Patients with a history of visual loss and recovery often have abnormal scores, especially when nervous or fatigued. It would appear that the test is affected by lesions outside the direct visual pathways, as well as within the direct visual pathways. The flicker-fusion test appears also to be concerned with perception. A *balance test* (43) developed in our clinic has also been used for five years. This test measures the sway of the body at its midpoint with the patient's eyes closed as well as open. Both tests are helpful in following the course of the disease. The flicker-fusion tests are very sensitive to impending "down-or-up turns" of the disease, and the balance test correlates closely with the overall progress of the disease. We have found both tests more sensitive than clinical acumen in judging changes in the course of the disease.

Standard X-ray examination of the head has been used in the past primarily to rule in or out diseases other than multiple sclerosis. With the introduction of *computerized tomography (CT),* it has been possible to take a more positive position with regard to radiology. Cerebral or brain stem lesions, which are enlarged or made denser by enhancement and then are no longer seen, or which have become significantly smaller a month later upon subsequent CT scanning, are most likely to be due to multiple sclerosis. Otherwise they could be due to metastatic malignancies or abscesses. An enhanced cerebral lesion in a patient with a clinically defined spinal cord lesion could constitute proof of a second relapse, and thereby confirm the diagnosis of multiple sclerosis.

The recently introduced *Nuclear Magnetic Resonance (NMR or MRI)* technique identifies much smaller lesions and shows promise of superior performance. However, our experience at present is insufficient to establish this, and in a number of early cases the test has failed to be confirmatory.

The *red-cell mobility test* developed by Ephraim Field and Greta Joyce (44) is performed on the blood of patients. After preparing the cells by several washings in saline solution, the addition of linoleic acid to the solution containing the red cells reduces the electric charge on the red cells. The electrical charge on normal red cells treated the same way is not altered.

This test is now used in England and on the Continent. In the United States it has been poorly received, primarily because the measurement of the electric charge on red cells is very tedious. Several studies have been unsuccessful in corroborating the test, primarily, it is believed, because of this problem. We were able to confirm Field's findings in collaboration with Dr. Geoffrey Seaman's laboratory and since then have used the test routinely (45).

The test has been positive for multiple sclerosis in about 95 percent of our M.S. cases and is positive in most early cases of the disease. We have seen a few very early cases with normal mobility tests when first seen, which in a few months became strongly positive for M.S., and also several cases of amyotrophic lateral sclerosis with mobility of red cells similar to what is seen in M.S. These results suggest that, like all the other tests, the reduced electrical charge on red cells is the result of the disease.

We are left with a series of diagnostic tests that are of interest, and to varying degrees helpful, in arriving at a diagnosis of multiple sclerosis. However, by themselves, none can rightfully be considered diagnostic.

CHAPTER 7

Multiple Sclerosis: Introduction to Treatment

The successful treatment of multiple sclerosis is dependent upon several factors, the crux of which is the Swank Low-Fat Diet. The degree to which this is adhered to, plus the avoidance of fatigue and nervous stress, determine the rate at which the disease will progress and whether disability will or will not develop. The low-fat diet allows a daily fat intake of fewer than 15 grams (three teaspoons) and encourages the intake of a minimum of 20 grams (four teaspoons) of oil (chiefly polyunsaturated) daily. The reduction in fat from an average diet is about 90 percent; the oil intake may be increased to as much as 50 grams per day.

It is important that the diet be adhered to strictly, and without fail. To neglect to do so will result in continued activity of the disease and ultimate serious deterioration (see Chapter 8).

For the convenience of the reader, the details of the diet are described in Section 4 of this book. Many useful recipes designed to make low-fat dieting both easy and savory are described in Section 5.

In the first year of dieting, patients are instructed to rest during the day for variable periods depending on the severity of disease. In early cases in remission, the midday rest should be for one to two hours. In the ensuing months and as the patient feels more energetic, this is gradually reduced to one hour. In working patients, the rest period, by necessity, is usually discontinued early. In more severely disabled patients, two rest periods each for one to two hours are required, one in the morning and the second in the afternoon. Eventually, one of the rest periods is discontinued. Patients in exacerbation remain in bed, except when eating or going to the bathroom. As they recover, the duration of rest is decreased.

Mild sedation is recommended during these periods. We have had good results with Phenobarbital or Butabarbital, 30 mg; Valium and related drugs in small doses; and antidepressants such as Amitriptyline, 25 mg, and Triavil, 2–25 mg, each, three to four times a day. As patients improve neurologically and psychologically, these drugs are discontinued and thereafter are used as needed to control nervousness. Addiction or even habituation to these drugs has not been a problem. Patients discontinue their use when no longer needed. We have not used stimulants to counter the fatigue. In the long run they are not helpful and can be harmful.

* * *

In addition to the low-fat diet and avoidance of fatigue and nervous tension, other problems must be considered and controlled if the course of the disease is to remain relatively smooth. *Keeping the patient on the diet* can be one of these major problems. To a variable extent, this is determined by how the patient is treated by the clinical staff and how he or she reacts, particularly during the first visit to the clinic. How we meet this challenge is described in this chapter.

There are additional problems that are apt to occur frequently and without warning. They cause fluctuations in the disease that are usually temporary and not cause for serious concern if treated early and adequately. These problems must, however, be understood by the patient and guarded against to prevent serious consequences. We will also consider these problems and the control of them in this chapter.

Finally, in this chapter we will describe our use of *plasma infusions* in patients with multiple sclerosis.

Keeping Patients on the Diet

Our program of treatment has been developed during the past thirty-six years. Following the initial visit and examination, those patients seen in Montreal between 1948 and 1954 were interviewed at the end of one month, then at two-month intervals during the first year. During the second year they were seen every three months, and thereafter every six months. On occasion, they were seen more frequently but usually small problems were handled by telephone. In the intervals between visits, the patients recorded their diets daily for one week in each month. At each visit their physical condition was evaluated. Their problems and questions received careful attention. The recorded diet was carefully checked by the dietitian and the next appointment was arranged. Periodic examinations were done, but emphasis was placed upon answering the patients' questions and teaching them how to care for themselves. For instance, if they experienced the beginnings of a relapse, they were to go to bed immediately and then call the office.

In recent years, however, we have found it necessary to see patients less often. The first visit is now followed three months later by the second visit, and subsequent visits have been six months apart for the first four to five years, and then extended to one year. The patients keep a record of their diets as before, and they receive the same care as before at each visit. As the result of less frequent visits, more small problems are handled by telephone and by mail. By these means, we have kept in close touch with the patients, and they have profited by learning to care for themselves.

We have found it essential to be honest and open with our patients. They are taken into our confidence, and our opinions regarding their disease are disclosed and explained in detail to them. If we believe that they have multiple sclerosis, we tell them. If the diagnosis is in doubt, we also tell them. In very early cases where the disease is suspected but cannot be diagnosed clinically, the patient is so informed, and we explain the reasons for our opinion. Husbands or wives of patients, or parents of young patients, are included in the assessment of the situation.

Initially, full disclosure was practiced because of the need to gain the patient's cooperation in what was then an experimental trial of dietary treatment. We soon learned that patients, with very few exceptions, were relieved by the disclosure, often having been frustrated for years by the lack of a diagnosis. Strangely enough, many patients already suspected the diagnosis and had wondered why it had been kept from them.

A paper (46) published in *Lancet* in July 1985 reported that 139 of 167 multiple sclerosis patients queried felt strongly that they should be told the diagnosis. Twenty-two patients were indifferent, and only 6 patients felt that the diagnosis should be withheld from them. In the same issue of that journal an editorial examined the issue and stated that "the bald diagnosis of a condition such as cancer, angina, or multiple sclerosis may be about as misleading as no diagnosis at all, unless the doctor is prepared to spend time explaining what that diagnosis implies for that individual patient. The explanation is as important as the diagnosis." We strongly endorse these observations and sentiments.

In the summing up to the patient the prognosis is included; in other words, the patient is told what he or she can expect in the future if he or she adheres to our dietary and other instructions faithfully.

When the diagnosis is made in our office, as much support as possible is given to the patient. This includes guidelines for him or her to follow to arrest the disease. We also advise the family that the patient needs additional rest and must avoid fatigue and stress.

This puts additional stress on the family. Roles change; for example, if the patient is female, her spouse may have to assume some of the responsibilities of cooking, cleaning, and added care of the children; if the patient is male, many times his spouse is faced with leaving the home and working while still maintaining her household. The children feel more pressure to help.

Since this adjustment period is as hard for the family as it is for the patient, it is necessary therefore that the family also have guidelines. Here are a few suggestions:

1. Sit down as a family and discuss the diagnosis and what it means.
2. Make lists of duties and divide them among the family, including the patient. It is important that the patient continue to be a working part of the family, even if he or she is to do only the dusting. The patient should be honest with the family as to what he or she can handle without becoming fatigued. If the patient becomes overtired, the family also suffers. If the patient reaches the point of crying or yelling, he or she can do the family a favor by going to the bedroom for a nap. It's difficult enough for them. They are trying to help, and the patient should do the same for them.
3. It is important that patients support their spouses and children. The patient should not dwell on, "Oh, I am so tired," and "I can't because I have multiple sclerosis." The family knows the patient has M.S. Once in a while they may need to be reminded, but no one wants to hear it on a daily basis. Remember the children's feelings; they may be embarrassed by the diagnosis, or feel guilty, or just plain resentful that their parent can't do as much as before.
4. Allow five to ten minutes periodically for the patient to air his or her complaints.
5. The patient's spouse may now be working full-time and has the added responsibility of taking care of many household chores. Usually the family does not mind the added responsibility if the patient is

also doing everything possible to maintain his or her health. The patient must stay on the diet and rest as directed. *It's frustrating for the family to be working hard knowing that the patient is not holding up his or her end of the bargain.*

Additional Problems

These additional problems can be precipitated by the patient's own actions or by circumstances beyond control, for example, weather changes. They cause no more than minor fluctuations of the disease if promptly treated; serious relapses can develop, however, if they are ignored. We shall discuss these problems individually and in detail because they vary widely in character.

Fatigue

Fatigue is the most frequent and persistent symptom of multiple sclerosis. It develops very early in the disease and usually precedes the first neurological symptoms. In a few patients fatigue pervades their entire life from early childhood, then intensifies as the actual clinical disease develops.

Fatigue is persistent, but this is not to say that it does not vary. In fact it varies a great deal, more or less spontaneously. Early in the disease, patients may have days, weeks, and even months in which they are not conscious of being fatigued, but these periods are usually followed by reappearance of their old unwelcome "friend." In longstanding or more advanced cases, there is little relief from the fatigue.

Periodically, a deeper fatigue which we have called lassitude may develop. These spells may develop quickly, and apparently without cause, and last for days and weeks, but rarely longer. This deep fatigue is often described as almost painful. During these periods patients are generally weak and may find it difficult to get out of bed or do the simplest chores. These spells of exhaustion usually lift or disappear suddenly, leaving the underlying persistent fatigue. The intensity of the fatigue may vary spontaneously, for no known reason, but its intensity can also be increased or decreased by specific circumstances or events.

Fatigue can be, and almost always is, intensified by illnesses such as the common cold or flu. If these illnesses are accompanied by fever, severe intensification of the fatigue almost always occurs. At the same time, many of the neurological symptoms of the disease increase or reappear. Urinary infections with fever are noteworthy for causing extreme severity of fatigue, general weakness, and intensification of neurological symptoms. Once the fever subsides the condition of the patient improves rapidly. *It is fortunate that our patients develop the common cold or flu less frequently than normal members of their family, and when present, the illness in patients is less severe.*

Fatigue accompanied by increased generalized weakness and deterioration of the neurological state usually follows the development of anxiety and mental agitation. If the stress causing the anxiety is of short duration, a quick recovery (one to two days) can be expected. If the stress is severe and prolonged, the fatigue and accompanied neurological symptoms are more marked and recovery can be delayed for months. Sometimes recovery is only partial or fails to occur under these circumstances.

Patients are exceedingly sensitive to weather changes and to exposure to very warm or very cold weather (32). Marked changes in the daily temperature will be followed within a week by deepening fatigue and weakness in many patients. For this reason, in the north temperate zone, we see many patients in October-November and again in April-May who complain of fatigue and weakness. The symptoms last for about two to four weeks, then disappear. Fatigue also occurs during the hot summer days. Fatigue from overwork, concern, and frustration develop in most women following the Christmas holidays.

Excessive work or exercise to exhaustion may also cause an increase and prolongation of fatigue, for example, running or jogging. The degree of change and its duration will depend upon how great the physical and mental exertion have been. However, it has been our observation that physical excesses are less apt to lead to severe and prolonged fatigue than are anxieties.

Fatigue is more evident, and is complained of more, in patients who are actively ambulant than by those who are inactive. Fatigue is complained of most vehemently early in the disease when the patients are most active. On the other hand, patients in wheelchairs register this complaint infrequently. Perhaps what we are dealing with is "easy fatiguability." Before the clinical onset of multiple sclerosis, most victims of it were very active and energetic. Many jogged, others were active hikers, and in general most were high physical and mental producers. The onset of multiple sclerosis brings with it reduced physical ability and endurance. Increasing fatiguability is the result. Even the act of ambulation through an eight-hour day may cause unusual fatigue.

The fatigue is not usually visible or obvious to the casual or even professional examiner. It is noticed and remembered by close friends and by members of the family. Deep fatigue, however, frequently is accompanied by a *drawn and pale countenance,* which is readily recognized by an interested observer.

It is difficult for people who have been active and aggressive all their lives to slow down to the speed of the average person. To have been driven all one's life by some poorly understood mechanism in one's body, and then be asked to cut the speed by a half or two thirds is asking a great deal. Obviously the slowdown cannot be done suddenly, and in practice most patients have found it very difficult to slow down, even gradually. Yet this adjustment is necessary for living a comfortable, exacerbation-free life.

Fatigue and easy fatiguability can be mild and not disabling or severe and disabling, to a very large extent due to the way the patient manages his or her own life, and in particular diet. There are two prerequisites to avoiding disability. First, the patient must understand the diet and other directions, such as the necessity for rest when tired, and the necessity to avoid psychological stress; second, the patient must be able to discipline himself or herself sufficiently to follow the rules. When the patient is tired, he or she must rest; when nervous and agitated, he or she must do whatever is necessary to correct the situation.

When the patient overexerts frequently or for long periods, and fails to allow sufficient time for recovery, deep fatigue may be prolonged. Several months of rest may then be necessary for recovery. Without sufficient recovery time, minor stresses such as prolonged exposure to the sun or to very hot weather or hot water, the *premenstrual period,* fever from any cause, and severe or fatiguing exercises —can cause a relapse. At these times the patient is like an automobile with less than one gallon of gasoline in the tank. He or she can travel fast for but a few miles, then stutter and stop.

The most practical advice to offer the patient is: pace yourself. Don't rush; don't attempt to be busy all the time; spend time relaxing and even meditating; avoid confrontations; and if you have a major task to perform, avoid the unimportant, tiring tasks, even if desirable. In other words, listen to your body, and very carefully monitor and control your desires. If you plan a major event, prepare for it by taking it easy for several days or weeks before and after the event.

With patients who are already to some extent disabled, the problem is somewhat different. Their endurance is already so low that they cannot extend themselves for more than a very short time. In order to do even a little, they are forced to almost continuously conserve their energy. Prolonged exertion will often precipitate an exacerbation and remissions from this are only partial.

The only effective treatment for fatigue in multiple sclerosis (not due to an infection with fever) is rest by lying down. Rest by sitting up is less helpful. If the fatigue is severe, go to bed for several days. If not severe, be sure to take your daily naps, or increase these naps to twice daily.

Mild sedation is helpful for those whose fatigue has resulted from anxiety.

Patients have frequently been observed to do very well when away from home on vacation. The fatigue and nervousness may lift and the patient returns rejuvenated.

Anxiety and Irritability

Everyone is to some degree anxious. A certain amount of anxiety is stimulating and zestful. It encourages alertness, it promotes striving for perfection and increased productivity. Anxiety of this degree is usually not detected by others and is well controlled. However, anxiety may be so near the surface in some individuals that, without an obvious cause, it often becomes evident to members of the family and to friends. When these people are exposed to real stress, the anxiety may become blatant. It is this sensitivity to stress that characterizes many patients with multiple sclerosis; few M.S. patients seem able to keep their anxieties under continuous control.

Anxieties tend to be self-perpetuating once they have been set in motion, and they are apt to lead to a growing or increasing anxiety reaction, and often to increasing fatigue, weakness, and neurological deterioration.

Serious anxieties are usually caused by recognizable stress. The stress may be due to many things, but usually at the root of the matter is the patient's belief that his or her security is threatened. In each case, however, dwelling on the insecurity intensifies the anxiety and leads to irritability. Unfortunately, in a number of people the source of the stress need not be real; it can be fabricated in the mind and amplified to the point that irritability results. When the stress is reduced or removed, the anxieties lessen, and patients usually recover their equanimity and the symptoms subside.

As anxiety increases, a characteristic series of symptoms develop that can forewarn the patient. The first symptom is usually a feeling of nervousness and difficulty sleeping. The next most common symptoms are headache, abdominal stress with heartburn, and/or backache. Less frequently palpitation, shortness of breath or hyperventilation, and night sweats occur.* At some point in the development of these symptoms, the patient gets irritable to the point of tears and frequent howling at the children. The patient refuses to compromise and insists that he or she is always right, and that everyone else is wrong. The patient is near exhaustion from lack of sleep and now worries that another disease is the basis of the many complaints. Hospitalization may result, but usually the workup is more tiring and stressful than the benefits.

Much of the material in this section also pertains to people not affected by M.S. Those with multiple sclerosis have a number of unique stresses to contend with. They fatigue quickly and have reduced stamina. They cannot always accomplish what they plan. In addition, they suffer from aching muscles and joints, especially when they are on their feet a great deal. They are also apt to have urgency and frequency of urination, and occasionally loss of control of the bowels. Some have lost their sex drive or are impotent, which is demeaning and a cause for marital discontent. Furthermore, they are an intense and sensitive group of people who have more than the usual problems in controlling their anxiety even without the added stress of a serious disease.

Stress cannot be avoided, but reaction to it can be improved. The spouse and family can help, but only if they understand the problem. If the patient attempts to do too much physically, the family can pitch in and help. It is especially helpful and rewarding to patients when children cooperate, both by being considerate and by helping with chores.

Patients must nap as often as necessary, but at least every midday. They should tell their families what they are experiencing without dwelling on it. This tendency to become isolated with their own problems intensifies and justifies the anxiety and the suspicion of those close to the patients. To ease tensions, meditation while practicing yoga has been used successfully, and counseling and vacations away from home are also often helpful.

Finally, it is often necessary to resort to the use of tranquilizers, sometimes for sleep alone, and often during the day. In either case,

* Dr. Swank observed similar symptoms in U.S. Army forces during prolonged air or ground combat (80).

tranquilizers and antidepressants should be used as sparingly as possible, but in sufficient doses to control the anxiety. Recovery from severe anxiety is slow and measured in months rather than days. For mild sedation, Butabarbital and Phenobarbital, 30 mg, three to four times daily, have proved to be most effective during the first twenty years of the study. It is of passing interest that practically all patients soon learn the value of these drugs and spontaneously stop them when they are no longer needed. When family problems or other sources of tension arise, they take the sedative again for several weeks or during the crisis. During severe nervous tension, the amount of these sedatives can be doubled for several weeks.

For a severely agitated patient or for a depressed patient, one of the newer tranquilizers is recommended. Several have been used successfully, but Triavil, 2–25 mg, and Elavil, 25 mg, have given good results. Valium, 5 mg, and Librium, 5 mg, also have been effective as intermediate sedatives, given three to four times a day. Many of the newer antidepressants and sedatives have proven useful under special circumstances, but in general we prescribe Butabarbital initially and then change to other drugs if necessary.

If not controlled, the irritability that accompanies the anxiety can result in the loss of cooperation by the family, and ultimately in separation and even divorce. Problems are then amplified and fatigue, general weakness, intensification of symptoms already present, and even the development of new symptoms result. Without question, if anxiety plus irritability are not controlled, they lead to estrangement of the patient from the family and ultimately to an increase in the seriousness of the disease.

Depression

During the prodromal and early stage of the disease, patients become very nervous and many experience mild depression. This reactive depression usually clears when the diagnosis is made and a treatment program is started. When necessary, antidepression medication such as Amitriptyline, 25 mg, or Triavil, 2–25 mg, four times a day have been helpful. Continued depression usually is attended by progressive deterioration.

Severe manic-depressive psychosis has been infrequent and has tended to develop in patients with a history of frequent severe mood changes. Treatment with Lithium has been helpful in these patients, without affecting the multiple sclerosis.

A few patients have been seen in the early stages of M.S. with very slow mentation, marked memory loss, and confusion. These patients have responded slowly, but satisfactorily, to the low-fat diet. They have responded rapidly to plasma infusions.

Divorce/Family Problems

Divorce has become an ever-increasing problem for multiple sclerosis patients. This has not always been the case. In Montreal from 1948 to 1954 divorces were rare. I can recall only 2 in 150 patients during this period. Divorces were also unusual from 1954 to 1970 in Portland, but since then they have become commonplace. Hardly a week goes by without new cases coming to light. Often these have been announced by the spouse without warning and without evident cause.

We discuss the problem here because it is an important cause of increased activity and exacerbation of multiple sclerosis. The feelings of rejection and of financial insecurity that develop in women being divorced lead to emotional tension, comparable to and in some cases exceeding, that which results from death of a loved one. Men suffer the same feeling of rejection, which can be complicated by preceding job and financial insecurity. We have also observed divorce proceedings in which women patients were financially secure. In these few cases, the tension from rejection alone has usually been well handled and significant aggravation of the disease has not occurred. In still others in which the marriage had been unsatisfactory for some time, the patients seemed to tolerate the divorce proceedings without hazard to their health, provided they were not subjected to severe financial deprivation.

We have also observed the flicker-fusion scores of patients during pending divorces and the period of rehabilitation that follows. Almost always, these scores progressively decrease during the three to six months preceding finalization of the divorce and then slowly recover, usually in about six months. Recovery may not be complete. The total period of depressed flicker-fusion scores is usually about one year, which agrees fairly well with the clinical evidence of aggravation of the multiple sclerosis. In a few cases, divorces are attended by increased disability, which is sometimes permanent. One would expect something good in return for such a price, but our observations over the years convince me that the gains are short lived and limited. In the long run, the spouse usually trades one burden for an equally unpleasant one.

Despite these considerations, there are cases in which divorce is practically unavoidable. In such cases, understanding, compassion, and consideration can smooth the transition.

Pregnancy/Major Surgery

A multiple sclerosis newsletter from a national M.S. chapter, released on April 12, 1984, suggested that the course of the disease is not affected adversely by pregnancies. It stated that the patients did well during pregnancy and that *disability* was not increased by pregnancy. The studies referred to were based on hospital records and neurological examinations of patients. We wonder if the majority of these patients were already seriously disabled when they became pregnant. Our experience with seriously disabled patients is that the degree of disability may not be significantly altered.

With active ambulant patients, however, our experience has been different. *The quality of life is affected adversely by pregnancies.* Although multiple sclerosis patients do very well during the pregnancy, in approximately 50 percent of them the disease exacerbated or became aggravated during the first three months following delivery. Six to twelve months of deep fatigue and general weakness, and often lingering neurological symptoms followed. Subsequently the disease stabilized, usually resulting in diminished patient activity. Similar observations by other investigators (47, 48) have been reported.

The conclusion we have reached, based upon observation of many patients before, during, and after pregnancy, is that disability is frequently made worse by pregnancy, and the quality of life is adversely affected as well.

Dr. Swank first became aware of this relationship about 1951 while still in Montreal. Dr. Primrose, head of Obstetrics and Gynecology at McGill Medical School, reported that he had had bad luck with pregnant multiple sclerosis patients shortly after delivery, even though they had done very well during the pregnancy. He had also witnessed severe relapses of multiple sclerosis after major surgical procedures. This agreed with a limited experience that Dr. Swank had had during his first three years directing an M.S. clinic.

Shortly before, it had been reported by Leo Alexander that blood transfusions prolonged remissions (49). Acting on this information, Dr. Swank suggested transfusing patients with one or two units of whole blood immediately after delivery and also after major surgery. This led to disappearance of the postdelivery and postoperative exacerbations, and it promoted rapid recoveries after both procedures.

Dr. Swank continued to transfuse patients with whole blood following delivery and major surgery until about eight years ago, when we found that similar results were obtained by infusion of two units of fresh-frozen plasma instead of the one unit of whole blood. Our entire experience with whole blood or plasma has shown that when plasma is given to postdelivery and postoperative patients while still in the recovery room exacerbations of their disease do not occur. When patients fail to receive the blood or plasma, a high percentage of exacerbations or severe aggravations do occur (approximately 50 percent). Although blood or plasma is advised in all cases, for a variety of reasons some patients have not received an infusion.* These patients have frequently suffered from relapses. We have also noted that transfusions that are delayed for several days are less effective in preventing aggravation of disease than when they are given promptly.

The type of exacerbations that occur in ambulant patients when blood or plasma is not given after delivery and surgery can be described as follows: either the patient has intensification of old symptoms, or new symptoms appear that take months to clear satisfactorily if at all, or patients develop deep fatigue and generalized weakness that lasts for six months to a year or longer.

Our advice to patients with multiple sclerosis who plan to become pregnant depends on the severity of their disease and the number of children that they already have. If they have two or more children, we usually advise against further expansion of the family. Also, if their financial situation is precarious our advice is the same, and if the disease is disabling and long-standing, our advice is still the same.

Needless to say, unplanned pregnancies occur, or patients choose not to follow our advice. Often therapeutic abortion comes under consideration. The factors we have already cited are taken into consideration. If termination of pregnancy is decided upon, it is mandatory, in our opinion, that a transfusion of two units of normal plasma be given. It is also frequently necessary to prescribe antidepressant medicine for some patients for up to six months.

We recommend that patients should be on the diet at least one year before attempting to get pregnant; that if possible they rest during pregnancy by lying down daily; and that they receive a transfusion of two units of fresh-frozen plasma immediately after delivery while

* Infusion refers to introduction into the body by way of a vein any solution. Transfusion usually refers to an infusion of blood, although it can refer to the infusion of plasma.

still in the recovery room. If fatigue develops in the next two weeks, the plasma transfusion should be repeated.

Since we have been giving blood or plasma following delivery, our patients on the diet have done well during pregnancy and have continued to do well after the baby is born. They have had very few minor fluctuations of disease and very little fatigue. The care of the baby (and of growing children), however, can be a real problem. If the mother has a relative or friend, or can hire help to assist in the daily chores and care of growing children, or if the children are old enough to help and are well-trained and willing, one can feel secure in recommending pregnancy if the other rules before and just after delivery are followed.

Our principle goal for multiple sclerosis patients is for them to maintain a satisfactory quality of life. Obviously this is not possible in all patients, but it remains our goal nonetheless. Increased disability is a sign of failure and it is to be avoided or prevented as long as possible. Exacerbations or aggravations of the disease, regardless of cause, push patients toward, or increase, disability and should therefore be avoided if at all possible (40).

Exercise/Physiotherapy/Rest

Patients in different stages of multiple sclerosis have different physical limitations that determine the types of exercise or physical activities they can tolerate. If this tolerance is exceeded to the point of exhaustion, the patient does not benefit and may be harmed. If the exercises are well tolerated, the patient usually benefits. To facilitate further discussion, it is convenient to divide patients into three general groups: those who are normally ambulant; those who ambulate with difficulty; and those who are nonambulant. This grouping is not rigid; patients may fit partly into two groups, and others may be in one group and later find themselves in another.

Patients who ambulate normally can engage in a wide variety of physical activities. However, they must observe the general rule—*avoid deep or continuing fatigue.* The few patients who can jog or run must observe this rule diligently. Fatigue or temporary symptoms, such as numbness, leg weakness or pain, dizziness, foggy or blurred vision, or double vision, that develop while running or jogging are warnings indicating that the patient is overdoing. Instead, they should indulge in less energetic exercise, such as aerobic exercises or dancing. A number of joggers have reported that aerobic exercises can be well tolerated when they cannot tolerate jogging or running. Even so, it is necessary to monitor heart rate while exercising, and to stop to rest when the rate exceeds 150 beats per minute, or when the heart rate fails to slow below 120 beats per minute after resting five to ten minutes, or if inordinate fatigue develops. Tolerance for physical exertion may vary from time to time, so that what is easily done at one time becomes difficult to do at other times.

Not all normally ambulant patients are willing or able to jog or exercise aerobically. Walking, swimming, calisthenics, or bicycling are more apt to agree with their limitations or tastes. The same rule governing exercise still applies—avoid lingering fatigue. Through experience, the patient should find out what his or her limitations are and carefully refrain from overdoing.

Patients who ambulate with mild or severe difficulty will be unable to either jog or aerobically exercise. They are still able to walk, swim, exercise lightly or perform stretching types of exercises (for example, yoga), and ride a stationary bicycle. If working, the physical exertion of the job may be all the exercise that patients need or can tolerate. Some will find that they quickly tire and can do very little, but that they recover from the fatigue quickly. Often these patients can repeat the exercise twice a day, each time for short periods. Most patients will find swimming several times a week satisfying. *The temperature of the pool should be no warmer than 82–84° F, otherwise exhaustion may occur from the heat of the water in the pool.* If this occurs, the patient should quickly get into cold water—take a cold shower or put a wet, cold towel around his or her neck and put the hands and feet into cold water.

A few patients in this group will benefit from massage of muscles and manipulation of the joints, particularly if they are suffering from aching or painful muscles or joints, or if movement of extremities is limited. No less than in the preceding group, these patients must avoid too strenuous exercise.

In the third group of patients, those no longer ambulant, active exercises are usually limited to the upper extremities, and upper back and neck. It is then that passive manipulation of all joints becomes important. All joints should be manipulated or they become frozen. Fixed or frozen joints become very painful and are accompanied by atrophy of the adjacent muscles. The shoulder joints most frequently become frozen. These are then very painful. Daily manipulation of these joints through a full range of movement will prevent this very painful complication.

Daily massage of the skin with lubrication solutions such as light baby oil, alcohol, or glycerine is advised to prevent breakdown of the skin and subsequent ulceration.

So far we have discussed patients whose disease is fairly stable—in partial or complete remission. *Additional rules are needed for patients whose multiple sclerosis is active.*

If first seen during exacerbation or in early phases of remission, patients are cautioned to rest as much as possible, avoid fatigue, and enter into very limited physical exertion. They are instructed to rest by lying down: at first, twice daily, morning and afternoon for one to two hours each time. Later, as they improve, they need to rest once daily, preferably after lunch. Forced rest is continued for six months to two years depending upon the severity of the exacerbation and the rapidity with which they recover. Once "recovered" they are to embark on an exercise program. There are no fixed instructions except that they are not to exceed their limitations. This means that they are to avoid fatigue. As they improve, however, their energy increases and they have less fatigue. They then find themselves able to do more. Many patients will find it necessary to rest by lying down an hour each day in order to remain reasonably vigorous the rest of the day.

Finally, we would like to discuss midday rest in ambulant patients as an important part of our therapeutic regime. *Rest by lying down restores needed energy far more effectively than rest by sitting.* Midday rest is needed by most, and desirable for all, multiple sclerosis patients because of the persistence of fatigue in all but a few. This fatigue usually lessens in three to five years in patients on the diet, but it almost never disappears. We continue to advise midday rest for as few as thirty minutes and as long as one to two hours, depending upon individual needs, in ambulatory as well as nonambulatory patients. A few very active patients may avoid the midday rest, but usually make up for the loss on weekends.

Physiotherapy is not a major part of our treatment. It is used in more advanced cases primarily to keep the muscles and joints supple and the skin in a healthy condition. In this way the severe pain of fixed joints is prevented. Vigorous physiotherapy or exercise leading to severe and prolonged fatigue is with few exceptions harmful to patients with multiple sclerosis.

Exposure to Heat and/or Sunlight

Hot baths and direct sunlight can quickly weaken most patients and can produce exacerbation of disease in many. *They are to be avoided by all sensitive patients.* Adjusting for hot weather can be accomplished by air-conditioning one or more rooms in the home. Temporary relief from heat can be gained by immersing hands and/or feet in cold water for five to ten minutes and wrapping a towel soaked in cold water around the neck. Another method of cooling the body was recently told to us by a patient. This patient uses a fine spray to mist her plants and finds that she can use the mister to mist herself. She mists her arms, head, neck, and upper chest. A cold bath or shower is even more effective, especially when general weakness develops from exposure to very hot weather or hot water. Total immersion in a swimming pool containing cool water is also effective and can be done to avoid getting overheated, regardless of cause. It is advisable to avoid sunburn.

Vision and Its Protection

Bright sunlight often causes fogginess of vision in patients who formerly suffered from visual loss. This can be partially countered by their wearing very dark glasses whenever in brightly sunlit surroundings. During exacerbations involving one's sight, television and the movies are to be avoided. Long trips by automobile may also be harmful at these times. When viewing television or the movies at any time, wearing dark glasses will usually prevent fatigue or foggy vision.

Pain

Painful, aching muscles and joints, especially in the lower extremities, are common symptoms of multiple sclerosis in active, ambulant patients. These symptoms can occur early, before there is weakness or alteration of reflexes, and may also be seen later in seriously disabled patients. These symptoms are precipitated or made worse by extended ambulation or exercise leading to fatigue. They occur during very warm and very cold weather, and during periods of severe nervousness.

Warm clothing (long, warm, or lightweight underwear) and warm bedding give some relief in cold weather, and keeping cool helps during warm weather.

No single medication has been generally successful in alleviating these pains. Baclofen, sedatives, quinine, calcium, and pain relievers have a few adherents. Local heat, however, gives most patients relief.

BURNING PAIN

Burning pain of the surface of the body is uncommon but can be the cause of intense and continuous discomfort for long periods of time. Limited relief is often obtained with mild sedation, and temporary relief may be obtained by applying cold water to the area. Plasma infusions may also give patients several months of relief from the pain. We have avoided narcotics because of their limited effectiveness in treating pain of long duration.

FACIAL PAIN

Facial pain (Tic Douloureux) occurs in a number of M.S. patients, and at any time or phase of the disease. It is usually severe and disabling, and often atypical. It may last weeks and then spontaneously disappear, or it may persist. In a few cases it will be relieved by Dilantin or Lioresal (Baclofen) or by a combination of these two drugs, but usually Tegretol is necessary for "complete" relief. It often becomes necessary to operatively treat the pain by severing or deadening the responsible nerve roots inside the skull. Because the standard operative procedure may not be successful, the operative treatment of this type of pain should be undertaken by a neurosurgeon who has had experience treating M.S. patients with Tic.

TRAUMA

Accidents, even those in which no physical trauma occurs, may cause the patient to become very nervous. This nervousness is apt to increase in the days following the accident and be accompanied by headaches and other symptoms of posttraumatic syndrome. This often results in aggravation of the disease and, if not controlled, can result in a permanent increase in disability. *Immediate* and *adequate* sedation to control the nervousness, and rest, are very effective in preventing disability after accidents (see pp. 47–49).

Urinary Problems/Infections/Constipation

Burning and discomfort of the urethra and frequency and urgency of urination are early signs of a bladder infection. Fever usually develops, and it may do so with very little warning. Fatigue and an increase in neurological symptoms and signs, and often the reappearance of symptoms long forgotten, may follow or accompany the fever. In some cases, inability to urinate will necessitate catheterization. Examination of the urine will reveal the signs of infection: bacteria, white blood cells, and epithelial cells.

Treatment with antibiotics for seven to fourteen days is usually sufficient to control the infection. This should be combined with a liberal intake of water. If infections recur, it is necessary to determine if the bladder is empty after urination. This is done by catheterization after urination. The urine remaining in the bladder after urination is referred to as residual urine, and the constant or even frequent presence of residual urine in the bladder predisposes one to urinary infections. One sign of failure to empty the bladder is the urge to urinate again some minutes after urination.

Residual urine in the bladder is much more common in women than in men. This is usually the result of childbirth, which weakens the support of the bladder and allows the bladder to sag, forming a pouch in which the urine collects and bacteria can grow. Residual bladder urine can be reduced and sometimes prevented by bending forward and pressing on the abdomen during urination. This simple postural-pressure exercise can often prevent urinary infection, but only if done routinely.

Some patients have repeated bladder infections. After a bladder infection has been cleared by daily antibiotic treatment for seven to fourteen days, we have found that a full day's dose of antibiotic one day a week is effective in preventing recurrences of infection. This one-day-a-week treatment should be continued for six to twelve months. This allows the bladder mucosa to become healthy and resistant to infection. The postural-pressure exercise during urination should be continued.

There are a number of treatments that patients have claimed to be effective in preventing urinary infection. One of these is cranberry juice. We cannot judge its efficacy, but we can see no harm in trying it.

Urgency and frequency of urination are common symptoms of multiple sclerosis. These symptoms, if not severe, can be managed well by keeping close to a bathroom while at home, but poorly when away from home. Several medicines are available to help control these symptoms—they actually delay the urgency, giving the patient more time to reach a bathroom. Two medications, Probanthine and Ditropan are recommended. Frequency is also increased by nervousness and can often be lessened by mild sedation. Urgency and incontinence of bowels is more difficult to control. They are sometimes helped by the same medications but more often are helped through bowel training—planning to empty the bowel at the same time each day.

Inability to urinate is another multiple sclerosis symptom, but it is less frequent and often temporary. It usually necessitates self-catheterization.

Constipation has not been a difficult problem early in the disease in patients on the low-fat diet, but with severe disability it may become a problem, often requiring assistance. Patients have solved this problem by adding bran to their diet, by the use of laxatives that, by trial, have proved effective, or by combinations of these methods. Some patients have found a tablespoon of mineral oil at bedtime helpful, others have used Agarol. In a few cases with a tendency to spastic bowel trouble, belladonna extract, 15 mg, at bedtime has been effective.

Here is a recipe for a safe and effective laxative.

1 pint water
1/4 pound senna leaves
1/2 pound prunes, pitted
1/2 pound raisins
1/2 pound figs

Heat water and pour over senna leaves, which can be purchased in any drugstore or specialty food store. Let this mixture stand for one half hour. Strain and save liquid. Put fruit through chopper, mix with liquids, and cook in double boiler for half an hour. Keeps well in refrigerator in an airtight container.

Take 2 teaspoons of this laxative daily for 4–5 days. If this is not effective, increase the dosage to 3 teaspoons daily for the next 4–5 days. The dosage can be increased in this way as necessary.

Sexual Problems

Sometimes both men and women suffering from M.S. lose their interest in or ability to have sexual intercourse. This change can occur early in the disease and to a large extent varies directly with the severity of fatigue. In early cases, sexual drive increases during remissions and lessening of fatigue, but often the full intensity of this drive is not restored. In more severely disabled individuals, sexual drive may be permanently lost. In males this decrease in sex drive is manifested by impotency, or inability to have or maintain an erection. In females a loss of interest or loss of sensations in the vaginal area can be a cause of reduced sex drive.

Impotency in males is due to lack of filling with blood of the vascular cavities (sinusoids) in the penis. Why this occurs with multiple sclerosis is poorly understood and treatment is often ineffective.

Fatigue is an almost continuous symptom of multiple sclerosis. It varies in intensity. During periods of deep fatigue, sex drive is apt to be absent. With recovery, sex drive improves. This suggests one of the more successful methods of treatment—REST. Testosterone (a testicular hormone) and similar drugs have been used as treatment. The results are usually disappointing, but on occasion they have been successful.

There are surgical procedures available for males that patients can discuss with their urologist.

Counseling for the patient and spouse with experts who deal with sexual problems is very important in some cases.

In both men and women, *sedatives* and *alcohol* are often the cause of reduced sex drive. Thus the use of sedatives in the treatment of nervousness in multiple sclerosis patients must be pursued cautiously and alcohol sharply reduced if lack of sex drive is a problem. Psychological stress leading to anxiety and deep fatigue are equally repressive to the sex drive.

Symptoms Upon Awakening

Patients occasionally awaken with sensory loss of extremities of the body and less often with weakness. In ten to fifteen minutes, when fully awake, these symptoms disappear. They are more apt to occur when the patient is worried or fatigued. One should consider them a warning and no more. Rest and tranquility are suggested at these times.

Steroids

We rarely use steroids, ACTH, or related drugs in the treatment of multiple sclerosis. These drugs have rarely been helpful and give the patient a false sense of security, which leads to abnormal activity and to further relapses. Undesirable side effects are not uncommon. Short-term steroid therapy (about two weeks) has not caused undue concern, but long-term continuous therapy is apt to bring about unpleasant complications. In any event, these medications *must* be withdrawn slowly, and the longer the period of therapy, the longer the period of withdrawal must be (sometimes a period of three to six months).

Hospitalization and Diagnostic Procedures

In general, patients are admitted to the hospital only if they cannot be cared for at home or if the diagnosis is uncertain. Diagnostic procedures such as pneumograms, arteriograms, myelograms, and even spinal punctures should be avoided unless absolutely necessary to establish the diagnosis. Too frequently they are followed by prolonged periods of increased disability.

Plasma Therapy

We discussed the use of normal plasma infusions after major surgery and deliveries earlier in this section. In the last five years, we have also used fresh-frozen normal plasma infusions in the treatment of acute and subacute flare-ups of the disease (120). Its use in the chronic stage of the disease has with few exceptions been disappointing. In acute relapses, however, a prompt beneficial response usually occurs. In subacute relapses, the response is beneficial, but the improvement is usually slower. The treatment consists of two units of normal plasma followed five to nine days later by an additional intravenous infusion of two units of plasma. Each infusion is preceded and followed by oral doses of 50 mg of Atarax (an antihistamine) the day before and after; and one hour before and after the infusion. Before the use of Atarax, allergic reactions consisting of hives occurred in 5 to 10 percent of patients, an incidence about twice what had been observed in nonmultiple sclerosis patients. With the addition of Atarax before and after infusion, the incidence of allergy has dropped to about 1 percent and the severity has also been reduced. Following the first infusion, most patients behave as if narcotized to a variable degree for several days. This was observed to occur before the antihistamine treatment. After Atarax the narcosis was somewhat deeper. After the second infusion of two units of plasma, narcosis was rarely noted by the patients until after we began premedicating them with Atarax.

In addition to the narcotic effect, in a few patients the focal neurological symptoms and signs were exaggerated, sometimes markedly, following the first infusion of plasma. However, after a few days rapid recovery occurred. For example, a weak and clumsy hand and forearm became almost totally paralyzed for a week and then recovered. After the second infusion five to nine days later, the narcotic effect or increase in symptoms has not been observed.

Fatigue and generalized weakness disappear rapidly, and the sense of well-being (remission) lasts for from two to eighteen months. Mental symptoms such as memory loss and clarity of thought are especially quick to improve. Other symptoms such as incoordination, imbalance, slurred speech, muscular and joint aching and pain, and weakness respond rapidly.

More than fifteen hundred infusions of plasma have been given since the beginning of 1983 with no long-term untoward complications except two mild cases of non-A non-B hepatitis. A number of early cases have received periodic infusions for up to three years as needed to maintain energy and prevent further deterioration.

Approximately 10 percent of our patients have required plasma periodically (approximately three times a year) to remain exacerbation-free. The remaining patients have remained exacerbation-free on the low-fat diet alone, supported by rest and tranquility.

The red-cell mobility test, which is positive before infusion, reverts to normal for six to eight weeks after infusion, then gradually becomes abnormal again (see Figure 16).

Despite frequent warnings, some patients receiving plasma have tended to become slack on the diet. They have assumed that the plasma was a substitute for the low-fat diet. These patients have ultimately failed to receive maximum benefit, and they finally receive no benefit from the plasma. Strict adherence to diet is necessary to receive significant long-term benefits from plasma.

The risk of hepatitis or AIDS should be considered when plasma or its products are infused for treatment of multiple sclerosis. The incidence of hepatitis or AIDS in the area from which the blood is obtained for subsequent infusions is now of primary importance. We have observed that the occasional allergic reaction can be promptly and successfully treated. It is advised that only activities of disease that might lead to disability should be treated with plasma and that the patient be made aware of the risks involved.

Treatment of the fluctuations of the disease while on the low-fat diet depends upon the severity of the aggravation. For example, the short periods of fatigue before and during menstruation in women can usually be controlled by a short midday rest and, when necessary, mild sedation. Fatigue, particularly when severe, can be overcome by rest alone. Exhaustion requires a prolonged period of rest and usually sedation. Severe anxiety, for whatever cause, requires rest and tranquility. The latter is obtained by meditation with or without tranquilizers. When severe irritability develops, sedation is usually required.

In those situations where rest and mild sedation are not sufficient, plasma therapy may be used as we have described.

CHAPTER 8

Results of the Swank Low-Fat Diet Therapy

Evaluation of treatment for multiple sclerosis is difficult because of the fluctuating nature of the disease and its variable duration and severity when the treatment is begun. In addition, the speed of recovery from attacks or relapses is usually rapid early in the disease and slow and incomplete later (see Figure 6). This has led to unjustified claims for a variety of treatments. In fact, in about 40 percent of cases, any treatment, even one medically ineffective, will be followed by improvement. This is the natural course of the disease no matter what treatment is used. Patients usually come to the investigator when in exacerbation and most periods of testing have averaged about two years. The observed improvement is probably due to the normal remission rate that occurs without treatment following exacerbations of the disease. For interested readers, this phenomenon has been explored elsewhere (40).

It also has been observed that many patients feel better for about two to three months while on any new regimen of prescribed therapy. This was seen with ineffective drugs, but it also may be true of other types of therapy including the use of acupuncture, histamine, and so forth that we have had opportunity to observe. Often these therapies relax the patient for short periods, which in itself is helpful. Finally, the desire to make the doctor and themselves feel good leads patients to overperform and favorably report.

However, a large number of patients, particularly those who began the Swank low-fat diet therapy in the early stages of the disease, have remained the same or improved during the entire period of our thirty-six-year study. Those who started the diet after becoming disabled have noted an increased feeling of well-being and a stabilization of their conditions, or a slowing down of deterioration, depending largely on the seriousness of the disability when treatment was started. Most patients have also been healthy, had fewer colds and gastrointestinal upsets, and have noted increased energy following an initial adjustment period ranging usually from three to six months, and occasionally up to one year.

The detailed results of treatment of multiple sclerosis with the Swank low-fat diet have been described in a series of publications. Two of the most important of these will be reviewed in detail in this chapter. The first, which was published in 1970 (51) covers the first twenty years of the study; the second is in preparation for publication. The reader is referred to this first publication for details not included here.

Materials and Methods

Our analyses include 150 exacerbating-remitting multiple sclerosis patients from the clinic and hospital of the Montreal Neurological Institute. Only six patients were lost to the study (their fate unknown) and could not be used to determine the death rates at the end of the study. For diagnosis, an exacerbating-remitting course from onset with two or more episodes was required, with evidence from history and examination that the central nervous system had sustained lesions disseminated in time and space. Only 6 percent of the patients were diagnosed alone by Dr. Swank. The remaining were first diagnosed in the Montreal Neurological Hospital and clinics or by neurologists in Veterans Administration hospitals in Canada or northern New York State, and then confirmed by Dr. Swank.

The neurological disability (neurograde) as defined before (40, 51) is used in the analyses. To understand the analysis, it is necessary to be acquainted with this method of grading.

0 Normal performance and normal neurological examination. Most of these patients suffered from periodic fatigue.

1 Normal performance physically and mentally, neurological signs present. These patients suffered periodic and occasionally continuous fatigue, but they usually worked full-time.

2 Mildly impaired performance but actively ambulant, neurological signs present; the patients usually worked part- or full-time. They suffered from almost continuous fatigue and were often exhausted. They displayed a marked reduction in endurance.

3 Severely impaired performance, but ambulant. A few patients worked part-time. Endurance was severely impaired and they were frequently exhausted. Neurological impairment was usually widespread.

4 Wheelchair. Often memory was impaired, but a few patients were still able to do sedentary work.

5 Confined to bed and chair.

6 Deceased.

In many cases the exact grade did not apply, so the intermediate grades 0.5, 1.5, 2.5, and 3.5 were used. This grading system, in use since about 1952, is similar to the scale developed by John F. Kurtzke (52). Each of the Swank neurological neurogrades equals approximately two grades on the Kurtzke scale.

The distribution of cases with regard to duration of disease, age of patients, and severity of disease upon entering the study is to be found in an earlier publication (51).

It was evident from the beginning of this study that keeping patients on a definite level of fat intake was difficult. This was shown by the wide spread in fat and oil intakes reported to us by patients. Even with the best of records, each weekly analysis was an approximation. However, the averaging of more than fifty diet reports for each patient soon revealed individual dietary patterns that deviated little in most patients. In those whose diet changed, this took place slowly and was revealed by the frequent dietary checks.

It has been suggested that patients deviated from their diets when they recognized that their disease was becoming more severe. To some extent, and in some patients, this was probably true. However, much more often we observed that the diet deteriorated several years before the patient's disease showed evidence of deteriorating.

The First Twenty Years

Frequency of Relapses or Exacerbations

Although the frequency of relapses varied from one person to another, in any one person there was usually a fairly definite pattern and rate of occurrence, as well as circumstances or seasons of the year when exacerbations occurred (see Chapter 5). The patient also tended to have relapses and remissions that were more or less characteristic for him or her. They were, in fact, predicted with surprising accuracy by many patients. These patterns tended to repeat themselves until late in the disease when the course of the disease became progressive.

The exacerbation rate (number per year) in our patients varied considerably from patient to patient, but on the average there was approximately one per year per patient for the three-year period before starting the Swank diet. This was slightly lower than determined in a study in Denmark (1.3 attacks per year) (53), and higher than in another study in the United States (.75 attacks per year) (54). The frequency of exacerbations dropped sharply the first year on the diet and thereafter gradually, to reach .05 attacks per year, a 95 percent reduction in frequency of exacerbation. In addition, the infrequent attacks while the patients were on the diet were very mild and of short duration (see Figure 3).

Performance

The ability of the patients on the low-fat diet to continue walking and working also helped to evaluate treatment when compared with an untreated group of similar patients. At the Mayo Clinic a large group of patients with multiple sclerosis, variously disabled but able to work and walk when first seen at the clinic, were followed for ten years (59). At the expiration of this period, during which no effective therapy was given, 50 percent of the patients had become unable to work or walk. Our own patients on the Swank low-fat diet were subjected to the same test. At the end of the first ten years, only 25 percent of our variously disabled, but working and walking, patients had become unable to work or walk. At the end of sixteen years of diet, only 33 percent had become disabled (see Figure 4). This comparison included all of the patients in the study, many of whom were

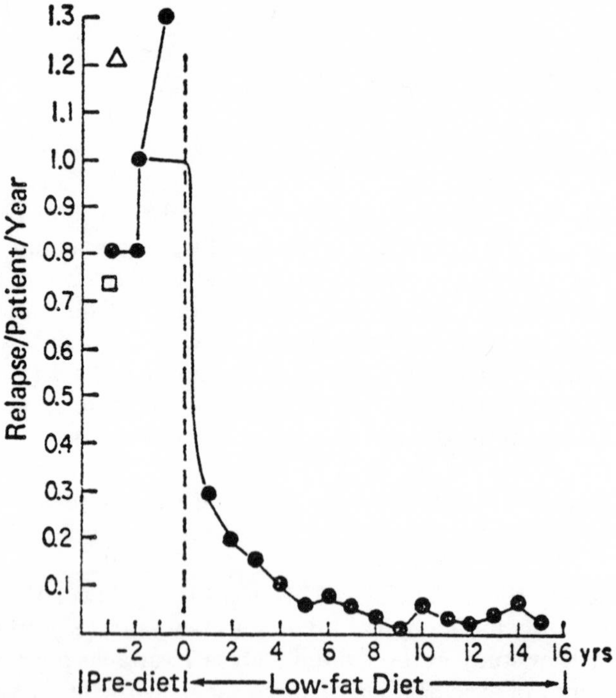

Figure 3. The exacerbation rate (number per year) before going on the low-fat diet and the decrease that occurred while on diet (●—●). △ is the rate computed in Denmark by Paul Thygesen (53), and □ the rate computed in Boston by Leo Alexander et al. (54). Note the decrease of approximately 95 percent in the exacerbation rate in patients on the low-fat diet. From Figure 3 of the 1977 edition.

moderately disabled when placed on the diet and only 12 percent of whom were considered early cases. Insofar as it was possible to judge, the Mayo control group and our low-fat diet-treated group of patients were comparable before treatment.

Mortality

Mortality rates showed the long-term benefits of the diet dramatically (see Figure 5A) (51, 55, 59, 60, 61). At the end of fifteen years of disease, the mortality rate in four untreated control groups was between 20 and 28 percent; for the Swank low-fat diet group it was 6 percent. After thirty years of disease, the mortality rate was 63 percent for untreated patients and 18 percent for those on the low-fat diet, and at thirty-six years and longer, 70 percent and 21 percent,

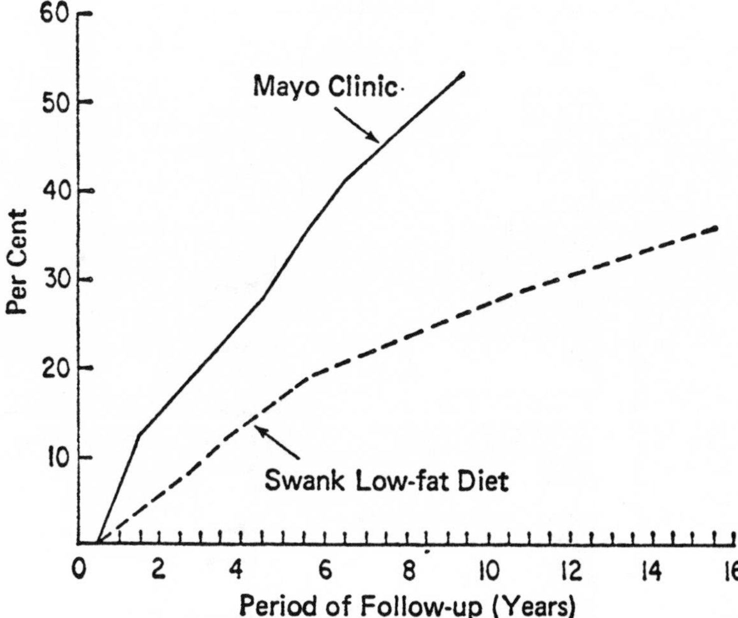

Figure 4. The rate at which working and walking patients when first seen at the Mayo Clinic (solid line) became unable to work or walk (percent disability), and similar data from patients on the low-fat diet (broken line)(51). Note that the rate at which disability increased in the Mayo Clinic group was twice that that occurred in patients on the low-fat diet. From *Archives of Neurology,* vol. 23, p. 640, November 1970. Reproduced by permission, copyright © 1970.

respectively. From these figures, one can assume an average reduction of the death rate of two thirds to three fourths as the result of our low-fat diet treatment for up to the first thirty-six years of the disease. For those interested in survival see Figure 5B.

Duration and Degree of Disability

It also was observed that when the treatment was started in the early stages of the disease when there was little or no evident disability 95 percent of the cases remained unchanged or actually improved during the following twenty years.

When the treatment was started later and definite disability was already present, deterioration of the patients' condition continued, but at a significantly slower rate (see Figures 6 and 7). In a few cases, the disability stabilized and remained unchanged. However, seldom did significant improvement for more than a few years result.

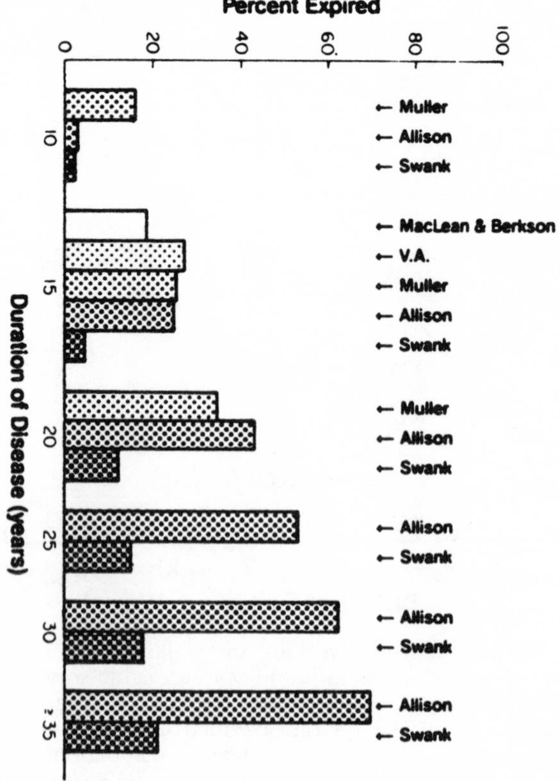

Figure 5A. The percentage of deaths at different duration of multiple sclerosis in each of four groups of untreated cases as compared with patients on the Swank low-fat diet.

It was clear that early diagnosis and treatment are necessary if disability is to be prevented or minimized.

Observations

Another index to the effectiveness of treatment was the change in deep fatigue of the patient. During periods of exacerbation, this symptom is usually marked. With improvement it lessens, but rarely disappears entirely. In the course of our studies of early cases, we have frequently observed the gradual lessening of fatigue during the first year of therapy. During the third year, these patients frequently noted a marked increase in their energy and often remarked, "I am beginning to feel like myself; I am much less fatigued." At this point

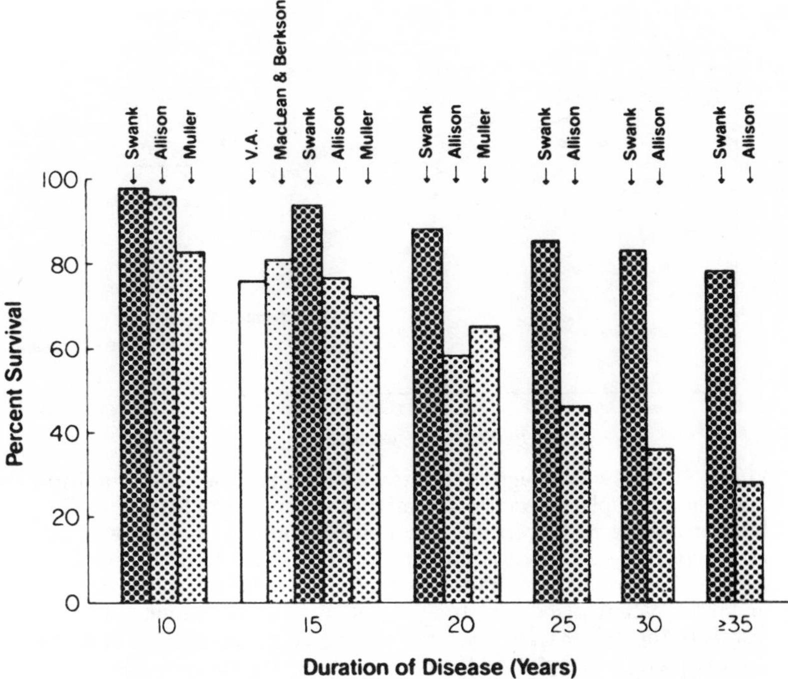

Figure 5B. The percentage of patients who survived over the same period of time in each group. Note the very low death rate and very high survival rate in those on the Swank low-fat diet.

one could feel reasonably secure that the patient would continue to do very well if he or she followed his or her diet carefully and did not overdo physically, or did not become unduly tense and agitated.

When the patients were first seen they could best be described as "fragile." Minor problems, a bit of effort, a hot bath, bad news, and operations or childbirth proved to be major stumbling blocks causing increased fatigue and aggravation of symptoms. In advanced cases in which the symptoms continued to be progressive, the "fragility" continued. However, in the patients started on treatment early it was different. The fragility began to disappear during the third year on the diet. As the years passed, the patients became progressively more stable. With each five-year period, the patients also became progressively more resistant to stress of overwork, worry, operations, and childbirth. But *it still was necessary for the patient to continue to follow the diet. If he or she failed in this, he or she slowly became disabled, sometimes without being aware of it. This downward trend was then most difficult to arrest.*

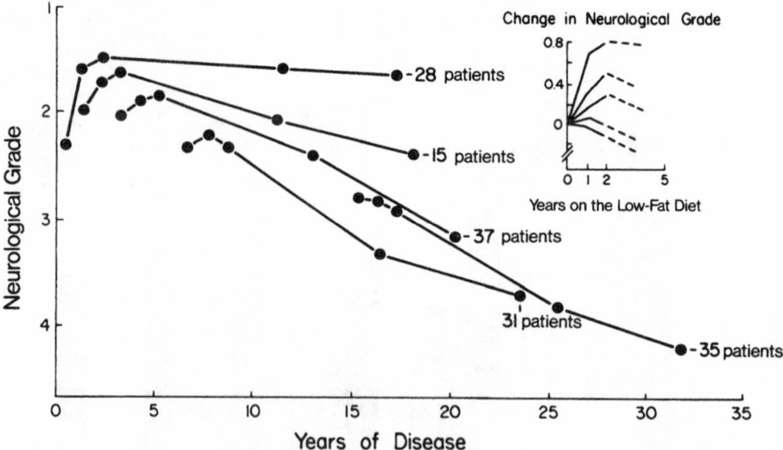

Figure 6. The twenty-eight patients with less than one year of multiple sclerosis when placed on the low-fat diet suffered very little deterioration during the first twenty years of observation. In patients with one to two years of disease, disability slowly increased even though relapses became infrequent, and in those with multiple sclerosis for three years or longer when placed on the low-fat diet, deterioration was even faster. In the upper right corner of the figure the remissions shown in the main graph are plotted together to show that they are more complete and occur more rapidly during the early phases of the disease. Most patients came to our attention shortly after or during a relapse. The neurological grades are defined under Figure 7 (51).

Relationship of Oil to Fat Intake

The relationship of fat and oil intake to changes in the performance of patients during the twenty-year period of study is shown in Figure 8. When the fat intake was reduced and the oil intake increased, the patients showed progressively less impairment of their performance to the point that virtually no change in their condition, except occasional improvement, occurred in the twenty-year period. On the other hand, as the fat intake increased, the oil intake simultaneously decreased and the patients' performance became impaired. The graph in Figure 8 is based on a linear regression equation correlating the average fat and oil intake with changes in performance that took place during the twenty-year period. It should be noted that high-fat consumers were almost always low-oil consumers, and that low-fat consumers usually were high-oil consumers. This was believed due to natural selection by the patient. However, it is not necessary to have a high-oil intake to have a good result. Many of our

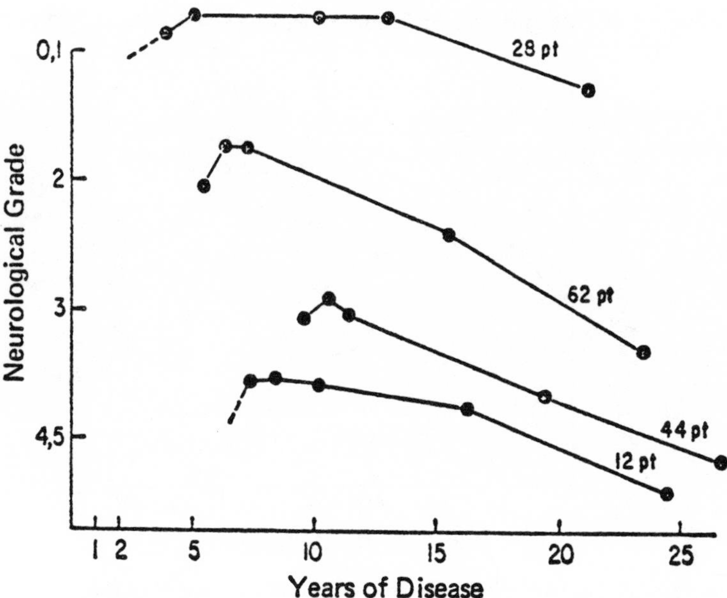

Figure 7. How the severity of multiple sclerosis when patients were placed on the low-fat diet affects its eventual course. The neurological grades range from 0 to 1 (normal performance) to 4 to 5 (confined to wheelchair or bed); 2 indicates slightly impaired performance; 3, seriously impaired performance; 4, confined to wheelchair. From Roy L. Swank, "Twenty Years on Low-Fat Diet." *Archives of Neurology,* vol. 23, p. 640, November 1970; copyright © 1970.

earliest patients did very well with a low-oil intake. On the other hand, very low intakes of oil (less than 5 grams) were often associated with fatigue. When the fat intake exceeded the prescribed level, however, the patients did poorly. Making more oil available to the patients made it possible to keep the fat intake at the desired low level, because as the oil intake increased, most patients automatically reduced their fat intake.

*Thirty-Four Years on a Low-Fat Diet**

The second study of the patients on the low-fat diet was recently finished. It is an analysis of the entire thirty-six-year* experience, and

* This book covers the entire thirty-six years of experience. The statistical analysis includes the first thirty-four years of experience.

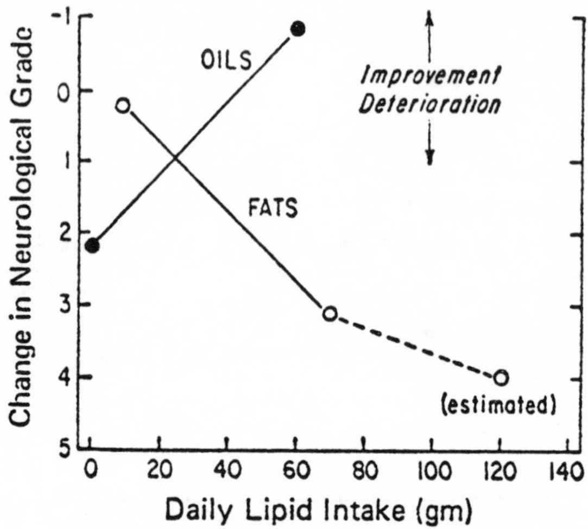

Figure 8. The relationship of average fat and oil intakes to the change in neurological grade or status that occurred during the twenty years on the low-fat diet. From Roy L. Swank, "Twenty Years on Low-Fat Diet." *Archives of Neurology,* vol. 23, p. 640, November 1970; copyright © 1970.

it concentrates on the relationship of the fat and oil intakes to deaths and the rate of deterioration of the patients. In general, it demonstrated that, as the fat intake decreased, the deaths and deterioration decreased. At the same time, the intake of oil increased. The details of this analysis follow.

Influence of Fat Intake on M.S.

A close, direct relationship of deterioration and death to the fat intake in the 150 patients is shown in Figure 9 (the solid lines). There was a 31 percent death rate in seventy of these patients whose fat intake was less than 20.1 grams per day (average approximately 17 grams) and an average neurograde decline of 0.7 during the thirty-four years of the study. The remaining 80 patients consuming more than 20 grams of fat per day (average approximately 38 grams). Eighty percent died and there was an average neurograde decline of 3.1.

A similar analysis was carried out in 66 of the patients who had had multiple sclerosis less than three years upon entry to the study. The deaths and deterioration rates were similar except for fewer deaths and less deterioration in both categories (those 35 patients consuming less than, and those 31 patients consuming more than, 20 grams of fat daily). These cases are represented by the broken lines in Figure 9.

In a smaller group of 11 patients, all of whom had multiple sclerosis less than two years and had consumed less than 20.1 grams of fat daily (average 18 grams), only one had died (9 percent) during the study. Each of these patients had an initial neurograde of 1, and an average final neurograde of 1.4.

The direct relationship of fat intake to deterioration and death was shown in another way. The 150 patients were subdivided according to whether their disease was mild or severe when the diet was started (see Figure 10). Those 90 patients with minimal to mild disease

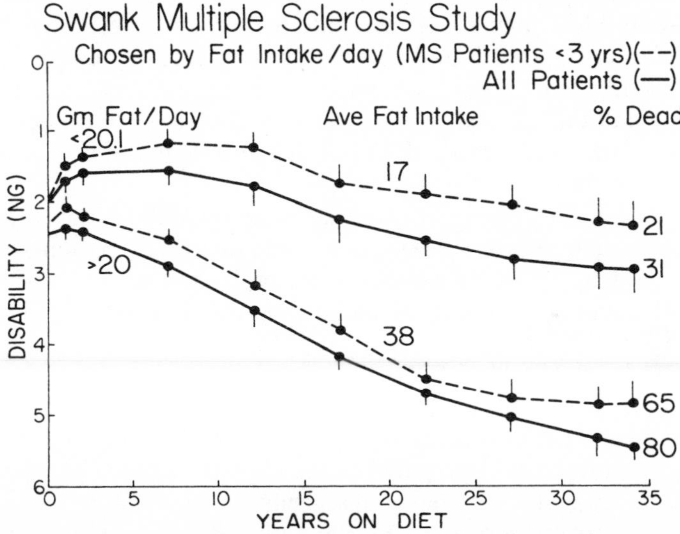

Figure 9. The relationship of fat intake per day to the rate of deterioration and percentage deaths during the thirty-four-year period of observation. All 150 patients (solid lines) and the 66 who were placed on the Swank low-fat diet less than three years from onset of the disease (broken line) were each divided into those who consumed less than (<) 20.1 grams daily, and those who consumed more than (>) 20.1 grams daily. In both groups, those who consumed less than 20 grams of fat per day deteriorated an average of less than one neurograde (Ng). Those consuming more than 20 grams of fat daily deteriorated an average of 3.1 neurogrades. Differences in the death rates are also shown.

(neurograde = 0, 1, 2) were further subdivided into those who deteriorated 1.0 neurograde or less (37 patients), and those who deteriorated more than 1.0 neurograde (53 patients) during the study. The average fat intake of those showing less than 1.0 neurograde deterioration was 20 grams per day, the average oil intake 16 grams per day. In those showing more than 1.0 neurograde deterioration, the fat intake averaged 34 grams per day, the oil intake was 13 grams per day. There were no deaths in those consuming 20 grams of fat per day, but 78 percent died in the 32-gram-per-day fat-consuming group. The change in disability was an improvement of 0.4 neurograde in the former, and deterioration of 3.8 neurograde in the latter subgroup.

The 60 severely disabled patients (neurograde = 3, 4, 5) on entry to the study were similarly divided between those showing 1.0 neurograde or less of deterioration (22 patients), and more than 1.0 neurograde of deterioration (38 patients) (see Figure 10). Those who deteriorated less than 1.0 neurograde had an average fat consumption of 21 grams per day and an oil intake of 16 grams per day. Those deteriorating more than 1 neurograde consumed an average of 29 grams of fat and 12 grams of oil per day. There were no deaths in those consuming 21 grams of fat per day, but 91 percent died in the group consuming 29 grams of fat per day.

Although most patients consuming more than 20 grams of fat suffered significant increases in disability and deaths, six patients (three female and three male) did not deteriorate and die. In this small group the average neurograde on entry to the study was 2.2. During the course of the study, two patients remained unchanged at neurograde 2.0 and 1.0, respectively; one deteriorated from neurograde 2.0 to 3.0; and three improved, one from neurograde 2.0 to 0.0, and two patients from neurograde 3.0 to 2.0, respectively. The average fat intake of these patients was high at 38 grams per day, the oil intake 13 grams per day. This group of six patients is about 4 percent of the entire group. The remaining 96 percent deteriorated rapidly on fat intakes of more than 20 grams per day.

Influence of Oil Consumption on M.S.

At the end of the study, there was a confirmed indirect (inverse) relationship of the oil intake to the intake of fat (see Figure 8), and consequently to the rate of clinical deterioration and percentage dead. It is our belief that the oil intake was increased by the patients to improve the palatability of their food. Patients appeared to desire

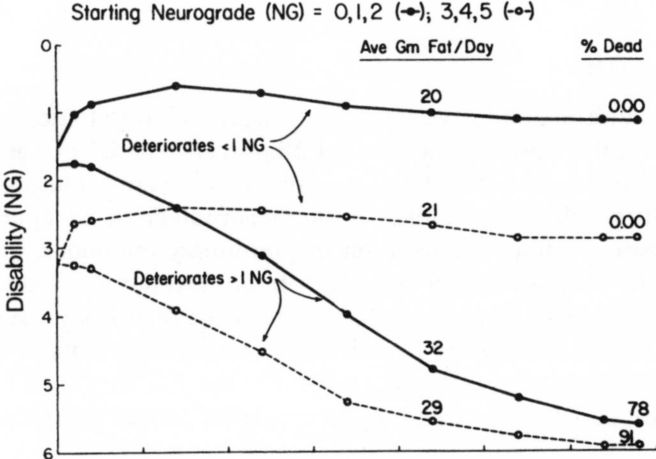

Figure 10. The effects of the fat consumption on early, mildly disabled (0, 1, 2; solid line), and late seriously disabled patients (3, 4, 5; broken line) in the Swank Study. Note the average fat consumption (Avg Gm Fat/Day) and percentage dead at end of the study (% Dead).

more than the minimum intake of lipid prescribed. If the fats were decreased, the shortage of lipid was made up by increasing the intake of oil.

Effect of Delay in Treatment with the Low-Fat Diet

At the end of twenty years, it seemed clear that delay in diagnosis and treatment of M.S. had a deleterious effect on the outcome (see Figures 6 and 7). This relationship of delay in treatment to deaths and rate of deterioration was even more evident at the end of thirty-four years of treatment. This was shown by comparison of three groups of patients in which the average duration of disease before start of the diet were 0.4, 0.8, and 3.5 years. There were 31, 50, and 37 patients, respectively, in each of these groups. The average ages in these three groups was 30.0 to 30.6 years. The average intake of fat was 23, 25, and 25 grams per day. The percentage of deaths at the end of the study was 26, 35, and 55, respectively. The average ages and average fat intakes per day were similar in these groups, and their neurogrades upon entry to the study were also similar. Yet the deaths and rates of deterioration steadily increased in direct relationship to the average delay from onset of the disease to the start of the low-fat diet.

Cause of Deaths

One hundred and forty-four patients were followed to death or to the end of the study. Eighty-one (or 56 percent) died. The causes of death as reported by their families or physicians were as follows: fifty-nine patients died from multiple sclerosis or infections complicating the disease, such as urinary tract or pulmonary infections. Twelve died from vascular disease of heart or brain; seven died of cancer of the bowel, breast, or prostate gland; and three died from M.S. complicated by tuberculosis in one, alcoholism in one, and a major operation in one.

Several observations deserve further consideration and emphasis.

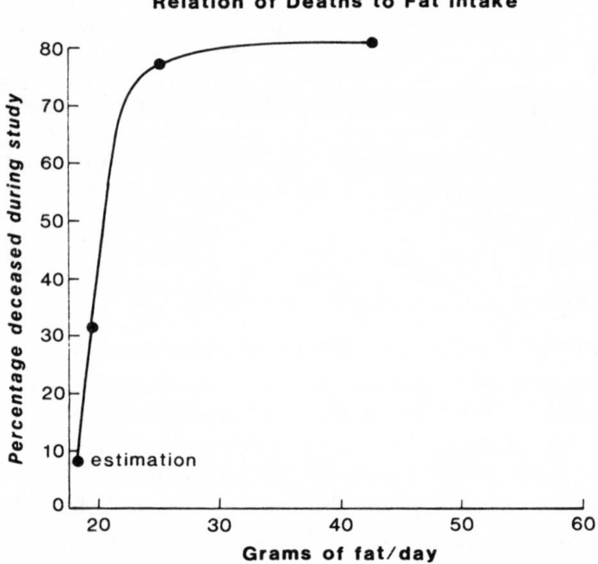

Figure 11. Number of deaths compared to the amount of fat consumed during the thirty-four years on the low-fat diet. This shows the sharp increase in deaths that resulted from the modest increase in fat intake from an average of 17 to 25 grams per day, and subsequent moderate increase in deaths following an additional increase in fat intake to about 42 grams per day. The estimated (□ - - Estimated) deaths at the lower left-hand corner refer to the group of twelve patients who were placed on diet less than two years after onset of the disease and consumed less than 20 grams of fat a day. At the other end of the graph, the estimate (Estimated - - +) refers to deaths of Allison's patients whose fat intakes were conjectural.

The clinical state, with few exceptions, stabilized *only* in those patients whose daily fat intake was less than 20 grams. Yet the rate of relapses decreased in those who consumed up to 40 grams of fat per day. It appears to be possible to reduce the frequency of relapses without fundamentally slowing the progression of the deterioration. This happened in patients in this study who consumed more than 20 grams of fat daily, and also probably occurred in other studies in which diets were supplemented by oils (16, 18). Our studies suggest that addition of oil to the diet, otherwise unchanged, would result in an undetermined reduction in the fat intake.

Further analysis of those eighty patients, shown in Figure 9, who consumed more than 20 grams of fat daily revealed that increasing the fat intake by nearly 10 grams to a total of 25 grams per day increased the death rate from 31 percent to 79 percent. An additional 16 grams of consumed fat to a total of 41 grams per day increased the death rate insignificantly (see Figure 11).

These results suggest a remarkable degree of sensitivity to or intolerance for saturated animal fats by patients with multiple sclerosis. They also emphasize the importance of reducing the fat intake as much as possible, and without question to well below 20 grams per day if the very best results are to be obtained. It is also necessary that the diet be adhered to without fail and that periodic "cheating" be discouraged. The results also indicate the importance of starting the diet early, before there is significant disability.

The six patients (4 percent of the entire group) who tolerated fat better than the remaining 96 percent may represent the small number of benign cases reported by Roland MacKay and Asao Herond (57) and by Pan Lehoczky and Tibor Halasy-Lehoczky (58). The latter authors estimated from their study of two thousand cases that about 4 percent of the cases fell into the benign category.

Our experience in the last few years has led us to advocate, as we do in this book, that the diet contain less than 15 grams (3 teaspoons) of fat daily. Oil supplementation of 20 grams or more daily is also beneficial. *It is also very important in order to obtain the very best results that patients be treated early before disability has developed.*

CHAPTER 9

Genesis of Multiple Sclerosis

The reader is advised that the material in this chapter is highly technical and may be of limited interest to many. It is not necessary for the patient to understand its contents to benefit from the treatment advocated in this book.

A viable hypothesis for the etiology of multiple sclerosis must integrate a number of facts and "near facts" with the clinical history, neurological findings, and pathophysiology of the disease. Two proposed hypotheses, the infectious (virus) and the autoimmune hypotheses have dominated the field for over fifty years. The infectious theory probably dates from the 1920s, when a spirochetal cause of M.S. was proposed. More recently, certain viruses, in particular the measles virus, have occupied the attention of virologists.

In the early 1930s, Thomas Rivers and Francis Schwentker produced focal inflammatory cerebral lesions in monkeys by repeated intramuscular injections of emulsified brain. This introduced the autoimmunity hypothesis, which has occupied the attention of immunologists in recent years. This hypothesis assumes that the patient's immunological system becomes sensitive to his or her own central nervous system myelin, which may or may not be in the process of degeneration. This tissue (myelin) is then targeted for destruction by the immunological system. It is usually assumed that the process is initiated by destruction of tissues by a virus infection.

Because of the numerous writing on and general awareness of these hypotheses, neither of which has managed to resolve the mechanism of multiple sclerosis, we feel it is unnecessary to describe them here. Instead, we will concentrate on, and present for consideration, two hypotheses based on fatty-acid metabolism that originated in the early 1950s from the work of Dr. Swank (9).

The random distribution of the symptoms and accompanying neurological signs, and the frequent location of the pathological lesions (plaques, or areas of demyelination) in the brain and spinal cord surrounding small venous channels, suggest that the small blood vessels (microcirculation), which include the arterioles, capillaries, and venules, play a role in the genesis of this disease. This contention has been supported by the observations that small arterioles and venules of the brain and spinal cord are thickened, often tortuous, nodular, and alternately constricted and dilated (62, 63), and by the occasional accumulations of platelets (thrombocytes) and small blood clots in small central venules inside the demyelinated lesions (64, 65). It should be added that a substantial number of multiple sclerosis relapses develop abruptly, in a manner similar to strokes.

An early observation that has recently received added recognition concerns the blood-brain barrier. Tore Broman (66, 67) first demonstrated that many microvascular blood vessels in the brains of multiple sclerosis patients were permeable to the dye trypan blue. This phenomenon is known as a "breakdown" of the blood-brain barrier. It does not occur in normal subjects. Although this phenomenon was confirmed by another method using bromide (68), it aroused little interest until it was repeatedly demonstrated by computerized tomography (CT) technique after intravenous injection of radio-opaque iodine solutions (69, 70). This barrier to passage of dye and other toxic molecules is thought to be due to the close proximity to one another of the inner lining cells (endothelial cells) of the blood vessels. Because of its importance, we shall give the blood-brain barrier further attention.

The vascular system, which nourishes the brain, has for some time been recognized as possessing properties that differ from those encountered in other organs. The classical observation of Felix Ehrlich that the brain was not stained when aniline dyes were injected intravenously, and the knowledge that certain toxins and bacteria did not penetrate the blood vessels to the brain, led to the concept that the brain vessels possessed a high degree of selective permeability. While some disagreement exists as to the anatomical representation of the barrier, there is increasing common agreement that the permeability of the brain capillaries is selective, and that many substances of physiological significance penetrate brain tissue from the bloodstream slowly.

Louis Bakay (71, 72) pointed out that the permeability of the capillary network is abnormally increased after a variety of cerebral injuries including those caused by heat, chemical agents, ultrasound, embolization, thrombosis, hemorrhage, and infection. As mild an alteration of status as exposure of the brain, especially if dura were removed, produced reversible permeability of the barrier (73). The permeability is also increased in tumor tissue. It has been stated that anoxia, ischemia, and passive congestion, the result of ligation of veins draining the brain, do not alter the blood-brain barrier unless they are associated with necrosis of tissues or physical damage to the brain or its blood vessels.

Of particular interest is the disturbance of permeability after embolization. Broman observed changes near solid particles (emboli*) after five to eight hours (74). Roy Swank and Raymond Hain found that paraffin emboli (particles) marked with carbon black of a size up to 17 microns in diameter produced lesions primarily in the white matter where most lesions in multiple sclerosis are found (75). Many of these lesions eventually were converted to glial† scars, resembling the lesions seen in postmortems in M.S. Larger emboli up to 35 to 60 microns produced lesions principally in the gray matter, most of which had a central core of necrosis,‡ similar to those frequently seen in postmortems in cerebrovascular disease (stroke). Increased permeability of the blood vessels appeared within thirty minutes of embolization, being at first more marked on the arteriolar and later more marked on the venular side of the capillary circulation. The permeability was maximal at about three hours. The permeability in and near the arterioles returned to normal in twenty-four to thirty hours, but around the venules it returned in forty-eight hours to as long as two weeks. After air and fat embolization, a disturbance of vascular permeability occurred in ten to thirty minutes (76, 74, 77).

In other studies (78), Revis Lewis and Roy Swank observed perivascular gliosis around the embolized capillaries, arterioles, and venules

* Emboli are small particles that occlude the circulation of smaller blood vessels. Embolization is the process of occlusion by emboli. Microemboli refers to any small emboli that predominantly occlude the microcirculation.

† Glial scars are produced by enlargement of the fibrils of astrocytes (a type of glia) that normally support the nerve cells and their nerve fibers. When a portion of the nervous system is damaged, these fibers enlarge and replace the damaged area. This process is referred to as gliosis.

‡ Necrosis is the death or decay of tissue in a part of the body which is the result of loss of blood supply, burning, and other severe injuries.

several days after embolization. One hundred days later, the perivascular gliosis enveloped the vessels completely and was quite dense. Jan Cammermeyer and Roy Swank noted thickening of vascular walls due to hyperplasia of the cells as early as four days after experimental fat embolization of the brain (79). It is of interest to recall that James Dawson and Giorgio Macchi observed perivascular gliosis and thickening of vascular walls in their histopathological studies of early as well as late lesions in the brains of multiple sclerosis patients (62, 63).

It is not clear why emboli have a more profound effect on the permeability than anoxia* and ischemia.† Normally the red blood cells flow near the center of the column of blood flowing in blood vessels and are surrounded by and separated from the endothelium by a layer of plasma. This relationship is probably not altered by ischemia and anoxia. Emboli, however, when larger, become wedged into a blood vessel, dilate the vessel and stretch its walls, mechanically traumatizing the endothelium (see Figure 12). At the same time, severe localized anoxia occurs and tissue metabolites accumulate. It would thus appear that trauma to the endothelium is a significant factor in the erosion of the blood-brain barrier. It seems likely that recovery of the blood-brain barrier at the venous end of the capillary is delayed by the relatively low oxygen tension of venous blood (75).

Chester Cullen and Roy Swank observed (98) striking and patchy increases in the permeability (breakdown) of the blood-brain barrier after injections of large-molecular-weight dextran, which caused marked aggregation of the blood cells which, in turn, occluded many of the smaller blood vessels for minutes at a time (see Figure 13). The aggregates also greatly reduced the speed of the cerebral circulation. It is felt that this effect on the blood-brain barrier was due to embolization of the cerebral arterioles and capillaries by the aggregates of blood cells.

It is important in our hypothesis that embolization has a more profound effect on the blood-brain barrier than does ischemia or anoxia. Embolization by aggregated blood cells or small solid paraffin emboli slows, but does not permanently stop, the blood flow. The flow was shown to be markedly retarded by paraffin emboli to the extent that most small emboli took from a few to thirty or more minutes to pass through the cerebral capillary bed (75). A similar

* Anoxia is a condition in which there is not enough oxygen for tissue oxygenation.
† Ischemia is an insufficient blood supply to an organ or tissue.

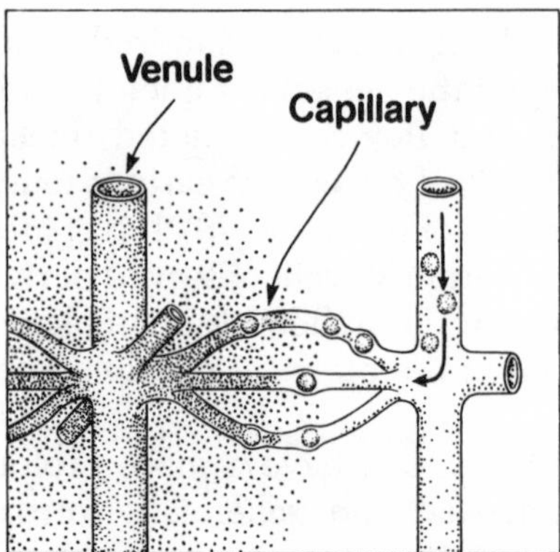

Figure 12. A schematic representation of aggregates (microemboli) flowing in the arteriole on the right into the precapillary arteriole and then into the capillaries. As the microemboli traverse the microcirculation, they dilate the capillaries, widen the endothelial junctions, and increase their permeability. The stippled black around the capillaries represents toxic materials that have escaped from the capillaries to the surrounding tissues. These materials flow to the area surrounding the venule where they become concentrated.

slowing of circulation occurred in a hamster's cheek pouch when the embolization was caused by aggregated blood cells (98), the result of large saturated-fat meals or intravenous injections of large molecular weight dextran or gelatin. It is felt that this patchy breakdown of the blood-brain barrier is an important link in the genesis of the lesions and symptoms of multiple sclerosis. We will discuss this more later in the chapter.

Recent study of cerebral blood flow (CBF) by Swank and his collaborators in seventy-seven normal women and fifty-three normal men of different ages as controls, and twenty-six men and forty-five women with multiple sclerosis, using the inhalation radioactive Xe-133 method, revealed significant reduction of the flow in the M.S. patients (81). In both normal and M.S. subjects, the CBF was high in teenagers but fell at first rapidly and then slowly in adult life. In normal subjects, the CBF was higher in women than in men, but when the differences in the red cell concentration (hematocrit) in men and women were adjusted, the flow of red cells to the brain was the same in the two sexes. In patients with M.S. there was a progressive, generalized decrease in CBF in both men and women before and after adjustment for hematocrit. The rates of decrease were significantly greater than in normals, and they correlated directly

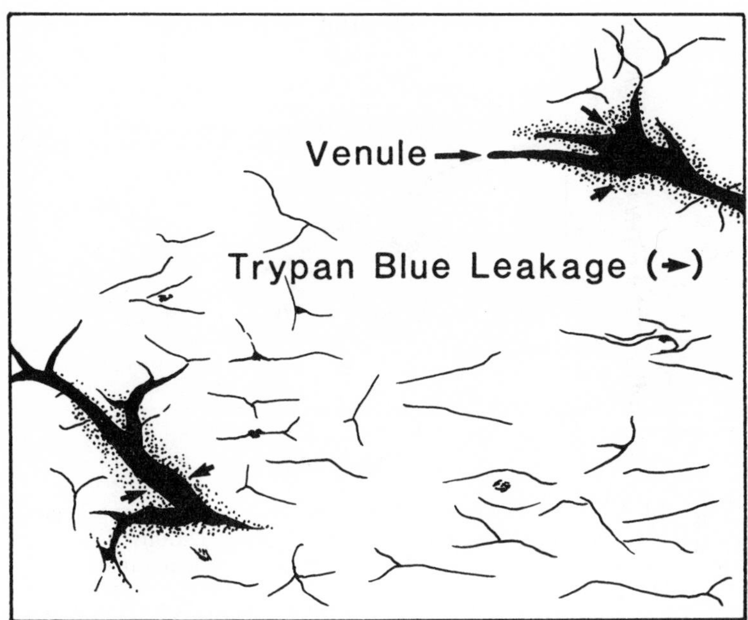

Figure 13. A drawing of the brain of a hamster showing trypan blue dye that has penetrated the broken blood-brain barrier of the microcirculation and become concentrated around venules after microembolism by aggregated blood cells (98).

with the speed of progress of the disease. These differences in females are shown in Figure 14.

Outside the nervous system, pathophysiologic changes have been observed in the general circulation of multiple sclerosis patients. Marked tortuosity, irregularities, and spasms of the small arterioles were described at the base of the nail beds (82, 83). Perivenular changes were seen around veins in the retina of the eye (84, 85, 86). Coldness of one or more extremities, weak pulsation of the arteries of the legs and feet, and subnormal skin temperatures of one or more extremities also were reported (87). These observations indicate a reduction of the general circulation as well as that seen in the brain of multiple sclerosis patients. Increased fragility of the subcutaneous (skin) capillaries (88) and small spontaneous hemorrhages in the subcutaneous tissues of the extremities, primarily of the legs, are frequently seen, particularly in women (89).

Physical changes in the circulating blood itself have also been reported. Aggregation (or clumping) of blood cells in the circulating blood of smaller arterioles of the conjunctiva and retina of the eyes

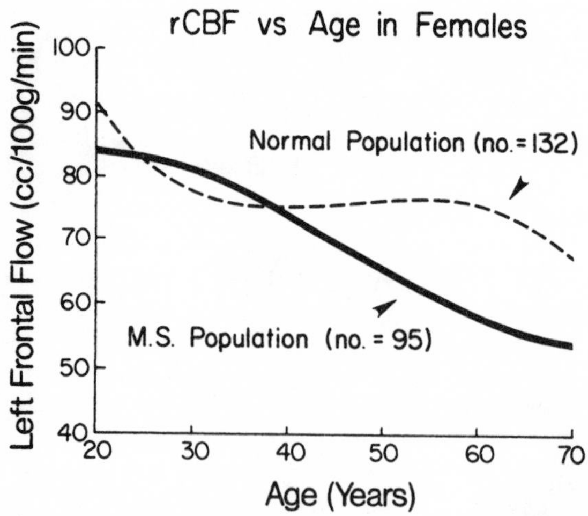

Figure 14. Changes in the blood flow of the brain with age in both normal (- - -) and in multiple sclerosis (——) populations. The blood flow decreases more rapidly in the multiple sclerosis population (81).

and at the base of the nail beds have been observed (64, 82, 83, 90, 91). The blood platelets, the smallest of the blood cells that control bleeding from damaged small blood vessels, have been closely linked to the disease. As early as 1951, platelet counts were reported to vary considerably in multiple sclerosis patients (92). Subsequently, the platelets were shown to be abnormally adhesive (93, 94, 95, 96) and thereby prone to clump together, combining frequently with polymorphonuclear leukocytes, a type of white blood cell.

A search for a mechanism that could cause both an interference with, and slowing down of, the cerebral and general body blood flow, and a breakdown of the blood-brain barrier in the central nervous system, leads to consideration of circulatory changes that have been observed in a number of species, including man, following large saturated-fat meals.

Swank and his collaborators observed that large saturated-fat meals caused marked aggregation of blood cells both in vitro and in vivo in dogs, humans, and hamsters (97, 98) and also increases in the viscosity of venous blood (99, 100) in dogs and hamsters. In hamsters, dogs, and rabbits, fat meals caused slowing of circulation (98, 99, 101) and decreased oxygen availability in the brain (102), and they also caused convulsions (103, 104) and marked increases in potassium and decreases in sodium excretion (105). Oil meals either produced no such changes or much lesser changes. In dogs intravenous injections of lipemic chyle also caused paralysis (100). Other investigators reported aggregation of blood cells in the blood vessels on the surface of the cerebrum in cats (106) and aggregation of blood cells in the conjunctival microcirculation of humans (107, 108, 109) after fat meals.

Swank suggested (97, 98) that the aggregation of blood cells (breakdown of the suspension stability of the blood) after fat meals was due to competition of all blood elements, including the massive entry of chylomicra (small fat globules) into the bloodstream, for emulsifying factors, that consequently became temporarily deficient. In still other studies, Swank and his collaborators demonstrated a breakdown in the blood-brain barrier (increase in its permeability) in hamsters by microembolism due to marked aggregation of blood cells caused by high-molecular-weight dextran infusions (98), and similar increases in permeability, the result of paraffin microembolism of the brain in dogs (75). (For details about the blood-brain barrier, see pp. 82–85.)

Aside from alterations already described, these aggregates in the circulation could cause severe focal areas of ischemia and hypoxia* and a shift of the acid-base balance to the acid side in the surrounding tissues. This in turn could activate the digestive enzymes contained in the lysosomes of the embolizing cells and surrounding nerve tissues. Erosion (digestion) of the surrounding tissues (110, 111) would result in demyelination (see Figure 15), destruction, and finally gliosis, similar to the lesions seen in postmortems on the brains of multiple sclerosis patients. In addition the "door" would be open to passage of substances in the blood that are toxic to nerve tissues in the brain and spinal cord as first suggested by Swank and his collaborators (14, 51) and later by Fredrick Seil (113). Either or both mechanisms could cause the lesions of M.S. as envisioned in this hypothesis.

A toxic substance that destroyed spinal cord myelin, the fatty sheath surrounding nerve fibers, was demonstrated by Arthur Weil in the urine of 115 of 165 patients (70 percent) with multiple sclerosis in the 1930s (114, 115). The urine from normal individuals (controls) did not contain this substance. The urine from 28 of 43 patients (65 percent) with a different destructive neurological disease, postencephalic Parkinsonism, also contained a similar myelin-destroying substance. Nearly thirty years later, these findings for multiple sclerosis were confirmed (116). In other studies, it was found that blood serum from multiple sclerosis patients (also from normal subjects) caused

* Hypoxia indicates a severe oxygen shortage in tissues.

reversible demyelination of cultured nerve fibers and also blocked the passage of nerve impulses through these fibers. Cortical evoked electrical responses were also reversibly blocked or attenuated by application of both normal and M.S. sera to the rat cortex (113, 117, 118, 119).

The possibility that normal plasma contains neurotoxins that can alter the function of the human brain in M.S. patients was indicated by the development of varying degrees of narcosis and occasionally by a temporary increase in the neurological deficit soon after infusions of normal plasma into M.S. patients in exacerbation (120). It was postulated that these symptoms were due to penetration of the barrier by toxic component(s) of the plasma. Recovery occurred in three to four days. After the second infusion of two units of normal plasma, no untoward effects occurred, and the patients rapidly improved and remained stable for several months to a year or more. The absence of narcosis after the second infusion suggests that normal plasma also contains substances essential to an intact blood-brain barrier, as well as substances toxic to nervous tissues.

In addition to the toxic component of plasma described in the preceding paragraphs, an abnormality in plasma, probably due to a deficiency, has been disclosed in multiple sclerosis plasma. Swank, Franklin, and Quastel, using a two-dimensional paper chromatography technique, found that normal and M.S. plasma differed (121, 122). In a few cases, these differences disappeared after transfusions of normal blood. Abnormalities were not observed in normal people (controls). It is of interest that, after butterfat meals, similar protein patterns were seen in the blood of dogs (123).

This observation was subsequently elaborated, using the Field's Red-Cell Mobility test (124, 125), which demonstrates a reduced red-cell mobility in multiple sclerosis. In a collaboration of Swank with Seaman and his laboratory (126), it was shown that the reduced

Figure 15. Drawings from two electron micrographs of lung tissues microembolized by platelet-leukocyte microemboli. Note the intact or normal inner lining (endothelium) of the normal blood vessel (capillary) above. The embolus has been present for but a few minutes in the vessel. Approximately one hour later the aggregate in the vessel below has begun to break up and has released its lysosomes. Their enzymes have already digested (eroded or destroyed) much of the endothelium of the blood vessel, and the parenchyma (surrounding tissues) are in the process of dissolution. Protein from the blood has already started to accumulate in the air space (AAS) above (110, 111).

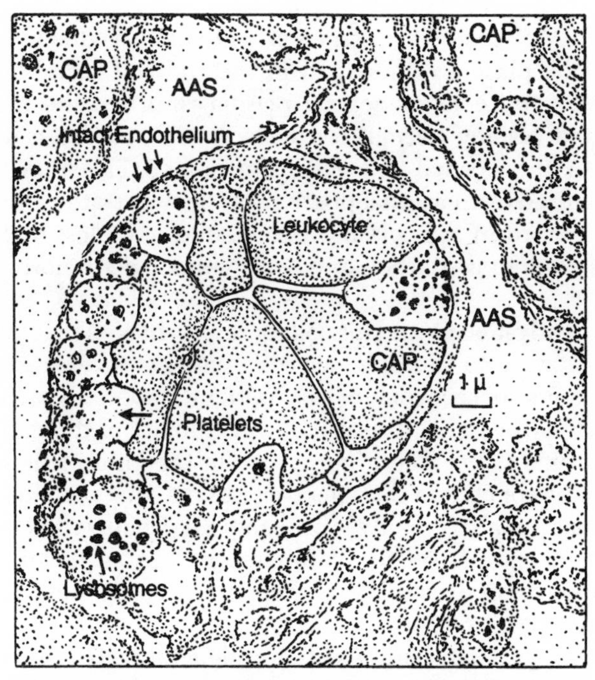
CAP
CAP
AAS
Intact Endothelium
Leukocyte
AAS
CAP
1 µ
Platelets
Lysosomes

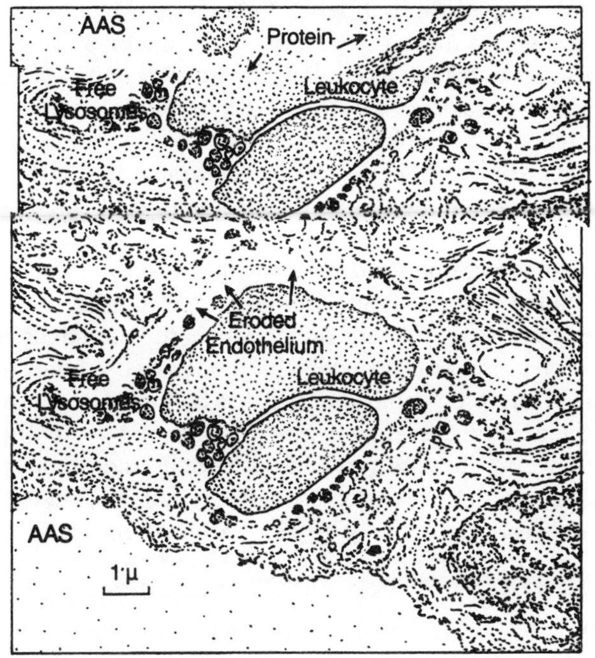
AAS
Protein
Free
Lysosomes
Leukocyte
Eroded
Endothelium
Free
Lysosomes
Leukocyte
AAS
1 µ

mobility of M.S. red cells in an electrical field was due to an abnormality in the plasma rather than in the red cell membrane, since placing M.S. red cells in normal plasma returned the mobility to normal, and placing normal red cells in M.S. plasma reduced the mobility of the normal red cells. Further confirmation that M.S. plasma differed from normal plasma was demonstrated when plastic beads immersed in M.S. plasma were found to be less mobile in an electric field than were the same beads immersed in normal plasma (127).

Subsequently, Swank and his collaborators showed that infusions of normal plasma into multiple sclerosis patients in exacerbation resulted in a rapid recovery of the patient, especially in the early phases of the disease, and return of the mobility of the patient's red cells to normal (120). (See Figure 16.) On the basis of these experiments, it was concluded that blood plasma of M.S. patients is abnormal and that this abnormality is probably a deficiency. This hypothetical deficient substance(s) will be referred to as *factor X* in the ensuing discussion. It is possibly the genetic component thought to be missing in M.S. (128).

With so many clinical and biochemical factors related to the circulating blood in a disease that seems to be related to a high-fat intake, it is reasonable to explore the possible ways in which these "facts and near facts" can be linked to explain the genesis of multiple sclerosis. One of these, *the saturated-fatty-acid* hypothesis, developed by the senior author of this book, is as follows:

The absence or shortage of a critical component in human plasma, the factor X, is fundamental to the production of the disease. This "surface active" material assists in preventing aggregation of the circulatory blood elements and is probably also essential to maintain an intact blood-brain barrier. When the circulation is stressed by certain environmental factors, factor X becomes deficient and aggregation of blood elements occurs. A high saturated-fat diet is the most important of these environmental stress factors. The large amounts of fat, periodically introduced into the circulation in the form of chylomicra, compete with red and white cells and other chylomicra for this factor, which when in short supply fails to prevent aggregation of the blood elements. The circulation then becomes sluggish and the microcirculation is microembolized. A breakdown of the blood-brain barrier in scattered areas of the brain results. Toxins in the blood penetrate to the nervous tissues, there is biophysiological impairment, and then pathological changes occur. Finally, gliosis

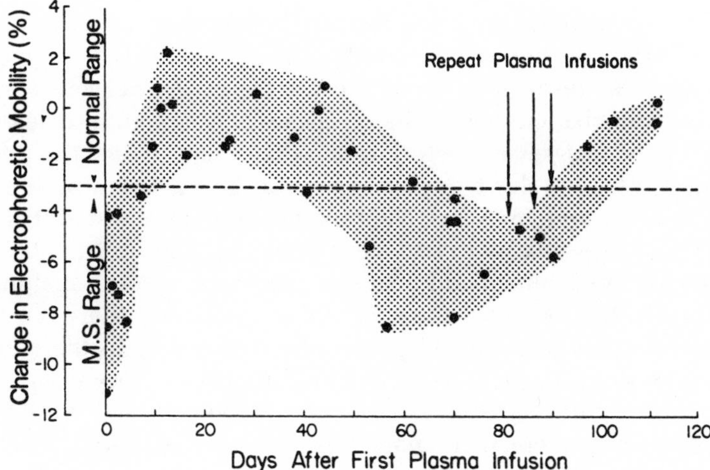

Figure 16. The effects of normal plasma infusions on the red-cell mobility test in multiple sclerosis patients. The broken horizontal line through the middle of the graph is the boundary between values for multiple sclerosis patients (below) and normal subjects (above). Note that after infusion of the plasma the red-cell mobility increases to become normal for 40 to 70 days, then returns to the multiple sclerosis range. Reinfusion repeats the cycle (120). This figure was modified from Figure 2 in Roy L. Swank et al (120).

results to form the sclerotic patches (plaques) characteristic of the disease.

This process may be accompanied by the digestion of the nerve tissues by enzymes released from cellular contained lysosomes following acidification of the surrounding tissues. These digestive enzymes could also be liberated from platelet-leukocyte aggregates embolizing the microcirculation. This mechanism was demonstrated in lung tissues by Reid Connell, Roy Swank, and Michael Webb (110, 111) and is illustrated here in Figure 15. Another possible mechanism of microembolism is as follows:

Platelets and leukocytes are also aggregated by adenosine diphosphate, which is liberated from red cells sequestered in the microcirculation, and by serotonin, adrenaline, noradrenaline, and other biogenic amines, which appear in increased concentrations in the blood during the stress of fatigue, nervous tension, and shock (112). In the acidified tissues surrounding the emboli, lysosomes could liberate their digestive enzymes and cause local destruction of tissues in patients under extreme psychic or traumatic stress. This hypothetical mechanism could explain the increased activity of multiple sclerosis during extreme stress.

In addition to destruction of focal areas of the nervous system during exacerbations, other mechanisms may account, at least in part, for the progressive deterioration that follows. First, the demyelinated areas are slowly replaced by glial fibers, which proliferate and harden into dense scars. Neuropathologists have stated that the glial fibers intermix with, and slowly envelop and destroy, the remaining nerve fibers in and near the glial scars. Second, anatomists have noted that between the ages of thirty and sixty there is a slow progressive loss of about 30 percent of nerve cells in the central nervous system. These two processes would result in a significant loss of functioning neurons and a steady progression of the disease. Such symptoms as increased memory loss, slowness of thought, lack of coordination, ataxia, visual loss, rigidity of extremities, and so on, would intensify even though the disease had become inactive.

* * *

Based on the data from Swank's low-fat-diet studies, a second lipid* hypothesis, the *unsaturated fatty acid hypothesis,* was developed by Hugh Sinclair (129). He suggested that an increased intake of essential fatty acids and improvement in their utilization by patients on the Swank low-fat diet was the important factor in patient improvement. He suggested further that these acids were essential for maintenance of healthy cell membranes in the body. If deficient, the membranes would tend to deteriorate. Myelin, in his opinion, would be one that would degenerate early in susceptible individuals. The development of the red-cell mobility test (124) seemed to bolster this hypothesis since this test is dependent on linoleic acid (an essential fatty acid), which when added to the solution of red cells reduced the electrophoretic mobility of multiple sclerosis red cells (the electrical charge on the red cell). It was thought that this was due to basic defects in the red cell membrane. However, this proposal was questioned by the observations of Roy Swank and Geoffrey Seaman and their collaborators (120, 121, 122, 126, 127) that the reduction in electrical charge on red cells was not due to impaired membranes on red cells, but to abnormalities in the plasma.

In the meantime Robert Thompson found reduced levels of serum

* Lipid is a general term that applies to all fatty substances, including saturated fatty acids and fats, unsaturated fatty acids and oils, and to other substances such as phospholipids and cholesterol.

linoleate in multiple sclerosis patients (130). Other investigators with Thompson (131, 132) found similar reductions in linoleate in platelets and red cells, and also a tendency for the concentration of linoleate to be lower, and that of oleate to be higher, in sera from M.S. patients than in controls during supplemental feedings of linoleate. These results suggest that linoleate is metabolized somewhat differently in patients than in control subjects.

Earlier in this book we showed that a reciprocal relationship of fat and oil consumption existed in our multiple sclerosis patients on the low-fat diet. Patients did best when the intake of fat was very low and oil relatively high, and poorest when the fat intake was high and oil low. We feel that the high oil intake in patients doing very well was increased by them to improve the quality of their food.

These considerations lead one to no definite conclusion regarding the importance of the oil intake for multiple sclerosis patients on the Swank low-fat diet. Sinclair's hypothesis (129) still remains alive despite what seemed earlier to be a serious setback.

Section III

ABOUT NUTRITION

CHAPTER 10

About Nutrition—Some General and Practical Points

In recent years there has been an increased interest in natural foods, food supplements, and vegetarianism. This originates largely from a growing feeling that the processing of foods, the use of chemical fertilizers, hormones, and pesticides, and the diminished use of organic fertilizers have caused a deterioration of the quality of food available to the consumer. To combat this perceived deterioration,

There are many opposing points people are turning to natural adherents. Unfortunately, many of these views are extreme and it seems likely that they will lead to unbalanced nutrition. We, however, consider our approach one of moderation.

This chapter on the practical aspects of nutrition has been included cal profession, poorly educated and uninformed on this subject, is being barraged with questions that many physicians are unable to answer satisfactorily. As a result, the patient is looking to questionable sources for guidance.

There are many opposing points of view and most have their adherents. Unfortunately, many of these views are extreme and it seems likely that they will lead to unbalanced nutrition. We, however, consider our approach one of moderation.

This chapter on the practical aspects of nutrition has been included to assist the reader in evaluating his or her own nutrition and some of the current assumptions. We will consider proteins, carbohydrates, and fats, and we will also discuss briefly vitamins, minerals, and the vegetarian diet. Those readers interested in a more detailed account may wish to consult the fifth edition of *Modern Nutrition in Health and Disease* by Robert S. Goodhart and Maurice E. Shils, published by Lea and Febinger, Philadelphia. A source of more current information is *Food, Nutrition, and Diet Therapy* by Marie V. Krause and Kathleen Mahan, published by W. B. Saunders and Co., Philadelphia, 1984.

Proteins

Proteins constitute about 75 percent of the dry weight of the tissues of the body when bones are excluded. These proteins make up the bulk of the muscles and organs of the body. They are also the basic ingredients of enzymes that, with the hormones, vitamins, and minerals, constitute the metabolic (or energy-making) machinery of the body. In emergencies, some of the protein mechanical and metabolic machinery can be converted to fuel for making energy, but this capacity is limited, as is survival, since the body cannot rely upon endogenous (its own) protein indefinitely after exhausting its fat stores.

Proteins consist of various combinations of amino acids, of which there are more than twenty. The way in which these amino acids are combined determines the way in which the protein molecule (basic building or metabolic unit) will be used in the body. For example, they can be used as a part of the composition of muscle cells with the ability to contract and exert a force, or as enzymes with the ability to supply energy from carbohydrates, fats, or proteins, or they can change carbohydrates into fat for storage.

During digestion, proteins are broken down into amino acids, first by the grinding of the food to small particles during chewing and then by enzyme actions in the stomach and intestines. The enzymes are supplied by special cells in the stomach, intestines, and pancreas. These enzymes rapidly break down the proteins first to peptones, which consist of several amino acids bound together, and then into the individual amino acids. As such, they pass through the intestinal walls into the bloodstream of the intestines. From there they reach the liver, which removes those amino acids it requires. The rest circulate to the entire body.

Tissues needing growth or replacement selectively remove those amino acids needed to produce the special proteins required by that tissue. In order to accomplish this, all the amino acids in the required amounts must be available or the special protein needed by that tissue will not be produced. In this event, the amino acids will be converted to carbohydrate and burned for energy, or converted to fat and stored. The tissues are able to store individual amino acids for only a few hours.

It is at this point that practical nutrition enters the picture. By accident or design, the consumer must supply to his or her tissues the more than twenty different amino acids at an interval little longer than six hours. Thus, if the amino acids supply from breakfast is incomplete in any one or more amino acids, for all practical purposes the missing amino acids should be supplied by lunch, about four hours later. If one must wait until dinner (eight to twelve hours after breakfast) for these missing amino acids, repair and growth based on breakfast amino acids might suffer.

The amino acids are divided into two main groups. The essential amino acids, of which there are eight or ten, cannot be produced in the body. They must be supplied by the food. The remaining fifteen or more nonessential amino acids can, within limits, be produced from other amino acids (both essential and nonessential) to make the required nonessential amino acids.

Eggs, milk, fish, poultry, and meat are easily digested and contain a fairly complete amino acid composition. They are considered to have high biologic value, which means they contain all essential amino acids and alone can support growth and metabolism. Most vegetable and grain proteins are low in some essential amino acids (have low biologic value), and when used alone in the diet do not support growth satisfactorily. If, however, a number of these foods of lower biologic value are used simultaneously, the overall biologic value of the protein meal is improved. For example, proteins in breakfast cereals are used more efficiently when milk proteins are included simultaneously. Corn and beans, the staple foods of Central American people, are better utilized when they are eaten together. Certain combinations of barley, wheat, and soy protein are good substitutes for milk in the diet when eaten together. This principle of supplementation of proteins to improve the biologic value of the daily food intake, only recently proven scientifically, has been practiced by the Orientals for centuries. Through experience they have learned to consume a number of vegetables and grains simultaneously, a nutritious way of eating that has become a part of their culture.

Among the nearly one quarter of the world's population who, because of poverty or lack of knowledge, consume a vegetable-cereal diet of low-protein biologic value and the growing minority of Westerners who are vegetarians by virtue of religion or conviction, the problem of mutual supplementation of proteins becomes of the first importance. A sensible mixing of a number of vegetables, fruits, and cereals, or supplementation by addition of small amounts of milk, eggs, fish, poultry, or meat becomes necessary if good health is to be maintained.

Mutual supplementation of proteins is not a problem to those residents of the industrial West who have a high animal-protein diet. Their total protein intake has a very high biologic value and is usually excessive. This leads to energy waste by the body; the excess of amino acids, both essential and nonessential, is used as energy or stored as fat at a certain loss of efficiency.

Another consequence of the high animal-protein diet, which bears directly on the main point of this book, is the accompanying high animal-fat intake. This factor is important in the high frequency of multiple sclerosis, stroke, heart disease, obesity, and probably other chronic diseases in the industrialized Western world.

If the trend away from animal proteins in the diet continues, accelerated in recent years by the rapid rise in their cost, we can expect the general diet to move toward a cereal-vegetable base. As this trend develops, the mixing of different protein foods at the same meal to make the different amino acids available to the tissues simultaneously will become essential, thus making possible complete utilization of the proteins for construction, repair, and metabolism. Rejection of a high animal-protein diet will increase the intake of complex carbohydrates from vegetables and cereals. This will further aid the efficiency of protein use since all energy requirements will be satisfied by carbohydrates, making protein breakdown for this purpose unnecessary.

It is inevitable that some protein will be metabolized for energy. In order to assure that all amino acids necessary for growth and repair of tissues and enzymes are available more or less simultaneously, some excess of protein must be consumed. However, this should not be an extreme excess as usually occurs among the majority who rely on meat and potatoes as their staple diet in the United States, Canada, and much of the rest of the industrialized Western world. It is also necessary that adequate vitamins, including C and all of the B vitamins, be available if structural proteins of good quality are to be produced; otherwise substandard tissues and enzymes will result.

The amount of protein intake that is desirable in a human being is debatable. If the protein intake is balanced so that all amino acids can be used constructively, the requirement is less than when the intake is unbalanced.* During moderate exercise there seems to be no need to exceed normal limits, but after severe exercise for prolonged periods there may be need to replace lost tissue proteins. During fever, after major burns, multiple fractures, and surgical procedures, there is a significant loss of tissue proteins and these need to be replaced by an increased protein intake.

Proteins are not stored or held in reserve, and one cannot "push" constructive protein metabolism by supplementing a normal diet with high-protein or amino acid additions unless disease or injury is present. Such supplements are a burden to the metabolic mechanisms since the amino acids must be degraded and burned as energy or stored as fat.

A high-protein intake, aside from the accompanying increase in animal fat, is not usually harmful. However, after periods of protein starvation, the protein intake must be increased slowly to avoid harm. Also, infants and young children not accustomed to a high-protein intake cannot tolerate such a diet. Excessive protein may lead to fluid imbalance and its retention in the body. This may occur when the total calories from proteins exceed 15 or 20 percent of the total caloric intake. Also, the end products from excessive protein metabolism may lead to accumulation of nitrogenous waste products in the bloodstream and place a burden on the liver and kidneys. It is clear that an overload of protein should be avoided.

Carbohydrates

Until the present century, more than 50 percent of the daily caloric intake of an average individual in the industrialized West was furnished by carbohydrates. The diet of cereals and vegetables provided a rich source of natural vitamins, minerals, essential oils, and proteins, and it was sufficient, with minimal protein supplementation (milk, eggs, poultry, fish, and meat), to ensure normal nutrition. During the present century, this natural balance of calories with other essential nutrients for growth, repair, and metabolism has suffered a near catastrophic change as the result of food-processing methods

* Under ideal circumstances, a minimum daily total protein requirement of 0.5 gm/kg weight has been found satisfactory for all adults of all ages under no stress. Because of variations in protein content of foods and irregularities of the daily food intake, most investigators seem to agree that about 1.0 gram total protein intake per kilogram of body weight in adult men and women on a fixed diet would safely guard one from protein deficiency and compensate for the periods of minor stress.

that delay spoilage of food, enhance its appearance, and prolong its shelf life. The refinement of flour has removed the wheat germ, which contains a number of important substances, including the richest natural source of the B vitamins available to Western man, essential oils, and vitamin E.

With the removal of the bran and the germ from brown rice, the disease beriberi became widespread in the Orient among those who, because of poverty or lack of information, failed to supplement their diet with fresh vegetables and other fresh foods. In the United States, removal of wheat germ from flour resulted in B vitamin deficiencies, causing polyneuritis, Wernicke's and Korsakoff's syndromes, heart failure, and pellagra. These deficiencies were frequently precipitated by a high intake of alcohol, the metabolism of which requires a generous supply of the B group of vitamins.

The frequent association of these diseases with a high intake of refined cereals and alcohol led to the discovery of thiamine (vitamin B_1) and soon after nicotinic acid, both members of the water-soluble B group of vitamins. In quick order, other members of this group of vitamins (riboflavin, pyridoxine, pantothenic acid, and biotin) were identified, all of which can now be synthetically produced. It is unlikely, however, that all of the vitamins removed during the refinement of cereals have been discovered. Therefore, when flour is enriched by adding synthetic vitamins, the enrichment fails to replace the oils and vitamin E, as well as unknown food essentials (vitamins).

Refining cereal also removes the bran. This material is helpful to the mechanical action of the intestines and to normal bowel elimination. It also slows down absorption of carbohydrates, thereby helping maintain the blood sugar at a more uniform level.

Cereals and vegetables, our main carbohydrate sources, have always been cheap. Because of the low spoilage rate, the highly refined carbohydrates have been the cheapest. It might seem that shifting from refined flour to whole grain flour would involve a cultural change of some magnitude, but even so, a trend in this direction seems to be developing.

During the present century the percentage of total calories derived from carbohydrates has dropped from 50 percent to approximately 42 percent. About 50 percent of these carbohydrate calories are from cereals and vegetables containing complicated starches and dextrins, which when consumed promote a moderately elevated and stable blood sugar level.

Another 43 percent of the ingested carbohydrates consists of single sugars, of which more than half is refined sugar (sucrose). These are rapidly digested and absorbed into the system, producing prompt high blood sugar levels. The occasional consequence of this is a massive release of insulin and a precipitous drop in blood sugar, a condition called hypoglycemia, which is attended by mental confusion, sweating, and marked weakness. This reaction is usually short-lived and self-correcting. Minor attacks of hypoglycemia are not uncommon.

The overall problem has been aggravated by the rapid increase in consumption of refined sugar, now supplying 25 percent of the total carbohydrate calories. These calories can only be metabolized with the generous addition of all the B vitamins to the diet.

Thus, there are three serious dietary deficiencies caused by the processing and "refinement" of our carbohydrate foodstuffs. One is a multiple vitamin deficiency due to removal of the naturally contained vitamins. The second is an increase in the relative amounts of simple, rapidly digested, and absorbed sugars in our diet, leading to a tendency of blood sugar levels to fluctuate wildly. The third is removal of roughage from cereals, leading to mechanical inefficiency of bowel function.

Digestion of carbohydrates breaks down the complicated starches and dextrins to simple sugars, principally glucose. These and other simple sugars are then absorbed into the bloodstream and go directly to the liver, which removes what it needs for energy and converts another portion of glucose to glycogen for storage there. The remaining glucose circulates to the other organs and tissues of the body for energy and is stored as glycogen in the muscles, heart, and smooth muscles of the intestines and stomach.

The circulating glucose in the bloodstream at no time is sufficient to meet the energy requirements of the body for more than half a day. The glycogen stores are the next immediately available energy source, and for sudden spurts of activity can furnish large amounts of energy more efficiently than any other source, including the circulating glucose. It is therefore important that the glycogen stores of both muscle and heart be adequate to meet the anticipated needs of the body. In well-trained athletes, very high levels of glycogen storage are maintained.

Healthy high levels of glycogen in the liver protect that organ from severe damage by toxins. Since all blood from the digestive organs passes directly to the liver before it reaches the general circulation of the body, and since one of the main functions of the liver is to neutralize toxic elements brought to it from that and other sources, it also is important that the glycogen stores in the liver be maintained at a high level.

Glucose efficiently transforms to glycogen. Protein is moderately efficient and fat poorly efficient in this respect. It would seem important, therefore, that the carbohydrate intake be adequate to supply all the energy and glycogen storage requirements of the body; that the secondary use of proteins as a source of energy be kept to a minimum consistent with good health and an adequate amino acid intake; and that the fats be used for energy only on an emergency basis, such as during a prolonged fast. Finally, it is absolutely necessary that a generous (not excessive) supply of the B group of vitamins be available for the transformation of glucose to glycogen or for the breakdown of glucose to give energy.

Under normal circumstances, energy used by the body comes from metabolism of glucose. During acute hypoglycemia the brain ceases normal function and heart function is soon impaired when its small stores of glycogen are exhausted. When these energy sources are used up, the fat stores are transformed to glucose, a process that can go on to complete depletion without harmful nutritional effects. As a last resort, proteins can also be transformed to glucose and metabolized for energy, but this process soon leads to serious consequences

glycerol, to which is attached three molecules of fatty acid. The glycerol is constant in structure; the fatty acids vary both as to their length (number of carbon atoms) and degree of unsaturation (number of double-valence bonds or points of easy chemical reaction).

Fats

Most fats or oils available for human consumption are classified as neutral fats or triglycerides. They are composed of one molecule of glycerol, to which is attached three molecules of fatty acid. The glycerol is constant in structure; the fatty acids vary both as to their length (number of carbon atoms) and degree of unsaturation (number of double-valence bonds or points of easy chemical reaction). As the fatty acids lengthen and the double bonds become saturated (exchanged for single bonds), the triglycerides become more viscous and the melting points increase. They are called "hard" fat because they are solid at room temperature. An increase in the number of double bonds (unsaturation) and the shortening of the carbon chain renders the triglycerides more fluid and lowers the melting point. In general, the term "oil" is applied to those triglycerides that are fluid at room temperature and even at ordinary refrigeration (about 4° C or 40° F).

You will often hear or read about mono- and polyunsaturated oils. The monounsaturated oils are predominantly made up of fatty acids with one double bond. A good example is olive oil. The polyunsaturated oils consist predominantly of fatty acids with two or more double bonds and have iodine numbers in excess of 90.*

In addition, some of the polyunsaturated fatty acids are essential to health. In a sense, they are vitamins and must be supplied with the food since the human body cannot produce them. Small amounts of these essential fatty acids are to be found in most oils and fats, but high concentrations are found in cod-liver oil, raw linseed oil, safflower oil, sunflower seed oil, and corn oil. Under normal circumstances only small amounts of these fatty acids are needed daily. The essential fatty acids (as triglycerides) are found in most tissues of the body since they are present in small amounts in all cell membranes. They are also present in cell membranes of plants. Therefore, if one were to eat a sufficient quantity of fresh unprocessed cereals and vegetables, the necessary daily requirement of essential fatty acids would be obtained.

Deficiencies of these essential oils are rare because of the widespread presence of them in nature. However, the consumption of very large amounts of saturated fats without polyunsaturated oils has produced the deficiency that, in animals, consists of skin and muscle lesions. In humans, only the skin lesions have been reliably described.

The polyunsaturated oils, including the essential oils, must be protected from oxidation in nature and in the body, otherwise they will become saturated and lose their essential character. This process is prevented by the presence in the oils of antioxidants. Two physiological ones are vitamins E and C. Vitamin E is normally present in vegetable oils in amounts sufficient to prevent oxidation of the oils,

* There are several convenient ways in which to measure the degree of saturation of fatty acids in triglycerides. Iodine readily combines at the points of double bonds of the unsaturated fatty acids. Under controlled conditions, very little iodine will combine with the more saturated fatty acids (contained in fats). The iodine number of some examples of saturated fats, such as coconut oil, is 8 to 10, butter 26 to 40, beef and sheep tallow 32 to 45, lard from pork 50 to 65. These triglycerides contain molecules that are relatively stable and combine with other elements (in this case iodine) in relatively small amounts. They have few available points for other molecules to become attached, hence the designation "saturation." The oils more readily react with iodine and other chemicals and have relatively high iodine numbers. For example, the iodine number of olive oil is 80 to 90, peanut oil 90 to 100, cottonseed oil 105 to 115, corn oil 115 to 124, soybean oil 130 to 138, safflower and sunflower seed oil 130 to 150, whale oil 166, cod-liver oil 155 to 175, and linseed oil 175 to 200.

but much of it is removed during processing of the oils for market. The remaining natural sources of antioxidants are vitamin C from vegetables and fruits, and vitamin E in wheat germ, plus the very small amounts distributed in all cells of animals and vegetables. For these reasons, it may be wise to supplement the low-fat diet with 25 to 50 I.U. of vitamin E in patients consuming a supplement of cod-liver oil and a relatively high intake of fish, seafood, and polyunsaturated oils. Most therapeutic multiple vitamin capsules contain about this much vitamin E. Also, refrigeration retards the oxidation of oils.

Not all polyunsaturated fatty acids are essential oils, but some scientists believe that degenerative ailments, particularly stroke and heart disease, are caused in some part by deficiencies of these fatty acids resulting from our changed dietary habits. These changes, plus new food-processing methods, they believe, have caused a reduction or deficiency of the polyunsaturated fatty acids compared with the amount of saturated fatty acids in the diet. Other investigators, however, consider the monounsaturated and polyunsaturated fatty acids as equivalents, especially important to the maintenance of health if the amount of saturated fat is reduced.

Chemical processing has also affected the oils, particularly the polyunsaturated and essential fatty acids. Many people think of margarine, shortening, and hydrogenated peanut butter as containing vegetable oils that may be better for them than butter and lard. It is true that the basic ingredients are vegetable oils; but, in the chemical process called hydrogenation, which turns these oils from liquid to solid, the oils become saturated and otherwise changed. Hence, in the low-fat diet, margarine, shortening, and hydrogenated peanut butter must be treated as "hard" fat. Hydrogenated oils are, in fact, a major source of fat in the average American diet today and have taken the place of the natural oils used by our ancestors.

Chocolate also is derived from a vegetable, but it is a vegetable with a difference. Unlike corn, wheat, and other vegetable oil sources, chocolate contains fatty acids that are about as highly saturated as those found in butter. For this reason chocolate, except plain chocolate-flavored syrup, is forbidden on a low-fat diet. Coconut "oil" and palm oil are also highly saturated and should therefore be treated as a fat. They, too, are not allowed on a low-fat diet.

Like proteins and carbohydrates, the triglycerides are broken down through digestion into their component parts, glycerol and fatty acids. They are then absorbed through the mucosa of the intestines. The short-chained fatty acids enter the bloodstream and go to the liver for metabolism; the longer fatty acids and glycerol enter the lacteals of the thoracic duct. In the process they are reunited to form triglycerides and flow with the lymph as small fat globules called chylomicra in the thoracic duct, finally to enter the venous system.

Excess fat is removed and stored in the fat cells as triglycerides. These fat cells are concentrated in an insulating pad under the skin, in the abdomen as a cushion for the intestines and kidneys, and diffusely in muscles and other tissues. In the muscles of beef the fat appears as marbling. The term "fat depots" is applied to these deposits or accumulations of fat. Ingested fat to a large extent is stored as saturated fat according to what it was when ingested. Fat converted from glucose or protein for storage is largely stored as "hard" fat (saturated).

Whenever the intake of food is inadequate to satisfy the energy metabolism demands, fat in the depots is broken down (hydrolized) into its component parts, glycerol and fatty acids, and released to the bloodstream. Both components are then metabolized primarily by the heart and muscles. As already mentioned, the brain relies almost entirely upon glucose for its energy needs.

It is of interest that women have survived periods of extreme starvation better than men. This was borne out by the higher survival rates of pioneer women after being snowbound during the winter on the way to California. This apparent advantage is probably due to the much greater body stores of fat possessed by females.

The presence in very small amounts of other, more complicated fats in the body, namely cholesterol and phosphatides (lecithin), has been mentioned. They are incorporated with proteins and carbohydrates to form cell membranes and they envelop, with proteins, the suspended fat globules (chylomicra) in the blood. In addition, both substances are required in small amounts for other functions. Cholesterol forms the basis for many hormones, and both lecithin and cholesterol are prominent constituents of the myelin sheaths that surround the central nerve fibers (axones) of the nervous system. The lecithins are present in the vegetable oils in particular, from which they are apt to be removed during the refining of the oil. Serious cholesterol and lecithin deficiencies must be rare, although very low levels of cholesterol have been observed, nor is there evidence that they cannot be synthesized or formed in the body.

Vitamins and Minerals

A number of vitamins are needed in very small amounts for nutrition. These consist of the fat-soluble vitamins (A, D, E, and K), the water-soluble B group of vitamins, and vitamin C. In general, all vitamins enter into a large number of metabolic processes. Their deficiency results in symptoms of a general nature such as fatigue, weakness, loss of appetite, and so forth. There are specific symptoms, such as drying of the cornea and eventual blindness in vitamin A deficiency, abnormal bone formation with vitamin D deficiency, and tendency to hemorrhage with vitamin K deficiency. The vitamin B group is especially important in carbohydrate metabolism. Symptoms such as polyneuritis (paralysis), heart failure, and confusion occur in extreme cases of deficiency of the vitamin B group, especially vitamin B_1, usually in chronic alcoholics. Vitamin C deficiency results in bleeding tendencies, especially found first in the gums, and in poor healing after injury.

Single deficiencies are impossible to produce outside a laboratory. Therefore, all deficiencies should be treated as multiple deficiencies. Furthermore, treatment of protein deficiency should be accompanied by a liberal (not massive) supply of all vitamins. On a well-balanced diet the intake of vitamins is quite adequate and supplementation is unnecessary except in unusual instances.

Minerals are needed also in variable amounts. Calcium and phosphorus with vitamin D are essential to bone formation. Other metals —iron, iodine, sodium, potassium, sulfur, chlorine, and the trace metals cobalt, copper, fluorine, manganese, and zinc are also essential as are vitamins, and are adequately supplied by a good diet.

Section IV

THE SWANK LOW-FAT DIET

Reasons—Rules—Recipes

CHAPTER 11

Low-Fat Diet Instructions

The following changes will be made in your diet.

1. You will eat NO RED MEAT FOR THE FIRST YEAR. This includes dark meat of chicken and turkey.
2. Following the first year, 3 ounces of red meat will be allowed once per week. The eating of red meat is discouraged except on special occasions.
3. Dairy products containing 1 percent butterfat or more will be eliminated with exception indicated on p. 112.
4. All processed foods containing saturated fat will be eliminated.
5. Your saturated fat intake must never exceed 15 grams (3 teaspoons) per day.
6. Your unsaturated fat intake (oils) should be maintained at a minimum of 20 grams (4 teaspoons) and a maximum of 50 grams (10 teaspoons) per day.
7. 1 teaspoon or 4 capsules of nonconcentrated cod-liver oil and one therapeutic-type multiple vitamin and mineral is recommended.
8. Measurement of all fats and oils will be expressed in teaspoons:

   1 teaspoon = 5 grams of fat or oil

Definitions to Remember

Saturated Fats: Those lipids* containing mainly saturated fatty acids found in animal fat, processed (hydrogenated) vegetable oils, coconut oils, and palm oils. Saturated or animal fats are solid or hard at refrigerator temperature (approximately 40° F).

Unsaturated Fats (Oils): Those lipids containing mainly unsaturated fatty acids which are found in vegetable and fish oils. These are liquid at refrigerator temperatures.

Rancidity: The exposure of fats and oils to warm temperatures over a period of time causes chemical changes to occur that produce an undesirable taste and foul odor. When oxidation of the oils occurs, vitamins A and E are destroyed. Vitamin E is an antioxidant and protects against rancidity, but when the oil is exposed to warm conditions this protection is lost. ALWAYS KEEP OPENED OIL IN THE REFRIGERATOR.

Hydrogenation: The addition of hydrogen to the double bonds of unsaturated fatty acids. Oleic acid, linoleic acid, and linolenic acid when completely hydrogenated become stearic acid. Vegetable oils are converted to solid fats by hydrogenation. Margarine is produced by hydrogenating oils. Hydrogenation decreases the polyunsaturated fatty acid content and increases the saturated fatty acid content. AVOID ALL HYDROGENATED OILS.

The following foods will be changed in your diet.

Dairy Products

PERMISSIBLE IN ANY AMOUNT

Nonfat milk, skim milk, buttermilk (without cream or butter bits added), evaporated skim milk, nonfat dry milk powder, rinsed low-fat cottage cheese, dry-curd cottage cheese, 99 percent fat-free cheeses (see p. 143), nonfat yogurt.

PERMISSIBLE IN LIMITED AMOUNTS

Dairy products containing 1 percent butterfat and *never* exceeding 1 gram of fat per serving. You are allowed 1 serving per day, not to exceed 1 gram saturated fat.

* Lipids is a general term used for unsaturated oils, saturated fats, cholesterol, and phospholipids.

FORBIDDEN

Whole milk, cream, butter, margarine (this includes margarine made from safflower oil or corn oil), sour cream, ice cream exceeding 1 percent butterfat, ice milk, cheese exceeding 1 percent butterfat, creamed or partially creamed cottage cheese, imitation dairy products containing palm, coconut, or any hydrogenated oil.

Fats and Oils

PERMISSIBLE

(Not to exceed 10 teaspoons per day)

Safflower oil, sunflower seed oil, corn oil, cottonseed oil, soybean oil, sesame oil, wheat germ oil, linseed oil, peanut oil, and olive oil. Although peanut oil clouds in the refrigerator, it can be used freely.

FORBIDDEN

All margarines, butter, shortening, lard, cocoa butter, coconut oil, palm oil, and all oils that have been hydrogenated (processed).

Commercial Mixes

PERMISSIBLE IN ANY AMOUNT

Any prepared mix made *without* hydrogenated oil, lard, butter, margarine, palm oil, coconut oil, or egg yolks. Any prepared mix indicating 0–1 gram of fat.

PERMISSIBLE IN LIMITED AMOUNTS

One cup per day from all dry soup mixes.

FORBIDDEN

All packaged commercial mixes for cakes, cookies, pastries, pancakes, biscuits, and dessert bread products if they contain saturated fat (hydrogenated or processed oils, palm oil, coconut oil).

Commercially Canned Foods

PERMISSIBLE IN ANY AMOUNT

All canned fruits and vegetables, sauces containing no hard fat (hydrogenated or processed oils, palm oil, coconut oil).

FORBIDDEN

Chili, soups, stews, spaghetti and meat sauces, pork and beans, hash, sandwich spreads, canned chicken and turkey.

Chips—Crackers—Breads—Cereals—Pasta

PERMISSIBLE IN ANY AMOUNT

Because of the minimal amount of shortening found in bread, most commercial breads are permissible. Whole grain breads—all varieties, enriched wheat bread, sourdough bread, pumpernickel bread, raisin bread, English muffins, bagels, French bread, melba toast, Ry-Krisp, all pasta, all grain cereals, matzo, pretzels (made from only flour, water, and salt), rice.

PERMISSIBLE IN LIMITED QUANTITIES

Saltines, graham crackers, wheat and vegetable thins, vanilla wafers, lemon and ginger snaps (all 2–3 per day).

FORBIDDEN

All commercially prepared chips, including potato, as well as fancy and flavored crackers, chow mein noodles, commercially prepared biscuits, and sweet muffins.

Pastry

PERMISSIBLE IN ANY AMOUNT

Angel food cake, any commercially prepared pastry made without hydrogenated vegetable oil, coconut oil, palm oil, or lard.

FORBIDDEN

Commercially prepared pies, cakes, pastries, doughnuts, cookies.

Fruits and Vegetables

PERMISSIBLE IN ANY AMOUNT

Except as indicated, all fruits and vegetables, all fruit and vegetable juices. All frozen or canned vegetables without butter or high fat seasonings.

PERMISSIBLE IN LIMITED AMOUNTS

Avocado—1/8 = 1 teaspoon unsaturated fat (5 grams)
Olives (ripe)—3 medium = 1 teaspoon unsaturated fat (5 grams)

Olives (green)—6 medium = 1 teaspoon unsaturated fat (5 grams)

Avocados and olives contain unsaturated fatty acids and are to be counted in your daily unsaturated fatty acid intake.

Eggs—Complete

You are allowed 3 whole eggs per week, but no more than one egg each day.

Egg Whites Only

Each egg white contains 3 grams of protein and no fat. You are allowed egg whites in any quantity.

Sugar Products

Sugar has a tendency to increase nervousness in patients. We suggest your intake be minimal and for taste only. The following high-sugar products can be eaten in minimal amounts: sugar, jam, jelly, marmalade, honey, molasses, maple syrup, corn syrup, gelatin and desserts made with egg whites; rice, tapioca, or cornstarch puddings, if made with skim milk.

PERMISSIBLE IN LIMITED AMOUNTS

Plain chocolate syrup can be used for making cakes, brownies, frosting, or chocolate milk (see recipe section). You are allowed the amount to equal 1 tablespoon per day.

FORBIDDEN

Chocolate and all products containing chocolates and fresh or flaked coconut.

Beverages

Caffeine-containing products increase nervousness and must be limited to 3 cups combined per day (see p. 28).

Coffee, tea, cola—No more than 3 cups combined per day.

Decaffeinated Products

Herb tea—Unlimited

Coffee—4 cups per day

Cola—Because of high sodium content, these products should be limited to no more than 16 ounces per day.

Alcohol—Moderate amount (see p. 28)

Meats and Fish

RULES

1. *You will eat no red meat for the first year on the diet. This includes dark meat of chicken and turkey.*
2. *Following the first year on the diet, no more than 3 ounces of red meat will be allowed once a week.*
3. *Always buy the leanest cuts of meats and use the best method of cooking to reduce the fat.*

The following meats are permissible in any amount as they contain only small amounts of saturated fat.

POULTRY

White meat of chicken and turkey with skin removed before cooking.

FISH—WHITE

Cod, abalone, halibut, snapper, smelt, flounder, sole, sturgeon, tuna canned in water, shark, mahimahi, haddock, perch, pollock, and so forth.

SHELLFISH

Clams, crab, lobster, oysters, scallops, shrimp.

For those patients with elevated cholesterol levels, shellfish should be eaten infrequently.

For those patients watching their weight, keep serving size at no more than 4 ounces.

The following fish can be eaten only in limited quantity because of the high unsaturated fat (oil) content.

The fish are listed in amounts to equal 1 teaspoon unsaturated fat (oil). You are allowed *4 teaspoons* (20 grams) minimum per day and a *maximum of 10 teaspoons* (50 grams) contained in fish, nuts, and oil products. Weigh the fish after cooking.

FISH	AMOUNTS TO EQUAL 1 TEASPOON OIL (5 GRAMS UNSATURATED FAT)
Tuna, canned in oil, not drained	2 ounces
Tuna, canned in oil, but rinsed and drained	3 ounces
Salmon—Chinook	1 ounce
Salmon—coho	2 ounces
Trout	2 ounces
Sardines, canned in oil	1 ounce
Herring and Mackerel	1 ounce

The following meats contain *saturated fatty acids* (fat) and are listed in amounts to equal 1 teaspoon (5 grams). You are allowed 3 ounces per week following the first year. Weigh the meat after cooking.

BEEF, POULTRY, AND GAME	AMOUNTS TO EQUAL 1 TEASPOON FAT (5 GRAMS SATURATED FAT)
Low Fat	
Lamb, leg	3 ounces
Liver: Beef, Calf, Pork	3 ounces
Kidney: Pork, Veal, Lamb	3 ounces
Heart: Calf, Beef (lean portion only)	3 ounces
Tongue: Calf only	3 ounces
Rabbit	3 ounces
Horsemeat	3 ounces
Venison and Elk	3 ounces
Liver—Chicken and Turkey	3 ounces
Gizzards—Chicken	3 ounces
Medium Fat	
Beef, lean only	2 ounces
Ham, lean only	2 ounces
Lamb, rib, loin, or shoulder	2 ounces
Pork, lean only	2 ounces
Veal	2 ounces
Heart—Lamb	2 ounces
Kidney—Beef	2 ounces

BEEF, POULTRY, AND GAME	AMOUNTS TO EQUAL 1 TEASPOON OIL (5 GRAMS UNSATURATED FAT)
Tongue—Beef	2 ounces
Chicken, dark meat, skin removed	2 ounces
Turkey, dark meat, skin removed	2 ounces
Hearts—Chicken, Turkey	2 ounces
Gizzard—Turkey	2 ounces
Pheasant, skin removed	2 ounces
Squab, skin removed	2 ounces

The following meats are forbidden because of the high fat content.

Spareribs, goose, duck, bacon, lunch meats, salami, frankfurters, ground turkey or chicken, weiners (including chicken and turkey), all sausages.

Unsaturated Fatty Acids (Oils)

Fats and oils deliver a concentrated source of energy; each gram supplies twice the amount of energy supplied by the same amount of protein or carbohydrate. The main source of this energy is the fatty acids. The average saturated fat intake in the American diet is between 150–200 grams per day. On a low-fat diet you may notice drying of your skin and hair, and easy fatiguability if you eat less than 4 teaspoons (20 grams) of unsaturated fat per day. Your lifestyle will dictate the amount of unsaturated fatty acids necessary in your diet. If you are working and exercising, you may need 4–10 teaspoons per day. If you are sedentary, 4 teaspoons per day will usually be sufficient.

Your weight can vary depending on the amount of oil in your diet. For weight reduction, keep your oil intake between 2–4 teaspoons (10–20 grams) per day. If you have difficulty gaining weight, increase your oil to 8–10 teaspoons (40–50 grams) per day.

The reduction of saturated fatty acids in your diet to no more than 15 grams will make it necessary to substitute unsaturated fatty acids to maintain a reserve energy level.

RULES

1. *Eat foods daily that contain unsaturated fatty acids.*
2. *Maintain a minimum of 4 teaspoons (20 grams) of unsaturated fatty acids per day and a maximum of 10 teaspoons (50 grams).*
3. *If you are sedentary or would like to lose weight, your unsaturated fat intake can be maintained slightly lower at 2–4 teaspoons per day.*
4. *If you are active, it may be necessary to maintain between 6–10 teaspoons of unsaturated fat per day.*
5. *Take 1 teaspoon or 4 capsules of cod-liver oil daily and count as 1 teaspoon (5 grams) unsaturated fat. If you are taking cod-liver oil capsules, the vitamin A should not exceed 1,250 I.U. and 135 I.U. of vitamin D per capsule.*

The following foods contain unsaturated fatty acids (oils) and are listed in amounts equivalent to 1 teaspoon (5 grams).

FOODS	AMOUNTS
Cod-liver Oil	1 teaspoon
Linseed Oil	1 teaspoon
Corn Oil	1 teaspoon
Sunflower Seed Oil	1 teaspoon
Soybean Oil	1 teaspoon
Peanut Oil	1 teaspoon
Cottonseed Oil	1 teaspoon
Wheat Germ Oil	1 teaspoon
Sesame Seed Oil	1 teaspoon
Olive Oil	1 teaspoon
Mayonnaise and Salad Dressing, Commercial	2 teaspoons
Mayonnaise, homemade	1 teaspoon
Peanut Butter and Other Nut Butters (old-fashioned, nonhydrogenated)	2 teaspoons
Peanuts, Almonds, Cashews	1/2 ounce
Any Other Kind (Walnut and Pecan halves, Filberts, Hazelnuts)	1/3 ounce
Sunflower Seeds	3 teaspoons
Sesame Seeds	3 teaspoons

FOODS	AMOUNTS
Pumpkin Kernels	3 teaspoons
Avocado—1/8	1 teaspoon
Olives (ripe)—3 medium	1 teaspoon
Olives (green)—6 medium	1 teaspoon

Fish containing unsaturated fatty acids must be counted in your daily oil intake (see p. 116–17).

Cod-liver oil contains highly unsaturated fatty acids and will give you more energy. It also aids in reducing the number of colds and flu you may have. It is high in vitamins A and D. Additional A and D should be restricted to only one therapeutic multiple vitamin and mineral capsule per day.

We would like to reemphasize the fact that oils derived from fish, vegetables, nuts, and seeds are liquid at refrigerator temperature, with the exception of coconut and palm oils, which are solid at this temperature and highly saturated. Coconut and palm oils are therefore forbidden. Since both of these oils can truthfully be labeled "pure vegetable oil," we must assume that a label that is not specific in identifying the kind (or kinds) of oils used could contain either of these oils, or a mixture containing them. Also, if the label specifies that the vegetable oils have "hardened," "hydrogenated," or in the contents it is noted that "diglycerides" or "polyglycerides" have been added, one should suspect that the virgin oil has been altered. *The amount of saturation can vary, but it is recommended that any product in question that carries a label with these terms should be avoided.*

Even though a product may indicate pure vegetable oil is used in cooking, it is not always permissible. If the product has been fried and the oil reused, such as potato chips, it is not permissible.

You are also cautioned against the use of imitation dairy products because these products are usually made with coconut or palm oil. Palm oil is being imported into the United States in increasing quantities each year because it can be produced more cheaply than the native vegetable oils. It is being used extensively as a substitute in the domestic manufacture of margarine, shortening, and for frying chips, crackers, and so on. READ YOUR LABELS CAREFULLY.

Converting to Oil

In addition to the recipes given in this book, you may easily convert your own favorite recipes for use in this diet. Just remember to count each whole egg or egg yolk used as 1 teaspoon of fat, use skim milk or nonfat dry milk powder (mixed with one part water to one part powder) where whole milk is called for, and substitute vegetable oil for shortening, lard, margarine, or butter. The following table has been worked out to assist you in substituting oil for shortening, butter, or margarine.

SHORTENING, BUTTER, OR MARGARINE	VEGETABLE OIL
1 tablespoon	1 tablespoon
2 tablespoons	1 1/2 tablespoons
4 tablespoons	3 tablespoons
1/3 cup	4 tablespoons
1/2 cup	6 tablespoons
3/4 cup	1/2 cup + 1 tablespoon
1 cup	3/4 cup

TABLES

Table of Measurements

1 tablespoon	3 teaspoons
1/4 cup (2 ounces)	4 tablespoons or 12 teaspoons
1/3 cup	5 1/3 tablespoons or 16 teaspoons
1/2 cup (4 ounces)	8 tablespoons or 24 teaspoons
3/4 cup	12 tablespoons or 36 teaspoons
1 cup (8 ounces)	16 tablespoons or 48 teaspoons
1 fluid ounce	2 tablespoons
16 fluid ounces	2 cups
2 cups	1 pint
2 pints	1 quart
4 quarts	1 gallon

30 (28) grams = 1 ounce = 2 tablespoons = 6 teaspoons

Table of Equivalents

16 ounces (2 cups)	1 pound
2 cups chopped cooked meat	16 ounces or 8 teaspoons fat
2 cups ground beef (measured before cooking)	12 ounces or 6 teaspoons fat (after being cooked)
1 cup commercial mayonnaise	24 teaspoons oil
1/3 ounce nutmeats (walnut and pecan halves, filberts, hazelnuts)	1 teaspoon oil

1/4 cup nutmeats (walnut and pecan halves, filberts, hazelnuts)	6 teaspoons oil
1/4 ounce nutmeats (peanuts, almonds, cashews)	1/2 teaspoon oil
1/4 cup nutmeats (peanuts, almonds, cashews)	4 teaspoons oil
1 tablespoon sesame seeds	1 teaspoon oil
1 tablespoon sunflower seeds	1 teaspoon oil
1 tablespoon pumpkin kernels	1 teaspoon oil

Keeping a Record of Your Diet

When starting the diet, be sure that you have accurate sets of measuring cups and spoons, as well as a food scale to weigh servings of meat and fish. You will soon be able to pour out oil and slice meat without measuring and weighing each time, but occasionally you should check yourself to be sure that your "eye" is still accurate. During the first year on the diet you will be weighing only those fish containing unsaturated fatty acids (oil). Remember, no red meats and dark meat of poultry.

During the first few months that you are on the diet, you should keep a detailed list of everything that you eat each day, noting the teaspoonfuls of fat and oil that you consume. This can be done conveniently on a form similar to that shown in Figure 17. You should keep these lists only as long as you feel that they are valuable to you as a guide to preparing meals and distributing your fat intake over the day. We then instruct patients to record all of the food they eat for one week every month. This will provide an accurate check of the amount of fat you eat. Soon you will be able to plan menus and prepare meals while remaining conscious of your fat intake, and without the feeling of actually being on a diet.

Midmeal Fatigue or Hunger (Low Blood Sugar)

How well will you feel when you go on this diet? You may experience a certain amount of weakness and irritability during the first few months, but your body will adjust and thereafter you will have as much or more energy than you had before. Fats hold food in the stomach. On the low-fat diet the stomach tends to empty rapidly. You will become hungry more often than before. Midmorning and midafternoon snacks will provide a light pickup and help you avoid the

NAME			F = Fats O = Oils		
Date -	F	O	Date -	F	O
Breakfast Snack Lunch Snack Dinner Snack			Breakfast Snack Lunch Snack Dinner Snack		
Total			Total		
Date -	F	O	Date -	F	O
Breakfast Snack Lunch Snack Dinner Snack			Breakfast Snack Lunch Snack Dinner Snack		
Total			Total		

Figure 17. Diet recording form.

weak periods. Try substituting a glass of skim milk, with or without a tablespoon of nutritional yeast, or a glass of nonfat dry milk, buttermilk, or fruit juice instead of coffee or tea. A cup of bouillon with a tablespoon of gelatin is also an excellent pick-me-up. For something a little more substantial, a cracker with fish or a teaspoon of peanut butter has more value than a cookie or a piece of hard candy. In time the body will adjust to the new diet and these hunger-weakness periods will subside. Remember, though, that you must eat at least three to four small nutritious meals a day to be sure of this.

Special Diets

If you are already following a special diet for obesity, diabetes, gall bladder disease, or some stomach or intestinal ailment, and you desire to go on the low-fat diet, the two diets can be successfully combined. The low-fat diet is also helpful in weight control during pregnancy, but you should consult your physician before starting it. The Swank low-fat diet is well tolerated by patients with long previous histories of stomach trouble.

Invisible Fats—Forbidden Foods

You may be surprised at some of the foods that are listed as forbidden or limited on this diet. Most of us are aware that such foods as milk, cream, and butter contain fat, and we may be conscious of this fact as we eat them. But these "visible" fats actually make up only about 25 to 50 percent of our normal daily fat intake. The remainder is made up of "invisible" fats—those added to our food in the cooking process, the butter, shortening, and eggs in cakes and pies, the cream and whole milk in ice cream, and the fat contained in the lean parts of meat, to name only a few. For instance, cheese is usually considered a protein food, but it may contain as much as 50 percent butterfat. To make this diet effective, you must become aware of the invisible fats that are contained in so many foods, as well as the visible ones, and judge your fat intake accordingly.

Virtually all foods contain some fat, but it would be impractical in day-to-day living to measure the small traces of fat in any of the foods we eat. It is quite possible that, even if you are careful, you could eat as much as 1, possibly 2, teaspoons of uncounted and unmeasured fat in a day. For this reason it is important that you weigh and measure accurately the accountable fats and that you abstain completely from foods included in the forbidden list.

Frying and Baking

Although we recommend broiling instead of frying, the use of a nonstick pan or vegetable spray is recommended when you want to panfry. If oil is required in the pan, such as in stir frying, then the oil that is used should be counted. (There are several stir-fry recipes in the chapter on Oriental cuisine.) If you feel that you must deep-fry, heat the oil to 350°–375° F and maintain this temperature during the cooking process, being careful that it does not reach the smoking stage. Because vegetable oils oxidize and become rancid after being heated, do not reuse the oil. It is not possible to measure accurately the amount of oil absorbed during deep frying.

Vegetable sprays or nonstick pans are also worthwhile for baking and we encourage their use, especially when baking cookies. Avoid those sprays that have been hydrogenated. When a vegetable oil is brushed on a cookie sheet, the oil will oxidize in a hot oven and become very "gummy" and extremely difficult to remove.

Vitamins

We advise that patients take one high-potency multivitamin-mineral capsule each day. Because of the relatively high oil intake by some patients, one must consider the vitamin E intake. Therapeutic multiple vitamins usually contain 30 I.U. of vitamin E, and this vitamin is contained in wheat germ and fresh vegetables. If followed faithfully, the Swank low-fat diet provides patients with all of the vitamin E they need. If desired, wheat germ or wheat germ oil can be added to the daily food intake or additional vitamin E can be taken. It is harmless if a moderate amount is taken (see Chapter 10).

We advise 1 teaspoon or 4 capsules of cod-liver oil daily. If taking the capsules, the vitamin A should not exceed 1,250 I.U. and 135 I.U. of vitamin D per capsule. If you find you cannot tolerate the cod-liver oil, raw linseed oil can be substituted. Both of these oils contain a very high percentage of essential fatty acids. Keep the oil in the refrigerator to prevent it from becoming rancid. This will also diminish the "fishy" taste of cod-liver oil and the bitterness of raw linseed oil. We recommend taking a gulp directly from the bottle and following it immediately with a few ounces of fruit juice or carbonated drink, or whatever you find the most palatable for you. We also recommend that you establish a regular time most suitable for you to take it: the first thing in the morning before breakfast or just before retiring at night. (We have observed that patients on the Swank low-fat diet have fewer colds than do other members of their families who are not following the diet and taking cod-liver oil.)

When traveling where you will be away from the conveniences of refrigeration, leave your cod-liver oil at home. It will become rancid rapidly if not refrigerated. Instead, take a supply of cod-liver oil capsules with you. Under these circumstances, we recommend taking four nonconcentrated cod-liver oil capsules per day.

Proteins—Oils—Fats

In assessing the value of your daily diet to assure normal growth and repair of tissues, it is important that the protein intake be adequate both in quantity and quality (see Chapter 10). Many foods, especially vegetables and cereals, contain proteins, and an adequate quantity of them could easily be obtained on a strict vegetable-cereal diet. However, without complete knowledge of the mixing of these foods, the protein quality would be inadequate for normal growth and replacement. Such a diet, though adequate in most other foodstuffs, would slowly lead to low levels of energy, less than normal growth, and general poor health, especially during the active growing period of life. By adding small amounts of high-value proteins, which contain relatively high concentrations of the essential amino acids (see Chapter 10) to a vegetable-cereal diet, the protein intake could be made adequate for a vigorous life. Animal foods such as meat, poultry, fish, milk, cheese, and eggs contain high-quality proteins. Soybean protein is a complete plant protein equal in quality to most animal proteins, and soybeans are high in protein content. Other legumes provide a good quality of protein but contain an insufficient amount of methionine. Nuts contain high amounts of protein, but the quality is not adequate.

Grain products are low in protein, lacking the amino acid lysine. Fruits and vegetables provide very little protein, and sugars, syrups, fats, and oils have none.

For Westerners accustomed to a diet containing a great deal of animal protein, the problem is different. They consume much more of the high-value proteins than needed, and the excess is consequently converted to carbohydrate and burned as energy or stored as fat. In either case, this is inefficient and places a burden on the liver and kidneys. One could continue to get all of the protein needed and simultaneously reduce the animal-fat intake by shifting to fish, seafood, white meat of poultry, one egg three times a week, and skim milk or buttermilk. At the same time, the amount of protein can be reduced to a level more compatible with efficient metabolism.

This excludes fat-containing red meat from your diet and reduces your fat intake. When reducing the fat intake, the oil intake can be increased to suit your needs. The fat and oil intake should be distributed over the course of the day, and a particular effort should be made to get some of your quota early in the day. Eat three or four relatively equal-sized meals daily instead of snacks here and there followed by a heavy meal at the end of the day. An egg for breakfast three times a week will give you one teaspoon of animal fat and a good start on your high-value protein intake of the day. A midmorning snack, nonhydrogenated peanut butter on whole grain crackers or bread, or a few nuts will provide you with some oil. A fish or seafood sandwich with mayonnaise included in your lunch will also help fill out your oil quota for the day. In this way your body is given an opportunity to utilize its food intake gradually over the course of the day when you are most active. This is particularly helpful when you are trying to lose weight.

Frequently patients starting this diet will unwittingly reduce their oil as well as fat intake to near zero. These patients often become tired and listless and remain so until they increase their consumption of oil. The chronic fatigue experienced by most patients with multiple sclerosis is not quickly cured by the oil intake, but a faithful and careful adherence to the diet will slowly restore a significant amount of energy to most patients over a period of a few years.

Eating Out

Eating out can be handled very effectively once you have mastered the basic concepts of the diet. More restaurants are adapting their menus to accommodate people on restrictive diets. We suggest, however, that you eat out no more than once a week because of the variable and often high amount of hidden fat in all restaurant food.

The following general rules may help you select the more appropriate restaurants and food on the menu.

1. Let your waiter know that you are on a restrictive diet and that you must avoid dairy products and saturated animal fats.
2. All fast-food restaurants are forbidden eating establishments. The high fat content of their food cannot be tolerated.
3. Moderately expensive restaurants are usually more accommodating and able to make adjustments to your needs. Lower-priced restaurants are not able to deviate from the menu and are generally not helpful.
4. Avoid gourmet-type restaurants because of the excessive use of butter, cream, and cheese.
5. Avoid Mexican restaurants because of the use of bacon, fat, and lard in the preparation of the food.

6. Oriental food can be eaten if you avoid all deep-fried or fried foods. Order only the vegetable and chicken dishes.
7. All deep-fried foods are forbidden. This includes even those foods prepared in pure vegetable oil.
8. Request that your meat be broiled, poached, or baked without butter—NEVER FRIED. Also, limit your meat intake to 3 ounces of very lean meat after the first year on the diet.
9. Request that your vegetables be steamed without butter.
10. Do not order sautéed vegetables or meat. Usually they are sautéed in (animal) hard fat.
11. Do not use salad dressings when the oil cannot be identified. Fresh lemon juice is a good substitute.
12. Order fresh fruit, gelatin, angel food cake, or fruit ices, all with no toppings, for dessert.
13. If there are no permissible items on the menu, order à la carte. A shrimp or crab cocktail and a salad can be complemented by a baked potato and roll to satisfy your hunger.
14. Do not be afraid to make special requests of your waiter.

Eating While Traveling

With a little planning your vacation can be adjusted to include the low-fat diet. After the first year on the diet you are allowed 15 grams of saturated (animal) fat each day. During vacation (two to three weeks only) you may increase your daily saturated fat intake to 20 grams, maximum. The increase in saturated fat for this short period of time should not alter the disease and will give you a little more flexibility while traveling. Upon returning from your vacation, we advise that you decrease your saturated-fat intake to no more than 5 grams daily for one month, then return to your basic low-fat diet.

Most airlines are accommodating and will prepare a vegetarian meal for you, if notified in advance. Many vegetarian meals are prepared with a large slice of cheese for protein. Since this is not permissible on the diet, we suggest that you carry a snack of fruit and nuts with you to complement your meal. If you are to be in the air more than three to four hours, plan ahead and bring several snacks. First-class accommodations are more expensive but can make following the diet easier. Upon leaving your hotel, request that a sack lunch be prepared to take with you on the plane.

Traveling by car will pose few eating problems if you keep the following suggestions in mind.

BREAKFAST

Your breakfast meal should not be difficult to find in any restaurant. If you are tempted to order the usual, hash browns and eggs or a plain waffle, thinking there is not much saturated fat, think again. The following list will give you some idea of the amount of saturated fat found in these foods.

1 egg—5 grams
1 piece French toast—3.3 grams
1 average pancake—3–4 grams
1 waffle—7.4 grams
1/2 cup hash browns—11.7 grams
1 cup whole milk—5 grams
1 baking powder biscuit—6 grams
1 buttermilk biscuit—4.1 grams

As you can see, it would not be difficult to exceed the maximum of 20 grams of saturated fat just at breakfast.

A simple breakfast of hot or cold cereal and dry toast or one poached egg, dry toast, and fresh fruit can be ordered easily in most restaurants. These suggestions keep your saturated-fat intake at no more than 5 grams for the breakfast meal.

LUNCH

Delicatessens can be found in most towns. They are terrific for nonfat, inexpensive lunches on the road. Usually they have sandwiches, pasta, and fruit and vegetable salads, which can be eaten in the deli or packed to take along for a picnic. If a deli is not available, most restaurants will be able to provide you with a turkey or tuna sandwich or salad.

The grocery store is always available when you grow tired of restaurants. Carry along a small cooler—ice is available daily in your hotel. Fresh fruit, smoked or canned fish, fresh vegetables, French bread, and something cool to drink make a delightful luncheon break. These lunches are inexpensive and a welcome change from restaurant food.

DINNER

Unlike lunch, your evening meal should be eaten at the more expensive restaurants. You will find the choices are much greater. The better restaurants will be happier to accommodate your needs. If you have been careful during the day and have not exceeded 1–2 teaspoons (5–10 grams) of fat, you should be able to order without problems. Always try to avoid red meat. This will help compensate for the hidden fats you have had to consume throughout the day.

Traveling Abroad

Although eating the low-fat way abroad is more difficult than at home, our experience indicates that it can be done.

Certain high-fat eating areas like Germany, England, Holland, Switzerland, and the Scandinavian countries offer very few low-fat dishes, and there is a high incidence of heart disease and multiple sclerosis in these countries. The following suggestions will help you avoid these problems.

Bed and Breakfast. We suggest that you avoid this way of traveling, unless the breakfast is the so-called continental breakfast; otherwise your morning meal will leave you no choice other than not to eat. Some typical breakfast meals you may encounter with this type of traveling are as follows:

England: Greasy eggs, bacon, toast with butter and marmalade, strong coffee or tea with cream.

Germany: Fresh cold cuts, cheese, bacon fat spread, dark bread, and strong coffee.

Switzerland: Croissants, cheese, strong coffee with cream.

It is advisable that you stay in a hotel with a restaurant. The menu will give you much more variety, such as fresh fruit, muffins, toast, and poached eggs.

When eating abroad you cannot apply home rules unless you have full control of the language. Even then it would be difficult, as nonfat products are not used in restaurants. Do not expect to find nonfat milk or low-fat cottage cheese. Fresh salads and fruits are always available. Usually a simple pasta dish with marinara sauce can be found.

If you are forced to order meat, ask for veal as it is lean. Usually the meat dishes are served with gravy. Simply scrape away the gravy and eat only 2–3 ounces of the meat.

Chicken is usually cooked with the skin. If you have no other choice, remove the skin when served and count this as 1 teaspoon (5 grams) of saturated fat. Fresh fish is usually available in most countries.

With the abundance of open markets, you can have fresh fruit, vegetables, and bread daily in your hotel room or on the road. Many markets in Great Britain have skimmed milk and low-fat cottage cheese. You must be careful to read the label. Skimmed milk may have vegetable fat added to it. "Light" milk is semiskimmed and contains some cream. Yogurt may be made with skimmed milk and also contains cream. In other countries it is more difficult to find non-fat dairy products.

Fast Foods

With the exception of the salad bar, it is not possible to eat in *any* fast-food restaurant and maintain the low-fat diet. The high-fat and high-sodium content of their foods are certainly conducive to heart disease, stroke, and multiple sclerosis.

The following list will give you an idea of what you can expect in a fast-food restaurant.

Fillet-O-Fish
22.7 grams of saturated fat
519 grams of sodium
373 calories

Fried Chicken (2 pieces)
46 grams of saturated fat
1,445 grams of sodium
720 calories

Peeling the skin off will not decrease the saturated fat content significantly. The fat of the chicken is under the skin and when cooked rapidly melts into the meat. Removing the skin after cooking helps very little in reducing the fat content of the meat.

Taco
8.0 grams of saturated fat
213 grams of sodium
194 calories

Hamburger (Small)
9.0 grams saturated fat

Hamburger (Large)
32 grams saturated fat

These are average figures. Some fast-food restaurants may have higher levels of saturated fat or slightly lower levels.

Shopping

1. READ ALL LABELS CAREFULLY. If you must buy prepared food, read the contents listed on the label carefully. *If for any reason certain contents are questionable, then avoid the product.*
2. Any product that does not specifically identify the kind of vegetable oil used should be avoided since it could be assumed to be either coconut oil, palm oil, or hydrogenated vegetable oil, all of which are saturated. Manufacturers often do not indicate that an oil has been processed. This is usually true of prepared foods. If a product is in question write to the company or avoid the product.
3. Dairy products vary from area to area. Therefore, it is necessary to check with your local dairy to be sure that the products you use contain less than 1 percent butterfat.
4. Buy whole grain and whole grain products as assurance that you receive the natural vitamins, minerals, proteins, and roughage.

Equipping the Kitchen

Because it is important to conserve your energy in the kitchen, we suggest you invest in a few helpful cooking aids. If you have a low energy level it is easy for one on a special diet to get discouraged and begin slipping off. Also, if you are at risk in the kitchen because of incoordination and loss of feeling in your hands, these aids will be much safer for you. These cooking aids are not NECESSARY to maintain your diet, they simply make it easier for you.

1. Food processor (good for making peanut butter, quick soups, quick breads)
2. Electric mixer (tabletop kind—always available for quick muffins, cakes, cookies)
3. Blender (for breakfast drinks)
4. Microwave (certainly not necessary, but safe and quick—good for those patients who have difficulty in the kitchen because of numbness in hands and risk of burning, also excellent for working patients and bachelors)
5. One heavy aluminum frying pan (easy to clean, does not stick, great for cooking fish)
6. One medium saucepan (aluminum)

7. One pair of stainless steel surgical scissors (very helpful for removing skin from chicken and less risky for cutting yourself)
8. One heavy oven mitt (for those of you who have difficulty telling when the oven is hot, this inexpensive item will save your hands)
9. Timer
10. Scale for weighing red meat and fish containing unsaturated fat (oil)
11. One nonstick muffin pan (cleans easily)
12. Two wooden spoons (that will not become hot when left in the pan—less chance of burning yourself)
13. Large spatula with wooden handle
14. Electric can opener (opening cans seems so easy—unless you have weakness in your upper extremities; then this chore can seem impossible—an electric can opener can be purchased very inexpensively now)
15. Oven Opener (a long wooden stick with curved fingers on the end for opening your oven without risk of getting burned—this can be found in most kitchen stores for under two dollars)

Herbs and Spices

The following section on cooking with herbs and spices is intended to help you improve the flavors and scents of your food.

STORAGE OF HERBS AND SPICES

Buy small quantities. The flavor and aroma are in the oils of the spices and herbs and will be destroyed by age, light, and heat. When the herb or spice has lost its aroma, it should be replaced. Old spices and herbs are left with a stale bitter taste. If you are growing your own herbs, the best method of preservation is freezing. Drying herbs must be done under the most optimal conditions. Spices and herbs lose their taste and scent in three to four months. Avoid commercial brands that have lost their fresh scent. Spice and herb shops or natural food stores carry a wide variety of these items in bulk, which are both less expensive and fresh. The amount of spice or herbs used is one's own individual preference. A good rule to follow is "season to taste." Recipes are seasoned for what will please the average person. Rarely should you use less than what the recipe calls for. You may want to add slightly more, but be careful of overseasoning. You should not be able to identify the particular spice or herb used in a recipe. The prepared dish should be such that people will ask what you have used to impart such a wonderful flavor.

Allspice is a berry of a West Indian tree. It is most flavorful when freshly ground. Its flavor resembles a blend of cinnamon, nutmeg, and cloves. It can be used ground with baked goods, puddings, relishes, stews, beef, lamb, pork, Indian and Middle Eastern dishes. When whole, it can be used for pickling vegetables and fish. It is also used with pepper to accent and give a spicy taste.

Arrowroot is a starch, a thickening agent. It can be used in place of cornstarch.

Basil is a member of the mint family. It is grown all over the world. Basil must be used sparingly as it can be overpowering. The longer it cooks, the stronger it tastes. It is used in Mediterranean foods, salads, soups, and sauces, and with tomatoes and fish.

Bay is the aromatic leaves of the laurel tree and comes from eastern Mediterranean countries. It should be used sparingly as it can also be overpowering. One leaf will flavor a dish for as many as eight to twelve people. It is excellent for pickling, stews, spiced vinegars, and soups. It combines well with fish, boiled or in chowder. Use with any tomato mixture, Italian tasting soups, and for marinades because of its preserving qualities.

Caraway Seeds are the dried seeds of a biennial plant which is grown in Northern Europe. The seeds are principally used in cakes, breads, stews, salads, marinades, and sauerkraut, and with cabbage.

Cardamom comes from small brown seeds that grow enclosed in a pod. Grown in Malay Archipelago, India, and Ceylon, it is a member of the ginger family. Ground, it is used in Indian dishes such as curries, Danish pastry, and coffee cakes. Whole, it is used in mixed pickling spices.

Cayenne is the hot, red powder made from several varieties of red pepper. The two most popular commercial varieties are Japanese, which is very hot, and Mexican.

Celery seed comes from a plant that is a member of the parsley family. Use it in dressings, soups, salads, and with vegetables.

Chervil is a member of the parsley family. Use it with soups, salads, and vegetables, or for marinades for fish and meat.

Chili Powder is made from Mexican chili peppers and blended spices. It can be purchased mild or hot. Chili powder is used in Mexican dishes, such as chili con carne, and also in shellfish and oyster cocktail sauces, gravy, and stews.

Chives are a member of the lily family. They are very delicate to the taste. Use in salads, sauces, and marinades, and with cheese and fish.

Cinnamon is the aromatic bark of the cinnamon tree. True cinnamon is grown in Ceylon; other varieties are grown elsewhere. Use sticks, as once ground the powdered cinnamon does not retain its flavor. Use in pies, cakes, drinks, and with fruits.

Cloves are a member of the myrtle family. They are the nail-shaped flower buds of the stately clove tree. It is grown in the East Indies, Madagascar, and Zanzibar. Cloves have a strong aroma and flavor. Use ground in baked foods, potato soup, and tea. Use whole in marinades and pickling, or with fruits and meats.

Coriander (Cilantro) is an herb of the parsley family. It is grown in Southern Europe, India, and Morocco. Both the leaves and dried fruit (seeds) are used in Mexican cooking, Spanish cooking, and Chinese cooking. Too, coriander is used in curries and most Indian dishes. Use very sparingly because of its strength.

Cumin is a member of the parsley family. It is a small dried fruit resembling the caraway seed in shape. It is grown in the Mediterranean islands, Morocco, and India. Cumin is used in Indian curries, Middle Eastern stews, hot Mexican chilis, chicken, rice, and vegetable dishes.

Curry is a blend of several spices. Use it for making curry sauces, in currying meat, fish, poultry, and eggs. Curry can also be used in soups and dressings.

Dill is an herb whose leaves and seeds (dried) are both used when preparing food. Dill is used with vegetables, salads, fish, rice, and soup.

Fennel seed is a small dried seedlike fruit with a flavor somewhat like that of anise. It is used for soups and breads, sweet pickles, candies, and liqueurs.

Garlic is an all-purpose herb of the lily family. Use it for Italian and French cooking, meat, fish, soup, salads, and dressings.

Ginger is the root of a tuberous plant grown mainly in Jamaica, West Africa, India, and the Orient. There are two varieties of ginger. Jamaican, which is light in color, is mild and has a sweet aroma. It is used in desserts. African is hot and much stronger. It is used in Indian curries and Chinese dishes. Ginger can be purchased ground and in this form is available in most markets. Fresh gingerroot is available in some markets. It spoils easily so it is best to use ginger quickly or freeze it. Use only a small slice to accent Chinese and Indian cooking. Dried gingerroot can be purchased in natural food stores or most spice shops. It must be ground. Use it for cakes, puddings, and with onions, zucchini, carrots, and sweet potatoes.

Mace and *Nutmeg* are from the same tree which is grown mainly in the East Indies. Because they are similar in taste they can be used interchangeably. Use for vegetables, sauces, soufflés, baked goods, and eggnog.

Marjoram is a member of the mint family. It is used with meats and vegetables, and in salads. The leaf can be used to flavor lamb. In combination with other herbs, use marjoram to flavor stews, soups, and poultry. Marjoram is grown in warm-climate areas. It cannot tolerate frost.

Mint is used in desserts, drinks, marinades, and salads. Spearmint is used frequently in Middle Eastern cooking.

Mustard is a spice made from the small seed of the mustard plant. It is widely cultivated but imported mainly from England, Europe, and the Orient. Some good varieties are grown in the United States. The black variety is used in Indian cooking. The yellow is used for meat, salads, curries, pickling, fish, vegetables, cheese dishes, and sauces.

Oregano is a member of the mint family and is grown in Greece and Mexico. It can be used in tomato dishes, vegetables, salads, dressings, stuffings, marinades for all fish and meat, Spanish and Mexican dishes, and, of course, Italian dishes.

Paprika is the powder of a dried sweet red pepper. Spanish paprika is used mainly for decoration because of its red color—it has little taste. Hungarian paprika is much stronger in taste and is used in, for example, goulashes. Paprika's flavor is good with shellfish, fish, and in salad dressings.

Parsley is used in soups, sauces, and stuffings.

Peppercorns come in three colors: black, white, and green. The green peppercorns are the mildest. The white peppercorns are the strongest. All three are used mainly in nonsweet cooking.

Poppy seeds are used with salads, fruits, vegetables, pastries.

Rosemary has a rather sweet taste and strong aroma. It is grown mainly in the United States, England, and Southern Europe. It is used with lamb dishes, shellfish, pork, chicken, beef, vegetables, sauces, fruit salads, and spiced wine or cider.

Saffron is a tiny stigma of a crocuslike flower grown in Mediterranean areas. It takes 80,000 flowers or 200,000 hand-picked stigmas to make one pound. It should be used sparingly as it has a very strong taste and is the most expensive of all the spices. Be careful that what you buy is not the imitation type made from safflower or marigolds. Use this spice for chicken, meat, sauces, tea, and rice.

Sage is the leaf of a low-growing herb. It has a strong aroma and strong flavor. The choicest comes from Yugoslavia and Greece. Use sparingly with meats, sausage, beans, lamb, duck, and pork.

Savory is a member of the mint family and is grown in many climates. It is used with turkey, chicken, trout, beef, and vegetables (especially beans), and for salads, and stews.

Sesame Seeds are usually small honey-colored seeds from an herb grown in Turkey, India, and the Orient. Sesame seeds and the oil made from them are used heavily in Chinese, Greek, Egyptian, and Indian cooking. The seeds are also used in pastry, rolls, salads, and as a coating for chicken or fish. The oil is used for stir frying and sautéeing.

Tarragon is an herb that should be used sparingly as its flavor can dominate. Since it will become bitter if overcooked, it should be added during the last five minutes of cooking. Use in sauces and salads, and with chicken, beef, seafood, and vegetables.

Thyme is grown in temperate climates. There are many varieties of it. Garden thyme enhances all meats and vegetables, soups, and stuffings for poultry. Lemon thyme is excellent with seafood and vegetables.

The following salt substitutes can be used in place of table salt for flavoring. Combine the spices and keep them in a closed container.

Salt Substitutions

1.	Thyme	1 tablespoon
	Sage	1 1/2 teaspoons
	Rosemary	2 1/2 teaspoons
	Marjoram	1 tablespoon
2.	Celery Seed	1 teaspoon
	Marjoram	2 1/2 teaspoons
	Savory	2 1/2 teaspoons
	Thyme	2 1/2 teaspoons
	Basil	1 teaspoon
3.	Thyme	2 teaspoons
	Savory	2 1/2 teaspoons
	Sage	1 1/2 teaspoons
	Rosemary	2 teaspoons
	Marjoram	2 1/2 teaspoons

CHAPTER 12

Milk Products and Dairy Substitutes

Since butter, margarine, sour cream, whole milk, whipped cream, and so on, are not allowed on the low-fat diet, we have included recipes for their substitutes. Nonfat yogurt can be used as a substitute in all recipes calling for sour cream. If nonfat yogurt is not available in your area low-fat yogurt can be used but must be counted in your saturated fat intake. Rinsed low-fat cottage cheese can also be blended to make a good sour cream substitute. Rinsing can be easily done by putting the cottage cheese in a colander and placing under cold water briefly to remove the fat.

Milk products are an excellent source of protein and calcium, and you are encouraged to use them whenever possible. A glass of skim milk as an in-between-meal snack makes a nutritious pick-me-up. The use of cottage cheese (or yogurt) in recipes will also increase your protein.

Dairy products vary from state to state, so it is advisable to check with your local dairy regarding the butterfat content of the milk products you use that are not so labeled. All dairy products must be less than 1 percent butterfat. Even buttermilk should be verified with your local dairy since there are some brands that contain more than 1 percent butterfat.

Table Spreads

Spreads to be used on bread, pancakes, waffles, or baked potatoes can be made in either of two ways. The first recipe is for a spread made with buttermilk. The second contains cornstarch, which is cooked before oil is added.

Each spread keeps well when stored in a covered dish in the refrigerator for two to three weeks.

SPREAD 1

2/3 cup instant nonfat dry milk
2/3 cup buttermilk
Few drops yellow food coloring
1/2 teaspoon salt
2 cups oil

Combine first four ingredients in small bowl. Mix smooth with rotary beater. Add oil, a little at a time, beating thoroughly after each addition. If using an electric mixer, blend on low speed; beat in oil gradually on high speed. Do not use electric blender. Yields 1 pound 7 ounces, or 3 cups

Fat: None
Oil: 1 tablespoon spread: 2 teaspoons

SPREAD 2

1 tablespoon cornstarch
2/3 cup instant nonfat dry milk
1 teaspoon salt
1 tablespoon lemon juice
2/3 cup water
2 cups oil
Few drops yellow food coloring

Mix cornstarch, instant nonfat dry milk, and salt together into top of double boiler. Combine lemon juice and water, gradually add to starch mixture, mixing until smooth. Cook over boiling water, stirring constantly, until mixture thickens, about 4 minutes. Remove from heat. Add oil, 1/4 cup at a time, beating with rotary beater after each addition. Add coloring to give desired shade. Do not use electric blender. Yields 1 pound 5 ounces or 2 2/3 cups

Fat: None
Oil: 1 tablespoon spread: 2 1/4 teaspoons

LOW-CAL SOUR CREAM SUBSTITUTE

1/2 cup cottage cheese (dry-curd or low-fat rinsed)
1/4 cup plain commercial nonfat yogurt
2 to 4 tablespoons skim milk

Blend all ingredients in blender. Stop blender when necessary and push mixture down into blades with spatula. Add more milk if mixture is too thick. For variety, add dry onion soup mix, chopped onion, parsley, chives, garlic salt or powder. Use on baked potatoes, vegetables, meats, or as a dip. Yields 1 cup

Fat: None
Oil: None

WHOLE EGG SUBSTITUTE

1 egg white
2 teaspoons oil
2 teaspoons nonfat dry milk powder
Drop of yellow food coloring (optional)

Combine all ingredients and beat well with electric mixer. May be stored in refrigerator for up to 1 week or frozen. Serves 1

Fat: None
Oil: Total—2 teaspoons; per serving—2 teaspoons

COFFEE CREAM SUBSTITUTE

2 tablespoons oil
1 cup nonfat dry milk powder
1 cup water

Put oil, nonfat dry milk, and water into blender. Mix at highest speed for 3 to 4 minutes. Refrigerate. Yields 1 1/2 cups

Fat: None
Oil: 1 teaspoon substitute: 1/8 teaspoon oil

WHOLE MILK SUBSTITUTE

1/4 cup nonfat dry milk powder
1 cup skim milk

Combine ingredients and mix well. Refrigerate. Yields 1 cup
Variation: This can also be made with equal parts of nonfat dry milk powder and water.

Fat: None
Oil: None

YOGURT CREAM CHEESE

Use this spread in recipes calling for cream cheese. The addition of sweet or savory ingredients provides a nice variety to the spread.

2 quarts plain, active-culture nonfat yogurt

SAVORY SEASONINGS

Freshly ground black pepper
1 cup finely minced scallions
Coarse (kosher) salt

SWEET SEASONINGS

Sugar
Fresh berries

1. Line a large colander or sieve with several layers of dampened cheesecloth, about 16 inches square, allowing the edges to overhang. Set the colander over a large bowl and pour in the yogurt. Let drain for about 30 minutes.
2. Pour off the liquid in the bowl. Tie the ends of the cheesecloth together with a long piece of string. Tie the string to a faucet so that the cheese is suspended over the sink or suspend the cheese over a large bowl. Let drain for at least 12 and up to 24 hours. (The cheese can be eaten after 12 hours, but it will not have as thick and creamy a texture.)

3. Turn the cheese into a medium bowl, cover with a dish towel, and refrigerate. The cheese will keep, refrigerated, for up to 4 days. Yields 2 1/2–3 cups

Fat: None
Oil: None

WHIPPED EVAPORATED MILK

1/4 teaspoon gelatin
2 teaspoons cold water
1/2 cup evaporated skim milk
3 teaspoons sugar
1/4 teaspoon vanilla
1/8 teaspoon salt

Soak the gelatin in the cold water. Scald milk in a double boiler, then add the soaked gelatin and stir until the gelatin is dissolved. Chill the milk until it is icy cold, then whip like cream. Add sugar, vanilla, and salt to taste. This will retain its whipped consistency for several days. Yields 2 cups

Fat: None
Oil: None

WHIPPED CREAM SUBSTITUTE

1/3 cup ice water
1 tablespoon lemon juice
1/2 teaspoon vanilla
1/3 cup nonfat dry milk powder
2 tablespoons sugar

Combine water, lemon juice, and vanilla in a quart bowl. Sprinkle nonfat dry milk powder over the top. Beat until stiff, 10 to 12 minutes, add sugar. Yields 2 cups

Fat: None
Oil: None

Nonfat Substitutes

Most imitation dairy products contain palm, coconut, or hydrogenated oil and are not allowed on the Swank low-fat diet.

The following products can be used as substitutes for dairy products.

Count Down, a processed cheese, is 99 percent fat free. It is very similar to Velveeta and can be purchased at some health food stores or ordered from the producer: Diet and Health Products, P.O. Box 1886, Lima, OH 45802.

Sap Sago is imported from Switzerland. It is a very hard 100 percent fat-free cheese that must be grated. It can be used in place of Parmesan cheese. It is excellent for flavoring salads or Italian dishes and can be purchased at specialty grocery stores and many natural food stores.

Pot Cheese is made from cottage cheese. This 100 percent fat-free cheese has the consistency of a smooth cheese spread. The flavor is very light, and the cheese can be spread on crackers or as a topping for a casserole. You will find this cheese in many grocery stores or specialty markets.

Nonfat Yogurt is an excellent substitute for sour cream. If suspended in a cheesecloth over the sink for several hours, it will develop into cream cheese. This product is not available in all areas. It can easily be found in most supermarkets and natural food stores in the Pacific Northwest. There are several brands; the most familiar are Weight Watchers and Dairy Lite.

Butter Buds, an imitation butter, has been defatted and is in powdered form. It can be reconstituted with water and used on vegetables, sauces, or as flavoring in place of butter. It also adds butter flavor when sprinkled on popcorn. It is available at most markets.

Butter Flavoring, which is an aromatic flavoring, can be found in the spice section of the grocery store. It is very concentrated and only a few drops will be necessary to maintain the flavor of butter.

Weight Watcher Frozen Dessert is an imitation ice cream. It is easily available in the Northwest in most markets. In other areas it is more difficult to find. You are allowed 1/2 cup per day.

Weight Watcher Fudge Bar, Chocolate Mint Treat, and Orange Vanilla Treat are easily available in most markets in the Northwest. In other areas they are more difficult to find. You are allowed one per day.

Baskin-Robbins Fruit Ice is available at your local Baskin-Robbins ice cream store. This product is 100 percent fat-free and is cool and refreshing. It is available in several fruit flavors. This product can be eaten freely, keeping in mind the high sugar content.

Hi Saf is an ice cream made with safflower oil and it is good. Although difficult to find in the Pacific Northwest, it is available in many places in California. Your local market may be able to order it for you.

Sorbet, a refreshing fruit ice, is available in most markets. You must watch the calories as it is high in sugar. This product contains no saturated or unsaturated fat and can be eaten freely, keeping in mind the high sugar content.

Rice Dream, a nondairy frozen dessert, can be found in many natural food stores. The base is made of a sweet milk derived from brown rice. Although low in saturated fat it contains 3 grams of unsaturated fat (oil) per 1/2 cup.

Section V

RECIPES

CHAPTER 13

Breakfast and Lunch

Breakfast

When following the low-fat diet, you will find that you are hungry more frequently. This is due to the reduction of saturated fat in your diet. Fat slows down digestion more than carbohydrates or protein do. When you remove saturated fat from your diet you may find it necessary to eat more frequently to maintain your energy. We suggest four to five small meals each day, rather than three large meals, until your system becomes adapted to the diet. To receive the maximum benefit from the low-fat diet, we stress the importance of starting the day with breakfast. Your morning meal does not have to be elaborate. If you are working or simply do not have the energy, keep it simple. This meal can be quick, easy to prepare, and enjoyable.

BANANA STRAWBERRY DRINK

1 cup buttermilk or skim milk
1 frozen banana
1/2 cup frozen strawberries
1 tablespoon wheat germ
1 teaspoon vanilla

Combine all ingredients in blender. Blend until smooth. Serves 2 (To freeze banana, peel and wrap in plastic wrap and freeze.)

Fat: None
Oil: None

BANANA PINEAPPLE DRINK

1 frozen banana
1 cup buttermilk or skim milk
1/2 cup crushed pineapple
1 tablespoon wheat germ
1 teaspoon vanilla

Combine all ingredients in blender. Blend until smooth. Serves 2 (To freeze banana, peel and wrap in plastic wrap and freeze.)

Fat: None
Oil: None

LEMON VELVET DRINK

1 8-ounce container lemon nonfat yogurt
1 6-ounce can frozen orange juice concentrate
2 1/2 cups skim milk
1 teaspoon vanilla

Combine all ingredients in blender and blend until smooth. Serves 4

Fat: None
Oil: None

BLENDER BREAKFAST

1 6-ounce can frozen orange juice concentrate, undiluted
1 can water
1 cup skim milk
1 teaspoon vanilla
1/4 teaspoon nutmeg
1 egg (optional)
12 large ice cubes

Combine all ingredients except ice cubes in blender. With blender on high speed, add ice cubes gradually. Serves 4

Fat: Total—1 teaspoon if egg is used; per serving—1/2 teaspoon
Oil: None

CAROB MILK

1 cup cold skim milk
1 tablespoon carob powder
1 teaspoon honey
1/4 teaspoon natural vanilla
2 ice cubes

Place all ingredients except ice cubes in blender container. With blender on High, drop in ice cubes and blend until mixture is frothy. Yields 1 1/2 cups

Fat: None
Oil: None

GRANDMA'S HOTCAKES

1/2 cup oatmeal, uncooked
1/4 cup cornmeal, uncooked
2 cups buttermilk
1/4 cup nonfat yogurt
2 teaspoons baking soda
3/4 teaspoon salt
2 eggs, separated
1/4 cup sugar (or less to taste)
1 cup all-purpose flour
3/4 teaspoon baking powder

Place oatmeal and cornmeal in mixing bowl. Add buttermilk, yogurt, baking soda, and salt. Stir until mixture foams. Add egg yolks and sugar and stir until blended. Mix flour with baking powder and add to batter. Beat egg whites until stiff; fold into mixture. Cook on hot nonstick griddle. Yields about 24 dollar-size or 16 4-inch pancakes (3 dollar-size or 2 4-inch hotcakes per serving)

Fat: Total—2 teaspoons; per serving—scant 1/3 teaspoon
Oil: None

PANCAKES

3 eggs
2 tablespoons sugar
1/4 teaspoon salt
1 cup buttermilk
1/2 teaspoon baking soda
1 tablespoon hot water
1 cup all-purpose flour
1 teaspoon oil (for brushing)

Mix eggs and sugar; beat well. Add salt and buttermilk. Dissolve soda in hot water and mix all ingredients except the oil. Batter should be the consistency of heavy cream. Allow to stand in the refrigerator for

1 or more hours. Brush griddle with oil lightly, pour batter onto the griddle a tablespoon at a time, and fry on both sides until nicely brown. Yields 18 5-inch pancakes

Fat: Total—3 teaspoons; per two cakes—1/3 teaspoon
Oil: Total—Negligible

GERMAN PANCAKE

1/4 cup all-purpose flour
1/2 teaspoon salt
2 eggs
6 tablespoons skim milk
1 teaspoon oil

Preheat oven to 450° F. Mix flour and salt. Whisk eggs until blended. Add flour in three additions, beating only until blended. Then add milk in two additions, then oil. Pour into heavy 8-inch skillet, either nonstick-coated or sprayed with vegetable spray. Bake 10 minutes at 450° F, then reduce heat to 350° F for 10–15 minutes. Yields 1 medium-sized German Pancake

Fat: Total—2 teaspoons; per serving—2 teaspoons
Oil: Total—1 teaspoon; per serving—1 teaspoon

OATMEAL PANCAKES

1 1/2 cups quick-rolled oats
2 cups buttermilk
1/2 cup all-purpose flour
1 teaspoon sugar
1 teaspoon baking soda
2 eggs
1 teaspoon salt

Mix together quick-rolled oats and buttermilk. Beat in remaining ingredients. Cook on nonstick or lightly oiled griddle until both sides are brown. Yields 12 4-inch cakes
Variation: Sprinkle a few blueberries on each pancake as they cook.

Fat: Total—2 teaspoons; per pancake—1/6 teaspoon
Oil: None

PUFFY OMELET

4 egg whites
1/4 teaspoon cream of tartar
3 egg yolks
3 tablespoons skim milk
Salt and pepper to taste
2 teaspoons oil
Creole Sauce

Preheat oven to 350° F. Beat egg whites and cream of tartar until stiff. Beat egg yolks until thick and lemon-colored. Beat in 1 tablespoon milk at a time, then the salt and pepper. Fold egg yolks into the egg whites. Pour into sizzling skillet in which the oil has been heated. Turn heat to Low. Cook slowly on top of stove until light brown underneath, about 10 minutes. Place skillet in oven. Bake until light brown on top and until when touched lightly with finger no imprint remains, about 10–15 minutes. Make 1/2-inch crease across omelet, halfway between handle and opposite side. Slip spatula under, tip skillet to loosen omelet, and fold in half without breaking. Roll omelet upside down onto hot platter. Garnish with Creole Sauce and serve at once. Serves 3

Fat: Total—3 teaspoons; per serving—1 teaspoon
Oil: Total—2 teaspoons; per serving— 2/3 teaspoon

Sauce

Fat: None
Oil: Total—6 teaspoons; per 1/4 cup—3/4 teaspoon

GRANOLA

Mix together:

4–6 cups rolled oats
2 cups raw bran
2 cups finely chopped or ground nuts and seeds (cashews, almonds, sunflower, and/or sesame)
2 cups wheat germ
1 cup nonfat dry milk powder
1 tablespoon salt

Mix together in separate bowl:

1 cup oil
1 cup water
11/2 cups honey
3 tablespoons vanilla
Raisins or other dried chopped fruit

Preheat oven to 250° F. Combine rolled oats, bran, nuts and seeds, wheat germ, nonfat dry milk powder, and salt, and set aside. Mix oil, water, honey, and vanilla together. With a large wooden spoon combine dry ingredients with honey mixture until oats are thoroughly coated. Spread about 1/2 inch thick on oiled cookie sheets. Place in the oven from 1 1/2–2 hours.

Turn mixture over after first 1/2 hour and every 15 minutes thereafter until oats are golden brown. Let cool. Add raisins or other dried chopped fruit. Store in tightly closed container in cool, dry place. Yields approximately 18 cups

Fat: None
Oil: Total—88 teaspoons; per one cup serving—5 teaspoons

The oil can be reduced in this recipe by decreasing the amount of nuts used.

BRAN MUFFINS

2 cups boiling water
2 cups whole bran cereal
1 1/2 cups sugar
1 cup oil
1 egg
3 egg whites
1 quart buttermilk
5 cups all-purpose flour
4 cups bran flakes or Raisin Bran cereal
5 teaspoons baking soda
2 teaspoons salt
Dates, raisins, chopped prunes, apples (optional)

Preheat oven to 400° F. Pour boiling water over whole bran cereal and let stand. Mix sugar well with oil, beat in eggs and buttermilk, and add bran mixture. Combine flour, bran flakes or Raisin Bran cereal, baking soda, and salt. Stir into liquid mixture. Add dates, raisins, chopped prunes, or apples. Fill desired number of muffin tins one-half full and bake for 20 minutes. This recipe can be kept covered in refrigerator for 3 weeks and used as desired. Yields approximately 4 dozen muffins

Fat: Total—1 teaspoon; per serving—negligible
Oil: Total—48 teaspoons; per 1 muffin serving—1 teaspoon

WAFFLES

2 cups all-purpose flour
4 teaspoons baking powder
1 teaspoon salt
1 tablespoon sugar
1 1/4 cups skim milk
1 whole egg
2 egg whites
2 tablespoons oil

Preheat waffle iron. Mix flour, baking powder, salt, and sugar together. Add milk. Separate eggs. Beat whole egg lightly and add to mixture. Mix thoroughly. Beat egg whites stiff and fold into mixture. Add oil. Pour small amount of batter in center of waffle iron. Bake waffle until golden brown. Serve with honey, maple syrup, or marmalade. Serves 6

Variations:

WHOLE WHEAT WAFFLES

Follow recipe for waffles, using whole wheat flour for white flour.

BERRY WAFFLES

Follow recipe for waffles, adding 3/4 cup washed blueberries or blackberries to batter.

APPLE CINNAMON WAFFLES

Follow recipe for waffles, adding 2 cups diced apple, 1 1/2 teaspoons cinnamon, and 2 tablespoons sugar.

Fat: Total—1 teaspoon; per serving—1/6 teaspoon
Oil: Total—6 teaspoons; per serving—1 teaspoon

WHEAT WAFFLES

2 cups skim milk
1/3 cup oil
1/3 cup maple syrup or maple blend syrup
2 eggs, separated, room temperature
1 1/4 cups all-purpose flour
3/4 cup whole wheat flour
1/2 cup crushed bran flakes cereal
1 tablespoon baking powder
1 teaspoon salt
1/2 teaspoon ground coriander
1/4 teaspoon baking soda
Pinch of cream of tartar
1 tablespoon sugar
1/2 cup finely chopped dates (optional)

Preheat waffle iron. Combine milk, oil, syrup, and egg yolks in large bowl and whisk to blend. Combine flours, cereal, baking powder, salt, coriander, and baking soda. Add to liquid ingredients and whisk until fairly smooth. Beat egg whites and cream of tartar in another bowl until soft peaks form. Add sugar and beat until stiff but not dry. Gently fold 1/4 of whites into batter to lighten, then fold in remaining whites and dates. Bake waffles until golden brown. Serve hot. Yields 8 waffles

Fat: Total—2 teaspoons; per serving—1/4 teaspoon
Oil: Total—16 teaspoons; per serving—2 teaspoons

SWEET SPICE WAFFLES

1/3 cup firmly packed light brown sugar
1 egg, separated, room temperature
3/4 cup buttermilk
1/4 cup molasses
3 tablespoons oil
1 cup all-purpose flour
11/2 teaspoons baking powder
1 teaspoon ground ginger
3/4 teaspoon cinnamon
3/4 teaspoon allspice
3/8 teaspoon baking soda
1/4 teaspoon dry mustard
1/4 teaspoon salt
1/3 cup chopped raisins
2 tablespoons ginger
Pinch of cream of tartar

Preheat waffle iron. Using electric mixer, beat sugar and egg yolk until light and fluffy, about 2 minutes. Mix in buttermilk, molasses, and oil. Combine flour, baking powder, spices, baking soda, mustard, and salt. Add to liquid ingredients and beat on low speed just until blended. Stir in raisins and 2 tablespoons ginger. Beat egg white and cream of tartar in another bowl until soft peaks form. Gently fold into batter. Bake waffles until golden brown and cooked through. Serve hot. Yields 6 waffles

Fat: Total—1 teaspoon; per serving—1/6 teaspoon
Oil: Total—9 teaspoons; per serving—11/2 teaspoons

BASIC BREAKFAST CRÊPES

1 cup all-purpose flour
11/2 cups skim milk
2 eggs
1 tablespoon oil
1/4 teaspoon salt

Combine all ingredients in small mixing bowl and beat on medium speed until well blended, or combine in a blender and blend about 45 seconds.

Heat a lightly oiled 6-inch nonstick skillet. Remove from heat and spoon in 2 tablespoons of batter. Lift and tilt skillet to spread batter evenly over bottom of pan. Return to heat and brown on one side only, 45 to 65 seconds. To remove, invert pan over paper toweling and remove crêpe by gently lifting one edge. Repeat with remaining batter, reoiling skillet occasionally. Yields 16–18 crêpes

Fill crêpes with your favorite fruit filling and sprinkle lightly with powdered sugar.

Fat: Total—2 teaspoons; per crêpe—trace
Oil: Total—3 teaspoons; per crêpe—1/5 teaspoon

Lunch

An appetizing lunch requires a little thought and preparation, as well as some consideration to its nutritive value. A bowl of soup, green salad, skim milk, and fruit or gelatin for dessert will make an excellent light lunch. If this is not enough, add a small sandwich. Packing a lunch to carry to the office will need a little more thought in order to avoid monotony. It is desirable for you to carry your lunch to work each day. In this way you will know the exact amounts of oil and fat that you have consumed and can plan the evening meal accordingly. Although eating out is not forbidden, it is not advisable as an everyday practice, since it is impossible to judge exactly how much fat is contained in restaurant meals.

SANDWICHES

You can choose from an endless variety of sandwiches. Because of the high fat content, many must be avoided, such as those with cheese or a quantity of meat. The nutritive value of a sandwich depends largely upon its bread. Many whole wheat breads are made commercially today, but unfortunately there is also a quantity of air-filled "sponge breads." Since the use of either butter or margarine is not allowed, we have included two recipes for spreads made with oil (see Chapter 12) or you can use mayonnaise and/or mustard for spreads. Crisp greens of many varieties, cucumbers, alfalfa sprouts, and so forth, make a delicious combination with whole wheat bread. All kinds of fish as well as the white meat of chicken and turkey can be mixed with mayonnaise and various seasonings for a very satisfying and tasty filling.

CHAPTER 14

The Cocktail Hour

With a few reservations alcoholic beverages are permitted on the low-fat diet. You can enjoy your preference whether it is scotch, gin, bourbon, rye, rum, vodka, tequila, liqueurs, wine, or beer. Drinks that are mixed with milk, cream, or butter are not allowed (see Chapter 4 for sensitivity to alcohol).

The caloric content of alcoholic beverages is so high that this is a factor for the weight watcher. For example, an ounce of whiskey, gin, or vodka will contain about 11 grams of alcohol, which furnishes the body nearly 45 calories (4 calories per gram). The usual drink at home will contain 2 ounces of beverage (90 calories), two drinks (180 calories), and so forth. Then one must consider the mixer. People on the low-fat diet tend to "feel" their liquor quickly, so drinking slowly is advised. Drinking during and after eating (on a full stomach) leads to a prolonged effect of the alcohol, a possible hangover, and fatigue for up to several days. Difficulty sleeping is also an unpleasant side effect from overindulging. White wine mixed with soda water or sweet vermouth mixed with one to two parts of soda water can be especially refreshing and is fairly safe.

Canapés, Hors d'Oeuvre, Appetizers

It is not possible to enjoy a cocktail party if the choice of appetizers is too restricted. At most parties many appetizers contain too much fat and must be avoided. Safety can be found with a relish tray of vegetables, olives, pickles, and nuts, fish and seafood dishes, and fruits. Dishes containing meat, cheese, sour cream, margarine, or shortening should be completely avoided since it is impossible to know just how much fat one is getting, and since tasty tidbits are hard to stop eating once started. One cannot possibly judge the fat content of these foods, especially when they are eaten away from home. The crackers usually served will also cause a problem since all commercially prepared chips and fancy and flavored crackers are forbidden. Only two to three saltines, tiny pretzel sticks, and Wheat and Vegetable Thins are allowed per day. However, melba toast, Ry-Krisp, and breads can be consumed with a fair amount of freedom. Hors d'oeuvre can be prepared at home that are tasty as well as fat-free. Here are a number of recipes for these.

Base for Dips

Whipped, rinsed low-fat, or dry-curd cottage cheese makes an excellent base. (To rinse cottage cheese, place curds in a colander and briefly wash with cold water.) Cottage cheese can be used in place of sour cream, table cream, and cream cheese. To obtain a more creamy consistency, mix in mayonnaise or nonfat yogurt. If nonfat yogurt is not available in your area, low-fat can be used. Low-fat yogurt will increase the saturated fat content to 2–4 grams depending on the brand used. Use dehydrated onion soup or ranch dressing mixed with a pint of nonfat yogurt or a pint of rinsed cottage cheese, or half yogurt and half cottage cheese.

Arrange fresh or blanched vegetables that have been chilled on a large platter. Such vegetables as cauliflower buds, mushrooms, broccoli, celery, turnips, carrots, and cherry tomatoes are delicious with the onion soup and ranch dressing. Also try shrimp, crab, anchovies, tuna, and salmon, each with appropriate seasonings. Add lemon or lime juice to fish or seafood dips.

BASE I

1/2 cup dry-curd or low-fat rinsed cottage cheese
1/4 cup plain commercial nonfat yogurt
2–4 tablespoons skim milk

Combine ingredients in blender and blend until smooth. Yields 3/4 cup

Fat: None
Oil: None

BASE II

1 cup dry-curd or low-fat rinsed cottage cheese
1/2 cup buttermilk
1/4 teaspoon salt

Combine ingredients in blender and blend until smooth. Yields 1 cup

Fat: None
Oil: None

MARINATED MUSHROOMS

1/2 pound fresh mushrooms or 2 3-ounce cans button mushrooms
3 tablespoons oil
1 tablespoon wine vinegar
1/4 teaspoon powdered dry mustard
1 tablespoon chopped chives
1/8 teaspoon coarsely ground black pepper

Clean the fresh mushrooms or drain the canned mushrooms. Combine remaining ingredients and pour over the mushrooms. Chill several hours in refrigerator, turning over occasionally to ensure the mushrooms are being well coated with marinade and cover tightly. Yields approximately 20 caps

Fat: None
Oil: Total—9 teaspoons

BROILED MUSHROOM CAPS

1/2 pound fresh large mushrooms
1/3 cup finely chopped green onion
2 tablespoons cracker crumbs
1/4 teaspoon salt
1/8 teaspoon pepper
1/8 teaspoon garlic powder
1 teaspoon oil
Paprika

Remove stems from mushrooms and chop the stems finely. Add onion, crumbs, seasonings, and oil. Mix thoroughly, then stuff into mushroom caps, top with paprika, and broil until slightly brown. Serve immediately. (The caps may be made the night before, kept covered in the refrigerator, and broiled the following day.) Yields approximately 20 caps

Fat: None
Oil: Total—1 teaspoon; per cap—negligible

MUSHROOM APPETIZERS

1 cup crabmeat
1 tablespoon fine, dry bread crumbs (unseasoned)
1 tablespoon each, finely minced onion, parsley, and chives
3/4–1 teaspoon seasoned salt
White pepper to taste
1 egg, slightly beaten
1 tablespoon oil
24 large mushrooms, stems removed

Preheat oven to 350° F. Shred crabmeat in food processor or by hand. Combine crabmeat, bread crumbs, onion, parsley, chives, seasoned salt, and pepper. Mix well. Add slightly beaten egg and mix well. Brush mushrooms lightly with oil, then spoon mixture into mushroom caps, mounding slightly. Sprinkle lightly with additional bread crumbs if desired. Bake on baking sheet for 2 minutes or until hot. Yields 24

Fat: Total—1 teaspoon; per serving—negligible
Oil: Negligible

GUACAMOLE DIP I

3 medium ripe avocados
2 teaspoons lemon juice
1/2 cup Sour Cream Substitute

Peel and mash avocados in small bowl or use food processor. Add lemon juice and Sour Cream Substitute and blend well. Yields 1 1/2 cups

Fat: None
Oil: Total—24 teaspoons; per serving of 2 tablespoons—2 teaspoons

GUACAMOLE DIP II

1 medium ripe avocado
Juice of 1/2 lemon
3 tablespoons mayonnaise

Peel and mash avocado in small bowl or use food processor. Add lemon juice and mix well. Add mayonnaise. Mix well. Yields 1/2 cup

Variations:

1. Finely minced tomatoes added last
2. Finely minced onion added last
3. 1–2 jalapeño peppers, seeded and minced

Fat: None
Oil: Total—12 1/2 teaspoons; per serving of 2 tablespoons—3 teaspoons

BEAN DIP

1 8-ounce can pinto beans
1/4 cup oil
1 small onion, chopped
1 small garlic clove, minced
1 4-ounce can green chilies
1/4 teaspoon cumin (optional)

Rinse pinto beans with cold water. Place in blender or food processor. Add oil and blend until beans are a smooth consistency. Add onion, garlic, and green chilies. Blend. Add cumin and blend well. Heat thoroughly. Yields 1 cup

Fat: None
Oil: Total—12 teaspoons; per serving of 2 tablespoons—1 1/2 teaspoons

SALSA

1 16-ounce can tomatoes, drained and finely chopped or 1 pound fresh tomatoes, peeled and chopped
1 4-ounce can green chili peppers, rinsed, seeded, and chopped (jalapeños if desired)
1/2 cup finely chopped onion
1 tablespoon vinegar
1 teaspoon sugar
1/8 teaspoon salt
1/2 teaspoon cilantro

In mixing bowl thoroughly combine tomatoes, chili peppers, and onion. Stir in vinegar, sugar, salt, and cilantro. Let mixture stand at least 30 minutes at room temperature. Store in refrigerator. Serve with homemade Tortilla Chips or as a relish. Yields approximately 1 cup

Fat: None
Oil: None

TORTILLA CHIPS

Tortilla chips can be made from commercial packages of tortillas. Using pure vegetable oil brush corn tortilla lightly. Cut into small pie-shaped pieces and place on cookie sheet. Bake 10 minutes at 400° F. Store in airtight container. Serve with *Salsa* or Bean Dip.

CRAB SPREAD

1/4 cup vinegar or fresh lemon juice
12 ounces fresh, frozen, or canned crabmeat
1/3 cup mayonnaise
3 tablespoons pimiento
2 tablespoons finely chopped green onion
1 teaspoon salt
1/2 teaspoon freshly ground pepper
1 tablespoon drained capers

Pour vinegar or lemon juice over crabmeat and chill 30 minutes. Drain. Mix together remaining ingredients except capers and add to crab. Garnish with capers. Serve with favorite bread or crackers. Yields approximately 2 cups

Fat: None
Oil: Total—8 teaspoons; per 2 tablespoons—1/2 teaspoon

QUICK ANTIPASTO

1 6-ounce can large ripe olives, well drained
1 8-ounce can tomato sauce
3 tablespoons white wine
1/2 pound fresh shrimp or 1 7 1/2-ounce can solid water-packed tuna
1 16-ounce jar giardiniera (mixed vegetables), well drained
1 12-ounce jar artichoke hearts in oil, well drained
1 8-ounce can whole button mushrooms or 1/4 pound fresh mushrooms

Combine all ingredients, mixing well. Place in covered casserole; refrigerate at least 24 hours. Mix well once or twice while mixture marinates. This dish is especially good when served at an informal meal, such as a barbecue. Serve with toothpicks and small slices of French bread. As an appetizer serves 24–30 people

Fat: None
Oil: Total—3 ripe olives—1 teaspoon; per serving—negligible

CURRIED APPETIZERS

1 cup crabmeat or shrimp
2 tablespoons minced fresh parsley or 2 teaspoons dry parsley
1 tablespoon finely minced onion or 1 teaspoon instant onion
3 tablespoons mayonnaise
1/4 teaspoon curry powder
1 tablespoon lemon juice

Combine all ingredients. Chill at least 15 minutes. If the dehydrated parsley and onions are used, cover and refrigerate at least 1 hour. Spread on toast or French bread and broil. Whipped dry-curd cottage cheese can be used in place of mayonnaise. Yields 1 1/2 cups

Fat: None
Oil: Total—4 1/2 teaspoons

Made with dry-curd cottage cheese:
Fat: None
Oil: None

SANDWICH SPREAD

1 cup fresh, frozen, or canned crabmeat
2 tablespoons finely chopped green onion
2 tablespoons finely chopped dill pickle
1 hard-cooked egg, finely chopped
1 tablespoon lemon juice
1/4 cup mayonnaise
1 teaspoon prepared mustard
1/4 teaspoon salt
Dash of cayenne pepper

Combine all ingredients and mix well. Yields enough filling for approximately 2 dozen small sandwiches

Fat: Total—1 teaspoon; per sandwich—negligible
Oil: Total—6 teaspoons; per sandwich—1/4 teaspoon

ZIPPY CHEESE SPREAD

1/2 cup rinsed low-fat or dry-curd cottage cheese
2 tablespoons mayonnaise
1/4 teaspoon curry powder (or to taste)
1/4 teaspoon dry mustard
2 tablespoons sesame seeds, toasted
Paprika

Combine all ingredients and mix well. Spread on pieces of bread, melba toast rounds, or small rolls. Garnish with a dash of paprika, or save the sesame seeds to sprinkle on top. Broil for a few seconds before serving. Yields 2/3 cup or enough for 32 melba rounds

Fat: None
Oil: Total—5 teaspoons; per 2 melba rounds—1/4 teaspoon

SPINACH SPREAD

1 10-ounce package frozen chopped spinach, thawed and well drained
1 small onion, finely chopped
1/4 cup minced fresh or 1 tablespoon dried parsley
1/2 teaspoon salt
Enough mayonnaise to spread

Combine spinach, onion, parsley, and salt. Add mayonnaise until mixture can be spread easily. Serve as a spread with crackers or melba toast. Yields 1 1/2 cups

Fat: None
Oil: Negligible

HUMMUS

1 15 1/2-ounce can garbanzo beans (2 cups), drained
1/2 cup tahini (sesame seed butter)
2–3 garlic cloves, finely chopped
2 small hot green peppers, finely chopped
1 teaspoon salt
Juice of 1 lemon
1/4 cup olive oil

Combine all ingredients and blend in food processor or blender until smooth. Serve with pieces of Middle Eastern bread. Yields 2 cups

Fat: None
Oil: Total—24 teaspoons; per serving of 2 tablespoons—1 1/2 teaspoons

EGGPLANT DIP

1 medium eggplant
2 garlic cloves, finely chopped
Juice of 1 lemon
1/4 cup olive oil
2 hot peppers, chopped
1/2 cup tahini (sesame seed butter)
Scant salt

Preheat oven to 400° F. Bake or boil eggplant until soft. Scoop flesh from peel. Combine remaining ingredients with eggplant and blend in food processor or blender. Serve cold or at room temperature as a dip with Middle Eastern bread. Yields approximately 2 cups

Fat: None
Oil: Total—24 teaspoons; per serving of 2 tablespoons—1 1/2 teaspoons

OATMEAL CRACKERS

1 cup quick-rolled oats
2/3 cup all-purpose flour
1/3 cup wheat germ
1 tablespoon brown sugar
1/2 teaspoon salt or seasoned salt or garlic salt or celery salt
1/3 cup water
1/4 cup oil

Preheat oven to 350° F. Combine dry ingredients. Knead in water and oil. Form dough into a ball. Divide in half. On oiled baking sheet roll each half into 12″ × 8″ rectangle. Cut into 2-inch squares. Bake for 20 minutes or until crisp. (Be careful—they burn easily.) Cool on wire rack. Store in tightly covered container. Yields 48

Fat: None
Oil: Total—12 teaspoons; per serving of 4 crackers—1 teaspoon

FRIED PRAWN BALLS

11/2 pounds prawns, shelled and deveined
2 garlic cloves, finely chopped
1/2 teaspoon cayenne pepper
1 stalk coriander, finely chopped
1 stalk green onion, finely chopped
1/2 teaspoon grated nutmeg
1 egg
Cooking oil for frying
Sprigs of coriander

Bring 2–3 quarts water to a boil in a large pot. Add prawns and cook 2–3 minutes until done through. Drain. Chop prawns finely and add remaining ingredients except oil and coriander sprigs. Mix well into a sticky paste. Form into balls. Heat 1/4 inch oil in deep pan. Fry prawn balls for about 5 minutes. Drain well and garnish with coriander sprigs. Yields 10 medium-sized Prawn Balls

Fat: None
Oil: Negligible

CHAPTER 15

Soups

Soups are as nutritious as are the ingredients that are put into them. A hearty soup can be used as the main dish of a meal and served with a salad, dressing, and hot bread. If soup is served as an appetizer before the main course, be sure it is a small serving and preferably a clear soup, otherwise you will be tempted to overeat.

Cream soups that have been canned commercially have a high fat content. It is for this reason that we have eliminated the use of all canned soups. You will notice that these are included on the forbidden list of high-fat foods. *All dry soup mixes, including cream mixes, are relatively fat free, so you are allowed 1 cup per day.*

Making your own soup stock is a simple procedure. After the soup has been strained and defatted, it can be frozen in ice cube trays or small containers so that small quantities can be easily available to use as a seasoning for cooked vegetables, sauces, or Oriental dishes.

Nonfat dry milk should be added to all homemade cream soups to improve the texture and flavor as well as the nutritive value. It is important that cream soup not be boiled, especially after the nonfat dry milk has been added.

SOUP CROUTONS

Cut stale bread in thick slices. Remove the crust and cut bread in small cubes. Fry in hot oil until delicate brown. Drain on paper towel. Flavor with your favorite spices. Serve a few croutons in each portion of soup.

BASIC SOUP STOCK

3 pounds soup meat (beef brisket, shinbone, veal bone, chicken, or turkey)
1 tablespoon salt
3 quarts cold water
2 or more cups chopped vegetables (onions, carrots, celery, etc.)
3/4 cup tomato purée
1/2 green pepper, chopped

Place the soup meat and bones in a soup kettle and sprinkle with salt to draw out the juices. Let stand for 1 hour. Add water and bring to a boil. Turn heat to simmer and cook for 3 hours. Chill soup until fat is set on top. Lift off fat. To the defatted liquid add the vegetables, tomato purée, and green pepper, and simmer covered for 1 hour or longer. Strain if desired. Serves 6

Bouillon: Use beef shinbone and vegetables.

Consommé: Use lean beef, veal bone, chicken, and vegetables.

Fat: None
Oil: None

BASIC CREAM SOUP

1 tablespoon minced onion
2 tablespoons oil
1 1/2 tablespoons all-purpose flour
1/4 teaspoon salt
Pepper to taste
1/8 teaspoon paprika
1 cup Basic Soup Stock
3/4–1 cup minced or sieved cooked vegetables
3 tablespoons nonfat dry milk mixed with 1 cup skim milk, scalded

Sauté onion in oil. Blend in flour, salt, pepper, and paprika. Stir in stock and heat to the boiling point. Add vegetables and scalded milk. Season to taste. Serves 4

Fat: None
Oil: Total—6 teaspoons; per serving—1 1/2 teaspoons

CREAM OF CHICKEN AND MUSHROOM SOUP

2 tablespoons oil
1/4 cup finely chopped onion
1 pound mushrooms, sliced
1/3 cup all-purpose flour
4 cups chicken broth
11/2 cups skim milk
1/2 cup nonfat dry milk powder
1/2 cup dry white wine
1 teaspoon salt
1/2 teaspoon hot pepper sauce
21/2 cups skinned, diced, and cooked white meat of chicken
1/4 teaspoon thyme
Chopped parsley
Paprika

Pour oil into a large saucepan and sauté onion over medium heat until tender. Add mushrooms and cook 10 minutes. Blend in flour. Gradually stir in chicken broth, skim milk that has been mixed with the nonfat dry milk powder, and the wine. Stir over medium heat until mixture thickens and comes to a boil. Add remaining ingredients except parsley and paprika. Reduce heat and simmer, uncovered, for 20 minutes. Garnish with parsley and paprika. Serves 6

Fat: None
Oil: Total—6 teaspoons; per serving—1 teaspoon

CREAM OF POTATO SOUP

3 cups boiling water
3 medium-sized potatoes, peeled and cut in bite-size pieces
1/4 cup chopped onion
1 rib celery, finely chopped
1/2 teaspoon salt
3 cups Thin Easy White Sauce
3 tablespoons chopped parsley

In a medium-sized saucepan bring 3 cups water to a boil. Add potatoes, onion, celery, and salt. Cook at medium temperature until potatoes are tender. Strain, reserving 1 cup stock. Prepare Thin Easy White Sauce and add to stock, stirring constantly. Add potatoes, celery, and onion to the sauce. Heat thoroughly. Sprinkle with parsley. Serves 6 generously

Variations:

1. Press potatoes through a sieve into stock. This makes a very smooth soup.
2. Add 1 61/2-ounce can chopped clams.
3. For a thicker soup prepare Medium Easy White Sauce.

Fat: None
Oil: Total—3 teaspoons; per serving—1/2 teaspoon

VICHYSSOISE

2 medium-large onions, finely chopped
3 ribs celery (yellow tops too), finely chopped
3 tablespoons oil
4 medium-sized potatoes, diced
4 cups chicken stock
2 cups skim milk, scalded and enriched with 1/4 cup nonfat dry milk powder
Salt and pepper
Chopped chives or parsley

In a medium-sized covered pot cook onion and celery in oil until transparent and tender. (Do not brown.) Add diced potatoes and stock to the onion and celery and cook 15 minutes until potatoes are tender. Put in food processor or blend in the electric blender until smooth, then add scalded milk and seasonings. Garnish with chopped chives or parsley. Serves approximately 6

Variation:

Try sweet potatoes or yams instead of white potatoes and a meat stock instead of chicken.

Fat: None
Oil: Total—9 teaspoons; per serving—1 1/2 teaspoons

BASIC NEW ENGLAND CLAM CHOWDER

1 cup diced onion
1 rib celery, minced (1/3 cup)
1 tablespoon oil
3 medium potatoes, diced (2 cups)
1 teaspoon salt
1/4 teaspoon black pepper
Pinch of thyme
1 teaspoon parsley
2 10-ounce cans clam juice
1 1/2 cups skim milk, scalded
3/4 cup nonfat dry milk powder
2 6 1/2-ounce cans minced or chopped clams
2–3 tablespoons all-purpose flour (optional)
1/3 cup skim milk (optional)

In large soup kettle brown onion and celery in oil for about 3 minutes or until onion becomes translucent. Add potatoes, seasonings, and clam juice. Bring to boil, then simmer until potatoes are tender. Add skim milk that has been blended with nonfat dry milk powder and clams with juice. If a creamy consistency is desired, mix flour with skim milk and blend into soup, stirring until thickened. Heat through but do not boil. Serves 6 generously

Fat: None
Oil: Total—3 teaspoons; per serving—1/2 teaspoon

MUSHROOM AND CLAM BISQUE

1/2 pound mushrooms
2 tablespoons oil
4 tablespoons all-purpose flour
2 8-ounce bottles clam broth (2 1/2 cups)
1 10 1/2-ounce can minced clams, drained
3/4 cup skim milk enriched with 1/4 cup nonfat dry powdered milk or 1 can evaporated skim milk
Salt
Paprika
Chopped parsley or chives

Sauté mushrooms in oil. Stir in flour, then slowly add clam broth and clams. Simmer for 5 minutes. Add milk and season to taste. Garnish with chopped parsley or chives. Serves 4

Fat: None
Oil: Total—6 teaspoons; per serving—1 1/2 teaspoons

OYSTER STEW

2 tablespoons all-purpose flour
1 1/2 teaspoons salt
1/8 teaspoon pepper
2 tablespoons water
1 pint oysters and liquid
4 cups skim milk, scalded and enriched with 1/2 cup nonfat dry milk
Paprika

Combine flour, salt, pepper, and water, and blend to a smooth paste. Stir in oysters and liquid. (This small amount of flour is the secret of the stew's perfection.) Simmer oysters over very low heat until edges curl, then pour into scalded milk. Remove pan from heat, cover, let stand for 15 minutes to improve the flavor. Reheat stew briefly to serving temperature. Dust with paprika and serve. Serves 4

Fat: None
Oil: None

GAZPACHO

2 small onions, chopped
2 cucumbers, peeled and chopped
1 garlic clove, minced
3–4 tomatoes, peeled and cut up
1 rib celery, thinly sliced
1 carrot, cut in lengthwise slivers
2 tablespoons olive oil
2 tablespoons lemon juice
2–3 drops hot pepper sauce
Tomato juice to make up 2 quarts

Mix vegetables and garlic well. Add olive oil, lemon juice, hot pepper sauce, and tomato juice. Chill for several hours or overnight. Yields 8 generous portions

Fat: None
Oil: Total—6 teaspoons; per serving—3/4 teaspoon

TOMATO SOUP

4 cups sliced ripe tomatoes
2 medium onions, thinly sliced
2 tablespoons sugar
Sprig of parsley
1 teaspoon salt
1/8 teaspoon pepper
1/8 teaspoon Worcestershire sauce
2 tablespoons cornstarch
1/4 cup water
2 tablespoons nonfat yogurt

Cook tomatoes, onion, sugar, parsley, salt, pepper, and Worcestershire sauce together until vegetables are soft. Blend until smooth in food processor or blender. Blend cornstarch and water, add to blended vegetables, and cook until thickened and clear. Serve hot or cold, each garnished with a teaspoon of yogurt. Yields 6 cups

Fat: None
Oil: None

PISTOU

2 cups sliced carrots
2 cups diced potatoes
2 cups sliced leeks or yellow onion
4 teaspoons salt
12 cups water
1 pound zucchini, trimmed and sliced
1/2 pound green beans, trimmed and cut in 1-inch pieces
1 cup spiral pasta
1 slice fresh bread, crumbled
1 16-ounce can red kidney beans, drained
1 16-ounce can white kidney beans, drained
1/4 cup tomato paste
4 garlic cloves, crushed
4 teaspoons basil
1/3 cup oil

In large kettle combine carrots, potatoes, onion, salt, and water; bring to boil. Reduce heat, cover, and simmer 1 hour, stirring several times. Add zucchini, green beans, pasta, and bread; stir to blend bread. Cover kettle; simmer 15 minutes or until vegetables are tender. Add kidney beans and simmer 10 minutes. Just before serving, in medium-sized bowl combine tomato paste, garlic, and basil. Drizzle oil in slow steady stream until combined. Add 1 cup hot soup to this mixture, then gradually stir mixture into soup; heat thoroughly. Serves 8

Fat: None
Oil: Total—16 teaspoons; per serving—2 teaspoons

EASY VEGETABLE SOUP

4 cups water
4 teaspoons beef bouillon powder
3 cups 1-inch potato cubes
2 cups sliced carrots
2 cups sliced celery
1/4 green bell pepper, cut in 1-inch cubes
1 1/2 cups chopped onion
1 8-ounce can corn
1 16-ounce can tomatoes, whole and peeled, or 2 cups peeled, sliced, and quartered fresh tomatoes

Combine water and bouillon powder in large saucepan. Add potato, carrots, and celery. Cook for 10–15 minutes. Add pepper, onion, corn, and tomatoes. Cook 25 minutes longer or until carrots are tender. Great reheated. Yields 8–10 servings

Fat: None
Oil: None

VEGETABLE BROTH I

2 cups diced potatoes
1 tomato, chopped
1 onion, chopped
2 cups chopped carrots
2 cups diced turnips
1 cup chopped cabbage or spinach
3 ribs celery, chopped
2 quarts water
2 sprigs parsley, chopped
1 1/2 teaspoons salt

In nonstick skillet brown vegetables with a trace of water. Pour into kettle with 2 quarts water, parsley, and salt. Bring to a boil; reduce heat and simmer, covered, 1 1/2–2 hours. Strain stock and use immediately or freeze. Yields 3 1/2 quarts

Fat: None
Oil: None

VEGETABLE BROTH II

2 cups chopped onion
2 cups chopped carrots
1 cup chopped and cleaned leeks
1 1/2 cups chopped celery
1/2 cup chopped turnip
2 quarts water or vegetable liquid
5 peppercorns
1 bay leaf
6 sprigs parsley
Sprig of thyme
Dash of salt

In nonstick skillet brown vegetables with a trace of water. Pour into kettle with 2 quarts water, seasonings, and herbs. Bring to a boil; reduce heat and simmer, covered, 1 1/2–2 hours. Strain stock and use immediately or freeze. Yields 3 1/2 quarts

Fat: None
Oil: None

CHAPTER 16

Salads and Dressings

A salad can be a complement to the main meal or a meal in itself. The success of any salad is serving the greens very dry and crisp and cold and adding the chilled dressing just before serving. Salad dressings can be an excellent source of oil. The use of a good dressing is encouraged as long as it does not contain cheese. Remember that the more colorful leaves or skin of vegetables contain much more vitamin A and slightly more vitamins B and C than the colorless parts. Also, the mineral content of the skin of many vegetables is relatively high. Consequently, washing them well may be preferable to peeling. A word of warning: in some commercially prepared salad dressings, the oil is fluid at room temperature but becomes solid when refrigerated. These dressings should be avoided. We highly recommend that you make your own dressings using high-quality vegetable oils.

When dining out, you should order the dressing in a side dish since some restaurants drench the rest of the salad with dressing, making it difficult to determine the amount of oil that it contains.

WALDORF SALAD

3 cups diced apples
1 cup chopped celery
1/2 cup chopped walnuts
3/4 cup mayonnaise
Lettuce leaves to serve 6
Whole walnuts

Mix apple, celery, and nuts, and moisten with mayonnaise. Arrange on crisp leaves of lettuce and garnish with nuts. Serves 6

Fat: None
Oil: Total—28 teaspoons; per serving—4 2/3 teaspoons

CABBAGE AND APPLE COLESLAW

2 cups shredded cabbage
1 cup diced apples
1/3 cup mayonnaise
Salt and pepper to taste

Combine shredded cabbage and apples. (For shredding cabbage a food processor is great.) Add mayonnaise and season to taste. Serves 6

Fat: None
Oil: Total—8 teaspoons; per serving—1 1/3 teaspoons

PASTA SALAD

2 cups broccoli flowerets
2 cups cauliflower slices
8 ounces spiral pasta
1 cup sliced celery
1 cup frozen peas, thawed
1 cup halved cherry tomatoes
1 4-ounce can sliced pimiento
1 garlic clove, pressed
1 cup mayonnaise
1 tablespoon wine vinegar
1 teaspoon salt
1/2 teaspoon crumbled sweet basil
Black pepper to taste

Steam broccoli and cauliflower 4 minutes. Submerge in cold water to stop cooking. Cook pasta according to package directions. Combine broccoli, cauliflower, pasta, celery, peas, tomato, and pimiento in a large salad bowl. Purée remaining ingredients in blender. Pour over salad and toss. Refrigerate at least 4 hours. Yields 6 servings

Fat: None
Oil: Total—24 teaspoons; per serving—4 teaspoons

ITALIAN VEGETABLE TOSS

2 cups shell macaroni (before cooking)
1 cup sliced fresh mushrooms
1/2 cup chopped green onion
1 medium tomato, seeded and chopped
2 cups broccoli flowerets
1/2 cup sliced pitted black olives
1/2 avocado, seeded, peeled, and sliced

Cook macaroni and drain. Combine remaining ingredients and add to macaroni. Prepare dressing and add to salad. Toss well. Yields 6 servings

DRESSING

1/3 cup white vinegar
2 tablespoons sugar
2 teaspoons salt
1/2 teaspoon basil leaves
2/3 cup oil
2 tablespoons minced onion
3/4 teaspoon oregano leaves
1/2 teaspoon garlic

Combine ingredients and mix well.

Fat: None
Oil: Total—44 teaspoons; per serving—7 1/3 teaspoons

LENTIL SALAD

1 cup dry lentils
2 1/2 cups water
1 teaspoon salt
1/3 cup mayonnaise
1/4 cup Italian dressing
1 tablespoon prepared mustard
1/2 teaspoon dillweed
1 cup chopped celery
1 tomato, diced
1 cup chopped zucchini or cucumber
3 green onions, chopped
2 tablespoons chopped parsley
2 hard-cooked eggs, chopped
2 teaspoons lemon juice

Rinse lentils, then combine with water and salt in saucepan. Bring to boil, cover, reduce heat, and cook for about 30 minutes or until tender. Drain. Combine with mayonnaise, Italian dressing, mustard, and dillweed. Add chopped vegetables and egg. Sprinkle with lemon juice. Chill for 2 hours, then serve. Great served with French bread and fresh melon slices. Use less lemon juice for a milder taste. Serves 8

Fat: Total—2 teaspoons; per serving—1/4 teaspoon
Oil: Total—8 teaspoons; per serving—1 teaspoon

LENTIL RICE CHICKEN SALAD

1 cup cooked lentils
1 cup cooked brown rice
1 cup skinned, cooked, and cubed chicken (white meat)
1/3 cup chopped green pepper
1/3 cup diced onion
1 1/2 cups chopped celery
1 tablespoon vinegar
2 tablespoons oil
3/4 cup mayonnaise
3 tomatoes, halved and scooped out
6 lettuce leaves
Curry powder (optional)

Toss together all ingredients except mayonnaise and refrigerate 3–4 hours. Just before serving blend in the mayonnaise. Serve in split, scooped out tomato cups on lettuce leaves. You may add curry powder for flavor if you like. Serves 6

Fat: None
Oil: Total—22 teaspoons; per serving—3 2/3 teaspoons

SHERRIED TOMATO SHRIMP ASPIC

2 envelopes unflavored gelatin
1/2 cup cold water
2 cups tomato juice
1 teaspoon salt
1 rib celery, chopped
1 small onion, chopped
4 sprigs of parsley, minced
1/2 cup dry sherry
1/4 cup finely chopped celery
1/2 cup cooked and shelled small shrimp

Soften gelatin in cold water. Combine tomato juice, salt, celery, onion, parsley, and sherry in saucepan. Cover and simmer for 15 minutes. Strain. Add softened gelatin, stir until dissolved. Cool. Stir in 1/4 cup celery and shrimp. Pour into individual molds or one large mold. Chill until firm, about 2 hours. This is good with any meat, poultry, or fish. Serves 4–6

Fat: None
Oil: None

THREE-BEAN SALAD

2 16-ounce cans kidney beans
1 16-ounce can wax beans
1 16-ounce can green beans
1 sweet Bermuda onion
1 whole green pepper
1 2-ounce can chopped pimiento
2 teaspoons salt
1/2 cup wine vinegar
1/2 cup sugar (or less to taste)
1/3 cup olive oil
Pepper to taste
Juice of 1 lemon
Lettuce

Drain kidney beans, reserve liquid from 1 can. Drain and rinse wax and green beans. Arrange beans in a deep dish or shallow glass dish approximately 13″ × 9″ × 2″. Slice onion and green pepper into thin rings and place on beans. Add pimiento. Combine remainder of ingredients with liquid from kidney beans and pour over the salad. Cover and marinate in refrigerator overnight or several days, stirring occasionally. Drain and serve on crisp lettuce. (Garbanzo or small lima beans can be used in place of one can of kidney beans.) Serves 12

Fat: None
Oil: Total—16 teaspoons; per serving—1 1/3 teaspoons

MACARONI SHRIMP SALAD

3 tablespoons wine or cider vinegar
8 teaspoons oil
1/2 teaspoon salt
Freshly ground pepper to taste
5 cups cooked macaroni or 3 cups uncooked macaroni
3 hard-cooked eggs, chopped
3/4 cup chopped celery
1/4–1/2 cup chopped green onion
1/4 cup chopped green pepper
1/4 cup chopped pimiento (optional)
1/2–3/4 cup thinly sliced water chestnuts
2–3 cups cooked shrimp
1/2 cup mayonnaise
1/2 teaspoon curry powder
1 tablespoon lemon juice

Mix vinegar, oil, salt, and pepper with the macaroni. Chill. Have remaining ingredients chilled. Mix macaroni with eggs, vegetables, and shrimp. Combine mayonnaise with curry powder and lemon juice, and add to salad. Toss and serve. This can be used as a main dish or a salad. Serves 10

Fat: Total—3 teaspoons; per serving—3/10 teaspoon
Oil: Total—20 teaspoons; per serving—2 teaspoons

SHRIMP RICE SALAD

1 cup rice
2/3 teaspoon salt
1 teaspoon marjoram
2 tablespoons oil
1/3 cup chopped onion
1 teaspoon basil
1 tablespoon lemon juice
2 ribs celery, chopped
1/3 pound shrimp
Parsley

Cook rice. Mix together remaining ingredients except shrimp. Cool. Add shrimp. Garnish with parsley. Serves 4

Fat: None
Oil: Total—6 teaspoons; per serving—1 1/2 teaspoons

SPINACH SALAD

1/2 pound fresh spinach
1 tablespoon olive oil
Lemon juice to taste
4 green onions, chopped
2 hard-cooked eggs, chopped coarsely
Omar's Special Dressing
1 tomato, sliced

Wash spinach thoroughly, trim, and discard stems. Blot dry. Tear leaves into a salad bowl. Sprinkle with olive oil, stirring thoroughly to coat all of the pieces. Add lemon juice, onion, and egg; toss. Serve with Omar's Special Dressing and garnish with tomato slices. Serves 6

Fat: Total—2 teaspoons; per serving—1/3 teaspoon
Oil: Total—3 teaspoons; per serving—1/2 teaspoon

RASPBERRY CHERRY GELATIN SALAD

1 10-ounce package frozen raspberries, thawed
1/2 cup currant jelly
2 cups water
2 3-ounce packages red-raspberry-flavored gelatin
1/2 cup dry sherry or port wine
1/4 cup lemon juice
1 16-ounce can pitted dark sweet cherries, drained (1 1/2 cups)
Mayonnaise or salad dressing to garnish
Celery

Drain raspberries, reserving the juice. Combine jelly and 1/2 cup of the water. Heat and stir until jelly melts. Add remaining 1 1/2 cups water and the gelatin. Heat and stir until gelatin dissolves. Remove from heat. Add sherry, lemon juice, and reserved raspberry juice. Chill until partially set. If desired, reserve a few raspberries for garnishing mayonnaise. Fold remaining raspberries and cherries into gelatin. Pour into a 6-cup mold. Chill until firm, 6 hours or overnight. Unmold on serving plate. Serve with mayonnaise or salad dressing and crisp celery. Serves 8–10

Fat: None
Oil: None

GRAPEFRUIT RING WITH SHRIMP SALAD

2 tablespoons unflavored gelatin
1 cup cold water
3/4 cup sugar
1 18-ounce can grapefruit juice (2 1/2 cups)
3 tablespoons strained lemon juice
1/4 teaspoon salt
Green food coloring (optional)

Soak gelatin in 1/2 cup water for about 5 minutes. Heat remaining water and sugar to boiling point, add soaked gelatin, and stir until gelatin is dissolved. Add remaining ingredients and enough green food coloring to tint a light green color. Pour mixture into an 8-inch ring mold and chill in the refrigerator at least 2 hours or until mixture is set. Unmold gelatin ring and fill center with Shrimp Salad. Pile remaining salad in small mounds around the outside of the ring. Serves 10

Fat: None
Oil: None

SHRIMP SALAD FOR GRAPEFRUIT RING

2 cups cooked shrimp
2 teaspoons lemon juice
2 cups diced celery
1 cup mayonnaise
1/4 cup diced green pepper (optional)
Salt and pepper to taste

Combine all ingredients and mix well. Serves 10 with grapefruit ring

Fat: None
Oil: Total—24 teaspoons; per serving—2 2/5 teaspoons

POTATO SALAD

1 cup mayonnaise
1 cup nonfat yogurt
1/3 cup prepared mustard
2 cups finely chopped celery
Pimiento and sweet pickle to taste
1 medium Spanish onion, finely chopped
10 large potatoes, boiled, cubed, and chilled
8 hard-cooked eggs, sliced and chilled
Salt and pepper to taste
Radish slices
Parsley

Combine first 6 ingredients. Refrigerate several hours to blend flavors. Add potato and egg. Toss lightly. Season to taste (this is a very moist potato salad). Garnish with radish slices and parsley. Serves 12

Fat: Total—8 teaspoons; per serving—2/3 teaspoon
Oil: Total—24 teaspoons; per serving—2 teaspoons

NORWEGIAN POTATO SALAD

4–6 large potatoes
Salt and pepper to taste
1/2 cup olive oil
1/2 cup dry white wine
1 tablespoon (or more) cider vinegar
1/2 cup chopped parsley
1/2 cup chopped chives or green onion

Boil potatoes in their jackets until tender. Peel while hot and slice into a bowl. Season with salt and pepper to taste, and pour the olive oil and wine over hot potatoes. Let cool, or refrigerate overnight. Just before serving, toss with the vinegar, parsley, and chives. Serves 8

Fat: None
Oil: Total—24 teaspoons; per serving—3 teaspoons

SCANDINAVIAN CUCUMBER SALAD

1/2 cup vinegar
2 tablespoons water
1/2 teaspoon salt
3 tablespoons sugar
1/8 teaspoon pepper
3–4 teaspoons finely chopped dill or half dill, half parsley
2 medium-sized cucumbers

Combine all ingredients except cucumbers and mix well. Slice cucumbers very thin. Pour dressing over the cucumbers. Cover. Let stand for at least 3 hours. Serve undrained in the dressing. Serves 6

Fat: None
Oil: None

QUICK KETCHUP

1 medium onion, chopped (about 1 cup)
1/2 garlic clove
5 tablespoons frozen apple juice concentrate
1 6-ounce can tomato paste
1/2 cup malt vinegar
1/2 teaspoon cayenne pepper
1/4 teaspoon cinnamon
1/8 teaspoon ground cloves

Place the onion, garlic, and apple juice in a blender and purée until smooth. Add the tomato paste, vinegar, cayenne, cinnamon, and cloves, and blend until smooth. Keep in an airtight bottle or jar and refrigerate. Yields about 1 cup

Fat: None
Oil: None

MAYONNAISE

1 egg or 2 egg yolks
1 teaspoon salt
1 teaspoon sugar
1 teaspoon mustard
1/2 teaspoon paprika
3 tablespoons lemon juice or vinegar
1 1/2 cups salad oil

In blender or mixer beat egg until light, add spices and lemon juice, and mix well. Very gradually add the oil, blending until it becomes very thick and smooth. Yields approximately 1 pint

Note: Homemade mayonnaise contains twice as much oil as commercial mayonnaise does.

Fat: Total—1 teaspoon per egg yolk used; per serving—negligible
Oil: Total—72 teaspoons; per 1 teaspoon serving—1 teaspoon

CURRIED MAYONNAISE

1/2 cup mayonnaise
1/2 teaspoon curry powder (or to taste)
Lemon juice to taste

Combine all ingredients and mix until curry powder is completely blended. Excellent for fish. Yields 1/2 cup

Fat: None
Oil: 12 teaspoons (when commercial mayonnaise used) per serving—2 teaspoons—1 teaspoon
24 teaspoons (when homemade mayonnaise used) per serving—1 teaspoon—1 teaspoon

PIQUANT DRESSING

1/2 cup mayonnaise
1/2 cup beer
1 tablespoon horseradish
2 teaspoons dry mustard
1/4 teaspoon garlic powder
1/4 cup vinegar
1/4 cup salad oil

Combine ingredients in order given. Beat with rotary beater or whirl in blender. Yields 1 1/4 cups dressing

Fat: None
Oil: Total—24 teaspoons; 2 1/2 teaspoons dressing—1 teaspoon

RUSSIAN DRESSING

1 8-ounce can tomato sauce
1/2 cup tarragon vinegar
2 teaspoons salt
1/2 teaspoon paprika
1 tablespoon Worcestershire sauce
1 cup oil
1/2 teaspoon dry mustard
1/2 teaspoon garlic powder
1 small onion, quartered
1 teaspoon sugar

Combine all ingredients in blender and blend to a smooth consistency. Good on crisp vegetables or fruit. Yields 2 1/2 cups

Fat: None
Oil: Total—48 teaspoons; 3 teaspoons dressing—1 teaspoon

FRENCH DRESSING

1/2 teaspoon mustard
1 tablespoon sugar
1/2 teaspoon salt
1/2 cup oil
1/4 cup vinegar or lemon juice
1 teaspoon onion juice
1 teaspoon paprika
1 tablespoon ketchup

Combine all ingredients in blender and blend to a smooth consistency. For a creamy dressing, slowly blend the oil into the rest of the ingredients. Yields 1 cup

Fat: None
Oil: Total—24 teaspoons; 2 teaspoons dressing—1 teaspoon

OMAR'S SPECIAL DRESSING

1 garlic clove
1 egg
1 teaspoon sugar
1/2 teaspoon salt
1/4 teaspoon paprika
1/4 teaspoon dry mustard
1/2 teaspoon Worcestershire sauce
1/4 cup ketchup
1/4 cup vinegar
1 cup oil
1/3 cup warm water

Rub blender container with cut garlic, add all ingredients except oil and water, and blend until smooth. Add oil slowly, blending into a thick dressing, and add warm water slowly. Keep refrigerated. Yields 2 1/2 cups

Fat: 1 teaspoon
Oil: Total—48 teaspoons; 2 1/4 teaspoons dressing—1 teaspoon

FRUIT SALAD DRESSING

1 teaspoon dry mustard
1 teaspoon celery seeds
1 teaspoon grated onion
2/3 cup sugar
1/2 cup honey
1 teaspoon paprika
5 tablespoons vinegar
1 tablespoon lemon juice
1/4 teaspoon salt
1 cup oil

Combine all ingredients in blender except the oil. Slowly add the oil while blending constantly. Yields 2 cups

Fat: None
Oil: Total—48 teaspoons; 2 teaspoons dressing—1 teaspoon

CHAPTER 17

Stuffing for Meat, Poultry, and Fish

The preparation of poultry or meat stuffing (dressing) is one of the few instances in which it is necessary to make a separate portion for the member of the family who is on the diet. The stuffing should not be placed in the fowl or with the meat because it will absorb too much fat in the cooking process. Place the stuffing in a separate baking dish and cook in the oven at the same time the main dish is baking.

BASIC STUFFING

1 tablespoon oil
1 large onion, chopped
1 cup chopped celery (with some of the leaves)
4 cups bread cubes
1 cup broth or consommé
1 teaspoon salt
1 teaspoon pepper
1 teaspoon thyme
2 teaspoons sage
1/2 cup chopped mushrooms or chestnuts or cooked giblets (optional)

Preheat oven to 350° F. Heat oil in saucepan and lightly sauté onion and celery. Toss together with other ingredients, using broth to moisten. Place in baking dish. Bake 1–1 1/2 hours. Cover with foil to keep from drying out. Serves 6

Fat: None (1 teaspoon if giblets are used [2 ounces])
Oil: Total—3 teaspoons; per serving—1/2 teaspoon

APPLE STUFFING

3 tablespoons oil
1/2 cup chopped celery
1/2 cup chopped onion
1/4 cup chopped parsley
5 tart apples
1/4 cup sugar
2 cups fine dry bread crumbs

In the oil sauté celery, onion, and parsley until tender. Add apples and sprinkle with sugar; cover and cook until tender. Remove lid and continue to cook until the juice evaporates and the pieces of apples are candied. Add the bread crumbs to the apple mixture. Serves 6

Fat: None
Oil: Total—9 teaspoons; per serving—1 1/2 teaspoons

CRANBERRY STUFFING

1 cup freshly cooked cranberries
1/4 cup sugar
1/4 cup chopped celery
2 tablespoons chopped parsley
4 tablespoons oil
4 cups stale bread crumbs
1/2 teaspoon sweet marjoram
1 teaspoon salt

Combine cranberries and sugar. Sauté celery and parsley in oil until celery is tender. Add to cranberries. Combine bread crumbs, marjoram, and salt. Add to cranberry mixture. This makes a nice side dish with sliced turkey or turkey sandwich. Serves 6

Fat: None
Oil: Total—12 teaspoons; per serving—2 teaspoons

PECAN STUFFING FOR TURKEY

1 1/2 cups skim milk, heated
2 cups bread crumbs
2 tablespoons chopped onion
1/2 cup raisins
1/2 cup chopped pecans
1/2 cup oil
1/2 teaspoon salt
1/8 teaspoon pepper
1 teaspoon sage
2 eggs

Pour hot milk over bread crumbs and add remaining ingredients. Mix well. Serves 8

Fat: Total—2 teaspoons; per serving—1/4 teaspoon
Oil: Total—36 teaspoons; per serving—4 1/2 teaspoons

RICE STUFFING

1 1/2 tablespoons chopped onion
1 tablespoon oil
3/4 cup uncooked rice
1 teaspoon salt
2 cups chicken soup stock
1/2 teaspoon poultry seasoning or bouillon base

Cook onion in oil until tender. Add rice and simmer until the rice has a golden tint, then add salt, soup stock, and poultry seasoning. Cover and steam for 20 minutes until rice is tender. Serves 4

Fat: None
Oil: Total—3 teaspoons; per serving—3/4 teaspoon

SPINACH STUFFING

1 1/2 cups drained cooked spinach
2 tablespoons grated onion
4 tablespoons oil
2 tablespoons lemon juice
2 cups soft bread crumbs
Salt and pepper to taste

Cut leaves of spinach from roots. Wash, making certain that all sand is removed. Put in saucepan. Heat gradually in own juice and cook until tender. Combine remaining ingredients and add spinach. Season to taste. Serves 6

Fat: None
Oil: Total—12 teaspoons; per serving—2 teaspoons

OYSTER STUFFING

3 cups soft bread crumbs
1 teaspoon salt
1/8 teaspoon pepper
Few drops of onion juice
1 teaspoon chopped parsley
25 oysters
2 tablespoons oil
1/4 cup oyster liquid

Mix bread crumbs, salt, pepper, onion juice, and parsley. Add oysters. Heat oil and oyster liquid. Add to mixture. Mix thoroughly. Excellent with turkey. Serves 8

Fat: None
Oil: Total—6 teaspoons; per serving—3/4 teaspoon

CORN BREAD STUFFING

6 tablespoons oil
1/3 cup chopped onion
2/3 cup chopped celery
3 tablespoons chopped parsley
4 cups corn bread crumbs
1/4 teaspoon thyme
1/2 teaspoon salt
1/4 teaspoon pepper

In the oil sauté onion, celery, and parsley until lightly browned. Remove from heat and mix thoroughly with remaining ingredients. Serves 6

Fat: None
Oil: Total—18 teaspoons; per serving—3 teaspoons

CHAPTER 18

Fish and Seafood

Fish contains as much protein and essential amino acids as meat does and should become an important part of your diet. This is especially so since we have limited or forbidden some of the fat-containing protein foods in common use. White fish contains only traces of fat, and the lipids contained in salmon, herring, mackerel, and trout are primarily unsaturated. On some diets shellfish such as crab, lobsters, and oysters are eliminated because they contain small amounts of cholesterol. We have not found this necessary because the blood cholesterol levels of patients on our diet usually varies from 120 to 175 mg/100 cc blood. For those cardiac patients who feel strongly about cholesterol-containing shellfish, these may be eliminated.

Be extremely careful when purchasing fish. Fish decomposes quickly so it must be *fresh* when purchased. It is much better to buy preserved or frozen fish when in doubt about the freshness. If frozen fish is purchased, it should be partially thawed slowly in the refrigerator and used immediately after thawing.

When purchasing a whole fish look for clear eyes. If the eyes appear cloudy, this indicates age. Also the texture of the body should be firm and there should be no odor to the fish. Once purchased, fish should be kept no longer than two days before cooking. After cooking it should be kept no longer than one day.

There are many ways to cook fish and we have included a wide variety and number of recipes in this book.

The most important rule to keep in mind when cooking fish is that *it must never be overcooked.* Properly cooked fish will never be dry. Cooking fish differs from cooking meat. Since some fish contains only small amounts of fat, heat penetrates it rapidly. Try combining two or more varieties of fish; experiment with different sauces and seasonings. You will soon develop an endless variety of dishes that are very tasty.

The following methods of timing fish cookery are offered to assist you in achieving the proper degree of doneness:

To Bake a Fish

Preheat oven to 300° F. A large piece of fish or a whole fish should be placed on a baking rack so that the oven heat can surround all surfaces. The fish can either be completely wrapped in a sheet of aluminum foil or heavy wrapping paper, partially covered by aluminum foil, or not wrapped at all. However, if the fish is stuffed or seasoned with a wine sauce, the wrapping is necessary. Allow fresh fish to attain room temperature before cooking. Frozen fish should be partially thawed and cooked immediately. Insert a meat thermometer into the thickest part of the flesh, usually just behind the gills. Brush fish with oil but do not salt. If the fish is not wrapped, place a pan or sheet of aluminum foil on a wire rack at least 3 inches below the fish to catch the drippings. Bake in a preheated oven until thermometer reading is 140° F. Allow approximately 20 minutes for heat to penetrate 1 inch, 30 minutes for 2 inches, 35 minutes for 3 inches.

For stuffed fish, insert a meat thermometer into the cold stuffing, cook to 135° F, and allow cooking to continue for another 10 to 15 minutes.

If you prefer faster cooking at a higher temperature, 400° F is advocated by many leading cooks. The thickness of the fish, and cooking time should be adjusted to 8 to 10 minutes per inch. At termination of cooking, the meat thermometer should still read 140° F when done.

To Bake Fillet of Fish:

Preheat oven to 375–400° F. Allow approximately 10 minutes for heat to penetrate fish or fillets 1 inch thick, 15 minutes for fish 2 inches thick, 20 minutes for fish 3 inches thick. Check thermometer reading frequently and remove from oven when internal temperature reaches 140° F.

To Broil a Steak or Fillets

These cuts should not be more than 1 1/2 inches thick. Turn fish after 8 to 10 minutes or when half the thickness has become opaque. Allow 15 minutes for cooking fish 1 inch thick, 18 minutes if 1 1/2 inches thick, but again the thermometer must be 140° F.

If fish is still frozen, then allow 20 minutes to the inch. Frozen fish should not be allowed to thaw completely.

To Fry Fish

Fish can be fried in a lightly oiled pan. Never cover the fish when frying as this will make it soft. Frying fish takes only a short time. Approximately 5 to 8 minutes at 375° F on each side for fish 1/2 to 1 inch thick. Do not overcook.

We repeat, the most important rule in fish cooking is not to overcook it. When a fish curls, flakes, pulls from the bone, or comes to the surface during deep frying, the fish is actually overcooked and the juices have been lost, the meat is dry, and the flavor diminished.

Fish odors in the house can be dissipated by pouring 1/2 cup of vinegar in the frying pan after frying and letting it boil, and authorities believe that only by overcooking fish (to internal temperatures over 150° F) do the unpleasant odors evaporate into the room. Probably the simplest method of deodorizing is the use of a fragrant candle manufactured for this purpose.

BEER BATTER FOR DEEP FRYING

1 tablespoon salt
1 tablespoon paprika (optional)
1 cup all-purpose flour
1 12-ounce can beer

Stir dry ingredients into the beer with a wire whisk until the batter is light and frothy. Batter will keep in the refrigerator for several days. This batter makes a light, crisp crust that absorbs very little oil. Yields 2 cups

Fat: None
Oil: None

CRUMB TOPPING MIX

2 cups well-crushed melba toast
1/2 cup wheat germ
2 tablespoons parsley flakes
1 tablespoon paprika
1 teaspoon dry mustard
1 tablespoon crushed tarragon leaves
1 teaspoon seasoned salt
1/2 teaspoon instant minced onion
1/2 teaspoon celery salt
1/2 teaspoon coarsely ground black pepper
1 tablespoon garlic powder (optional)

Combine all ingredients and mix well. Sprinkle on casseroles or use for cooking fish or poultry. Refrigerate in tightly covered container. Yields enough for 3 or 4 1 1/2-quart casseroles

Fat: None
Oil: None

BREAD STUFFING FOR Fish

1 1/2 cups chopped celery
1/4 cup water
1 tablespoon grated onion
1/2 teaspoon salt
1 tablespoon lemon juice
2 cups bread crumbs

Partially cook celery in water. Add onion, salt, and lemon juice to celery. Combine with bread crumbs and mix well. Yields enough for 2–2 1/2 stuffed fish fillets

Fat: None
Oil: None

HERBED FISH FILLETS

1 vegetable bouillon cube
1 cup hot water
1/4 cup diced green pepper
1/4 cup diced celery
1/2 cup diced carrot
2 pounds fillet of sole or other white fish fillet
1 cup skim milk
Dash of pepper
1/4 cup all-purpose flour
1/8 teaspoon ground marjoram
1 tablespoon chopped parsley

Preheat oven to 350° F. Dissolve bouillon cube in water in small saucepan. Add vegetables and simmer for 10 minutes. Drain and save liquid for sauce and vegetables for stuffing fish. Wipe fillets with paper towel. Place vegetables on fillets, fold up, and secure with toothpicks. Place in a shallow baking dish. Add milk and pepper, bake for 30 minutes, basting occasionally. Remove fish to platter, reserving remaining hot milk. Keep fish warm while preparing sauce.

SAUCE

Combine flour and vegetable liquid in a saucepan, mixing until smooth. Gradually stir in hot milk from baked fish and cook, stirring over moderate heat until thick. Remove from heat, add marjoram and parsley, mixing well. Pour over fillets and serve. Serves 6

Fat: None
Oil: None

FISH BAKE

2 2.3-ounce packages dry mushroom soup mix
2/3 cup water
1/4 cup sliced ripe olives
1/4 cup slivered toasted almonds or cashews
2 tablespoons chopped green peppers
2 tablespoons chopped pimiento
1 tablespoon minced onion
1 4-ounce can mushrooms, with liquid
2 cups drained cooked noodles
1 cup cut-up cooked fish or seafood
Crumb Topping Mix or toasted bread crumbs

Preheat oven to 350° F. Combine soup and remaining ingredients except fish and crumbs. In a 2–3-quart casserole add half of the noodles, cover with fish, and add remaining noodles. Cover with soup mixture. Sprinkle with Crumb Topping Mix or bread crumbs. Bake 40–50 minutes. Serves 6

Fat: None
Oil: Total—9 teaspoons; per serving—1 1/2 teaspoons

SPANISH BAKED FISH

6 4-ounce slices white fish
1/4 teaspoon salt
1/4 teaspoon black pepper
1/4 teaspoon mace
1 large onion, thinly sliced
2 tablespoons diced pimiento
6 thick slices of tomato
3 tablespoons snipped green onion tops
1 cup thinly sliced mushrooms
1/2 cup dry sherry or white wine
1 cup toasted bread crumbs

Preheat oven to 350° F. Wipe fish with damp cloth. Sprinkle with salt, pepper, and mace. Arrange onion slices and pimiento in well-oiled baking dish 12″ × 8″ × 2″. Top with seasoned fish slices arranged side by side. Top each piece of fish with a tomato slice; sprinkle with green onion. Scatter mushrooms over all; add wine and bread crumbs. Bake uncovered about 35–40 minutes. Serves 4–6

Fat: None
Oil: None

QUICK BAKED FISH

2 pounds fish fillets or small fish cut into serving pieces
2 teaspoons salt
1 cup skim milk
2 cups fine bread crumbs (do not use flour, cornmeal, or cracker crumbs)
2 tablespoons oil

Preheat oven to 500° F. Dip fish into salted milk and coat thoroughly with crumbs. Place in shallow baking pan. Dribble with oil. Bake for approximately 10 minutes. Do not add liquid and do not turn fish. Serves 6

Fat: None
Oil: Total—6 teaspoons; per serving—1 teaspoon

INDONESIAN BAKED FISH

2 garlic cloves, minced
2 teaspoons salt
1/2 teaspoon freshly ground black pepper
4 pounds fish fillets
1/4 cup oil
3 tablespoons lemon juice
1/4 cup soy sauce
1/4 teaspoon chili peppers or cayenne pepper

Preheat oven to 375° F. Mix the garlic, salt, and pepper to a paste; rub paste into the fish. Place fish in baking dish and bake for 15 minutes. Mix oil, lemon juice, soy sauce, and chili peppers. Pour half the mixture over the fish. Bake 15 additional minutes. Then add remaining mixture and bake 10 more minutes, basting and turning fish. Serve with rice cooked in vegetable bouillon. Serves 10–12

Fat: None
Oil: Total—12 teaspoons; per serving—1 teaspoon

SCALLOPED TUNA

2 cups finely crumbled bread sticks or very dry bread
1 cup finely diced celery
1/2 cup finely diced onion
2 garlic cloves, finely chopped (optional)
2 6 1/2-ounce cans water-packed chunk tuna, well drained
2 eggs, beaten
1/2 cup oil

Preheat oven to 325° F. Toss first five ingredients together until well blended. Turn into well-oiled shallow baking dish. Combine eggs and oil and pour over tuna mixture. Mix. Bake for 25 minutes. Serve with rice or noodles. Serves 4

Fat: Total—2 teaspoons; per serving—1/2 teaspoon
Oil: Total—24 teaspoons; per serving—6 teaspoons

TUNA-CASHEW ORIENTAL

1 tablespoon oil
1 medium onion, sliced
1 cup chopped celery
1/3 cup chopped green pepper
1/4 cup water
2 2.3-ounce packages dry mushroom soup mix
2/3 cup water
1 7 1/2-ounce can water-packed tuna
1/2 cup raw cashew nuts

Heat oil in heavy skillet. Add onion and celery and sauté, stirring constantly to keep from browning, for 2–3 minutes. Add green pepper and water; cover and steam for 5 minutes. Mix mushroom soup with 2/3 cup water. Add to skillet with tuna and heat. When ready to serve, garnish with cashew nuts. Serve over rice or noodles. Vegetables should be crisp and crunchy. Serves 4

Fat: None
Oil: Total—13 teaspoons; per serving—3 1/4 teaspoons

TUNA POT PIE

1/4 cup oil
1/3 cup all-purpose flour
1 1/2 teaspoons salt
1/4 teaspoon pepper
1/4 teaspoon marjoram
1 2/3 cups skim milk
2 7 1/2-ounce cans water-packed tuna, drained and flaked
2 cups frozen peas and carrots, thawed
1 1/2 cups frozen small whole onions, thawed
2 teaspoons Worcestershire sauce
Pastry for Single-Crust 9-Inch Pie

Preheat oven to 425° F. In large saucepan heat oil. Blend in flour, salt, pepper, and marjoram until bubbly. Gradually add milk, stirring constantly until mixture boils and thickens. Add tuna, vegetables, and Worcestershire sauce. Stir gently to combine. Spoon into a shallow 2-quart baking dish (or into 6 individual 10-ounce baking cups). Roll out pastry to fit top of baking dish or, 6 5-inch circles for individual pot pies. Place on top of dish, flute edges, and cut slits for steam to escape. Place on baking sheet. Bake 35–40 minutes or until crust is golden and mixture is bubbly. Serves 6

Fat: None
Oil: Total—24 teaspoons including crust; per serving—4 teaspoons

TUNA BALLS IN WINE SAUCE

1/3 cup fresh bread crumbs
1/2–3/4 cup plus 3 tablespoons chicken stock or canned broth
1/3 cup plus 1 tablespoon dry white wine
1 6 1/2-ounce can water-packed white meat tuna, drained and flaked
1 hard-cooked egg, finely chopped
1 egg, lightly beaten
3 tablespoons minced parsley
2 large garlic cloves, minced
1/4 teaspoon salt
Pinch of freshly ground pepper
Flour for dusting
2 tablespoons olive oil

In a medium bowl, moisten the bread crumbs with 3 tablespoons of the chicken stock and 1 tablespoon of the wine. Mix in the tuna, hard-cooked egg, raw egg, parsley, garlic, salt, and pepper. Form the tuna mixture into 1 1/2-inch balls and dust with flour. Heat the oil in a large skillet. Add the tuna balls and sauté over moderately high heat, turning until browned all over, 15–20 minutes. Add the remaining 1/3 cup wine and 1/2 cup of the chicken stock. Cover, reduce the heat to Low, and simmer for 30 minutes. If all the liquid has evaporated, pour in 1/4 cup more stock and simmer, scraping up any browned bits on the bottom of the pan, for 2 minutes. Serve hot or at room temperature. Skewer on toothpicks if desired. Serves 4–6

Fat: Total—2 teaspoons; per serving—1/2 teaspoon
Oil: Total—6 teaspoons; per serving—1 1/2 teaspoons

If served to six:
Fat: Per serving—1/3 teaspoon
Oil: Per serving—1 teaspoon

EASY SALMON PATTIES

1 6 1/2-ounce can salmon
1 egg
3/4 cup cracker crumbs
1 green onion, chopped
2 tablespoons mayonnaise
1/2 teaspoon tarragon
Oil

Drain and flake salmon. In small bowl combine all the ingredients. Shape into patties and fry in oil until lightly brown on each side. Yields 6 patties

Fat: Total—1 teaspoon; per serving—1/6 teaspoon
Oil: Total—6 1/4 teaspoons; per serving—1 teaspoon

GRILLED SALMON WITH TARRAGON SAUCE

SAUCE

2 cups mayonnaise
1/4 cup chopped fresh tarragon or 2 teaspoons dried and crumbled tarragon
3 tablespoons finely minced green or red onion
2 tablespoons fresh lemon juice
2 tablespoons chopped capers
1/4 teaspoon coarsely ground pepper
Salt

Combine all ingredients together in blender and blend well. Cover and chill 2–24 hours.

Oil
6 salmon steaks, 1/2 pound each, cut 1 inch thick
Lemon or lime slices, halved (for garnish)
Tarragon sprigs (for garnish)

Arrange rack over grill or in broiler pan about 5 inches from heat. Brush rack with oil. Preheat coals or broiler. Place salmon steaks on rack and spread on each 2 tablespoons of tarragon mayonnaise. Broil 6 minutes. Turn fish and spread on remaining sauce. Broil another 4–6 minutes. Fish should be barely opaque with a touch of deeper pink color. Arrange on serving platter. Garnish with citrus slices and tarragon sprigs. Serves 6

Fat: None
Oil: 2 teaspoons sauce—1 teaspoon; 2 ounces salmon—1 teaspoon

SALMON LOAF I

1 16-ounce can salmon, with liquid
2 eggs, beaten
1/2 cup soft bread crumbs
1/4 cup oil
1 1/2 teaspoons salt
1/2 teaspoon pepper
1 tablespoon minced parsley

Preheat oven to 350° F. Flake salmon, add eggs, and mix well. Add remaining ingredients. Place in oiled 3 3/8″ × 7 3/8″ loaf pan. Bake for 40 minutes. Serve with Easy White Sauce. Serves 4

Fat: Total—2 teaspoons; per serving—1/2 teaspoon
Oil: Total—20 teaspoons; per serving—5 teaspoons

SALMON LOAF II

1 16-ounce can salmon
1 egg
1/4 cup nonfat yogurt
1/2 cup soft bread crumbs or cracker crumbs or cornmeal
1/2 teaspoon salt
2 teaspoons lemon juice
1 teaspoon Worcestershire sauce
1 teaspoon mustard
1 tablespoon oil
3 tablespoons chopped parsley
1/4 cup finely chopped celery
2 tablespoons chopped onion
2 tablespoons chopped green pepper
Creamy Fish Sauce or Curried Mayonnaise

Preheat oven to 400° F. Drain and flake salmon. Combine the remaining ingredients and mix well. Add salmon. Place in a 4″ × 8″ loaf pan and bake for 30 minutes. If individual baking dishes are used, bake for 20 minutes. Serve hot with Creamy Fish Sauce or cold with Curried Mayonnaise. Serves 4

Fat: Total—1 teaspoon; per serving—1/4 teaspoon
Oil: Total—11 teaspoons; per serving—2 3/4 teaspoons

WHOLE BAKED SALMON WITH WINE SAUCE

1 7- to 10-pound whole fish (or large piece)
3/4 cup dry white wine
1/4 teaspoon thyme
1/2 teaspoon basil
1/4 teaspoon tarragon
1/4 teaspoon rosemary
Celery leaves
3 shallots, minced
2 slices lemon, with peel
Salt to taste

Preheat oven to 375° F. Place fish lengthwise on a large piece of heavy foil. Let fish reach room temperature. Combine remaining ingredients in medium saucepan. Cook on low temperature for 1/2 hour without boiling. Pour wine mixture over the fish and inside the cavity. Fold foil and crimp edges. It is not necessary to wrap the fish completely. Place fish on rack so that it does not rest directly on the roasting pan. This will allow the heat to circulate completely around the fish. Insert a meat thermometer into the thickest part of the fish, usually just behind the gills. Bake until thermometer registers 140° F. This should take between 1–2 hours. (See detailed baking instructions on p. 191.) Serve with White Wine Sauce. Serves 12

Fat: None
Oil: 2 ounces salmon—1 teaspoon

WHITE WINE SAUCE

2 shallots, finely minced
1 tablespoon oil
6 tablespoons all-purpose flour
1 cup water
1 1/2 cups skim milk, enriched with 1/4 cup nonfat dry milk powder
1 1/2 cups dry white wine
3 tablespoons mayonnaise
Salt and pepper to taste (optional)

While fish is baking, sauté shallots in oil. Let stand until fish is done. Blend flour and water and set to one side. When fish is done, pour off liquid into saucepan with the shallots; add the milk and wine and bring to a scald. Add the flour-water mixture and stir until thickened. If not thick enough, blend a little more flour and water. Beat in the mayonnaise until well blended. Add seasonings if needed. Yields approximately 5 cups

Fat: None
Oil: Total—7 1/2 teaspoons; 1/3 cup sauce—1/2 teaspoon oil

SEAFOOD STROGANOFF

1–1 1/2 pounds salmon steaks or fillets
1 medium-sized onion, thinly sliced
2 tablespoons oil
1/4 pound mushrooms, sliced
1 15 1/2-ounce can pear-shaped tomatoes
1/2 teaspoon salt
1 teaspoon Worcestershire sauce
1 tablespoon lime juice
1 tablespoon ketchup
1/2 pound medium-sized shrimp, shelled and deveined
1 cup nonfat yogurt or rinsed low-fat cottage cheese
2 tablespoons all-purpose flour

Remove any bone or skin from fish and cut into bite-size pieces; set aside. Sauté the onion in the oil, stirring until golden; add mushrooms and mix until coated with oil. Add the tomatoes, salt, Worcestershire sauce, lime juice, and ketchup; crush tomatoes with a spoon. Cook, stirring until liquid is reduced and the consistency of heavy cream. Stir in shrimp; cover and simmer 1 minute. Stir in fish and simmer for 2 additional minutes. Blend yogurt or cottage cheese with flour until smooth. Add to fish mixture and cook, stirring until it boils and thickens. Serve spooned over rice, or regular or spinach noodles. Serves 6

Fat: None
Oil: Total—14 teaspoons; per serving—2 1/3 teaspoons

HALIBUT IN FOIL

Aluminum foil, 4 pieces about 9" × 12" each
1 teaspoon grated lemon peel
1/4 cup lemon juice
1/4 cup finely sliced green onion tops or chopped chives
1/4 teaspoon white pepper
1/4 teaspoon crumbled dried marjoram leaves
4 halibut steaks (2 pounds)
Parsley
Lemon slices
1/4 pound fresh small shrimp

Preheat oven to 350° F. Turn up edges of foil paper to make a container for fish. Combine lemon peel and lemon juice, green onion, white pepper, and marjoram. Pour 1/8 of the sauce into each foil container. Place fish on top of sauce in foil and cover with remaining sauce. Sprinkle with parsley. Fold foil securely around fish and place in flat baking pan. Bake 20–25 minutes. Open foil and spread into attractive shape; garnish with lemon slices, parsley, and shrimp. Fish may be prepared and wrapped 1–2 hours ahead and refrigerated until time to bake. Serves 4

Fat: None
Oil: None

HALIBUT STEAK

2 halibut steaks (1 pound)
Lemon juice
Salt
2 2.3-ounce packages dry mushroom soup mix
2/3 cup water
1 6-ounce can mushrooms, drained (save liquid)
1/2 cup dry sherry or white wine
2 tablespoons cornstarch
1 teaspoon lemon juice

Preheat oven to 425° F. Arrange fish in baking dish and sprinkle with lemon juice and salt. Bake for 10 minutes. While fish is baking, prepare sauce.

SAUCE

In saucepan combine soup mix, water, liquid from mushrooms, sherry, and cornstarch, and bring to a boil. Add mushrooms and lemon juice. Remove fish from the oven and cover with sauce. Reduce oven temperature to 375° F and continue baking another 10 minutes. Serves 2

Fat: None
Oil: None

SAVORY HALIBUT

2 1/2 pounds halibut
1 medium onion, chopped
3/4 cup diced celery
1 tablespoon oil
3/4 cup rice
2 1/2 cups boiling water
1/2 teaspoon chili powder
1/4 teaspoon salt
Dash of pepper
2 16-ounce cans whole tomatoes
1/4 pound shrimp
1 10-ounce package frozen mixed vegetables
2 tablespoons chopped parsley

Cut fish into 1-inch chunks. Sauté onion and celery in oil. Add rice, boiling water, and seasonings. Cover and simmer 15 minutes. Add fish, tomatoes, shrimp, and frozen vegetables. Bring to boil. Cover and simmer 10–12 minutes or until halibut is firm but not dry. Sprinkle with chopped parsley. Yields 6 generous servings (may easily be cut down to suit individual needs)

Fat: None
Oil: Total—3 teaspoons; per serving—1/2 teaspoon

VEGETABLE-STUFFED HALIBUT

1/3 cup chopped onion
1 rib celery, diced
1/4 pound fresh mushrooms, sliced
1 carrot, grated
1 tablespoon oil
2 tablespoons water
1 tablespoon chopped parsley
2 tablespoons lemon juice
1/2 teaspoon salt
1/2 teaspoon rosemary
2 halibut steaks (1 pound)
Pepper to taste
Parsley
Lemon slices

Preheat oven to 375° F. Simmer onion, celery, mushrooms, and carrots in covered saucepan with oil and water for 5 minutes. Add parsley, lemon juice, salt, and rosemary. Mix thoroughly. Season fish with salt and pepper. Place one halibut steak in baking pan. Cover with vegetable stuffing and second steak. Bake approximately 20–25 minutes; garnish with parsley and lemon slices. Serves 6

Fat: None
Oil: Total—3 teaspoons; per serving—1/2 teaspoon

OVEN-POACHED HALIBUT

2 pounds halibut steaks
1/2 lemon, thinly sliced
3 slices onion
1 teaspoon salt
4 peppercorns
1/2 bay leaf
3 whole cloves
1 1/2 cups boiling water
Tangy Tomato Sauce

Preheat oven to 375° F. Place halibut in baking dish. Arrange lemon and onion slices over halibut. Add salt, peppercorns, bay leaf, cloves, and boiling water. Cover, using foil if dish has no cover, and bake for 20 minutes. Drain halibut and arrange on heated serving platter. Spoon a portion of Tangy Tomato Sauce over halibut. Serve remaining sauce on the side. Serves 6

Fat: None
Oil: None

HEARTY HALIBUT

2 pounds halibut steaks or other white fish
2/3 cup thinly sliced onion
1 1/2 cups chopped fresh mushrooms
1/3 cup chopped tomatoes
1/4 cup chopped green pepper
1/4 cup chopped parsley
3 tablespoons chopped pimiento
1/2 cup dry white wine
2 tablespoons lemon juice
1 teaspoon salt
1/4 teaspoon dill seed
1/8 teaspoon pepper
Lemon wedges

Preheat oven to 350° F. Cut fish into serving size portions. Arrange onion in bottom of 12″ × 8″ × 2″ baking dish. Place fish on top of onion. Combine remaining vegetables and spread over fish. Combine wine, lemon juice, and seasonings. Pour over vegetables. Bake 20–25 minutes. Serve with lemon wedges. Serves 6

Fat: None
Oil: None

BAKED HALIBUT WITH HERBED DRESSING

3 cups dried bread crumbs
1/4 cup chopped parsley
1 teaspoon salt
1/8 teaspoon pepper
1/2 teaspoon sage
1/2 teaspoon rosemary
2 tablespoons oil
1/2 cup chopped onion
3/4 cup chopped celery
2 tablespoons vinegar
2 tablespoons water
1 1/2-inch-thick slice halibut (about 2 pounds)

Preheat oven to 350° F. Combine bread crumbs with parsley and seasonings. Set aside. Heat 2 tablespoons oil. Add onion and celery and sauté until tender. Add vinegar and water, and heat. Pour mixture over bread crumbs and toss thoroughly. Place dressing in oiled baking dish. Place halibut over dressing. Bake 20–25 minutes. Serve with Easy White Sauce. Serves 6

Fat: None
Oil: Total—6 teaspoons; per serving—1 teaspoon

BAKED FISH AU CHABLIS

2 pounds halibut or white fish (slices or fillets)
Salt and pepper to taste
1 large onion, sliced
1 cup Chablis or dry white wine or sherry
2 tomatoes, sliced, or 1 8-ounce can tomato sauce
1/2 green pepper, sliced (optional)
2 tablespoons Worcestershire sauce

Preheat oven to 375° F. Place fish in baking dish, sprinkle with salt and pepper, and cover with onion slices. Pour wine over fish and marinate 1 hour. Remove fish and onion slices to large shallow baking pan, cover with tomatoes, green pepper, and sprinkling of salt. Bake until fish is tender, about 20–30 minutes. Mix remaining marinade with Worcestershire sauce and use this to baste fish during baking. Serves 4–5

Fat: None
Oil: None

BAKED TROUT

4–6 medium-sized trout (about 1/2 pound each)
Juice of 1 lemon
1 teaspoon salt
1 garlic clove, minced
1 cup dry white wine
2 tablespoons chopped parsley
2 tablespoons chopped green onion
2 tablespoons dry bread crumbs

Preheat oven to 400° F. Wash and dry trout with paper towels; rub outside with lemon juice and sprinkle with salt. Arrange the minced garlic in the bottom of a shallow baking dish large enough to hold trout in a single layer. Place trout in dish; pour wine over the top. Sprinkle the parsley, green onion, and dry bread crumbs over trout. Bake, uncovered, in oven for 20 minutes. Serve hot. Serves 4–6

Fat: None
Oil: 2-ounce trout—1 teaspoon

FLOUNDER BAKE

4 6–8 ounce fillets of flounder
12 small white onions, peeled
1/2 pound small fresh mushrooms, sliced
2 small carrots, thinly sliced
Salt and pepper to taste
2 tablespoons chopped parsley
1/4–1/2 teaspoon rosemary
8 thin slices lemon
1/3 cup dry white wine

Preheat oven to 350° F. Place fish in oiled shallow casserole and arrange onions, sliced mushrooms, and thinly sliced carrots around fillets. Season with salt, pepper, parsley, and rosemary. Arrange lemon slices and pour wine over fillets. Bake for 20–30 minutes. Serves 4

Fat: None
Oil: None

CREAMED FINNAN HADDIE

1 pound salt haddock fillets
2 cups skim milk
4 tablespoons all-purpose flour
1/2 cup cold skim milk
1 teaspoon salt
1/2 cup mayonnaise
2 hard-cooked eggs, chopped

Preheat oven to 300° F. Place fish in saucepan. Add water to cover. Bring to boil and simmer covered for 15 minutes, but do not boil. Drain and rinse well in hot water. Drain again. Heat skim milk to scalding. Mix flour with cold milk until smooth. Add to heated skim milk and cook gently until thickened. Add salt and mayonnaise, and blend until smooth. Place fish in baking dish, cover with sauce, garnish with hard-cooked eggs, and bake 10 minutes. Serves 4

Fat: Total—2 teaspoons; per serving—1/2 teaspoon
Oil: Total—12 teaspoons (sauce); per serving—3 teaspoons

SPICY SNAPPER

2 pounds snapper or other fish fillets
2/3 cup tomato juice
3 tablespoons vinegar
2 tablespoons oil
1 5/8-ounce envelope French dressing mix

Clean fish; cut into serving-size portions. Place in single layer in shallow baking dish. Mix together remaining ingredients and pour over fish; let stand 30 minutes. Remove fish from baking dish. Broil 4 inches from heat 4–5 minutes on each side, basting with remaining sauce. Serves 6

Fat: None
Oil: Total—6 teaspoons; per serving—1 teaspoon

CURRIED FILLETS

2 pounds snapper or perch or other white fish
1 cup thinly sliced celery
1 cup thinly sliced onion
1 tablespoon oil
1 teaspoon curry powder
1 teaspoon salt
Dash of pepper
3/4 cup skim milk
Paprika

Preheat oven to 350° F. Place fish in a 12″ × 8″ pan. Cook celery and onion in oil until tender. Stir in curry powder, salt, pepper, and milk, and spread over fish. Bake for 20–25 minutes. Sprinkle with paprika. Serves 6

Fat: None
Oil: Total—3 teaspoons; per serving—1/2 teaspoon

SOLE WITH HERBS

4 fillets of sole (1 1/2 pounds)
Salt
1/4 teaspoon paprika
1 tablespoon all-purpose flour
1 tablespoon oil
1/4 teaspoon each, dried chives, parsley, tarragon, and chervil
1 tablespoon lemon juice
1/2 cup dry white wine or sherry

Wipe fillets, season, and dust with flour. Heat oil in skillet and add fish. Brown on one side and turn. Sprinkle with mixed herbs and add lemon juice and wine. Cover and simmer 5 minutes. Serve at once. Serves 4

Fat: None
Oil: Total—3 teaspoons; per serving—3/4 teaspoon

SOLE MARINARA

2 tablespoons oil
1/4 cup chopped celery
1/4 teaspoon garlic salt
1/4 teaspoon salt
1 No. 2 can tomatoes
1/4 teaspoon cayenne pepper
1/4 teaspoon sugar
1 tablespoon oregano
1/2 teaspoon dried basil
1 teaspoon dried parsley
4 fillets of sole (1 1/2 pounds)
1/4 cup dry white wine or sherry
Cooked rice

Heat oil in heavy skillet. Add celery and cook until tender. Add remaining ingredients except fish, wine, and rice, and simmer until mixture is reduced or somewhat thick, about 30 minutes. Place fillets in large skillet and add wine. Cover and bring liquid to boil. Reduce heat and simmer 5 minutes. Lay fillets on serving platter, surround with cooked rice, and pour sauce over fish. Serves 4

Fat: None
Oil: Total—6 teaspoons; per serving—1 1/2 teaspoons

TERIYAKI SHRIMP

1 pound large shrimp
Teriyaki Sauce

Peel the hard cover from the shrimp. Remove the dark sand vein from the center back of each shrimp and wash the meat in cold water. Marinate shrimp for 1–2 hours. Broil 3–4 minutes per side or until tender, basting shrimp with Teriyaki Sauce.

Serve with rice and an assortment of fresh stir-fried vegetables. Serves 3–4

Fat: None
Oil: None

BOILED SHRIMP

1 pound large shrimp
Salted water
Cocktail Sauce

Peel the hard cover from the shrimp. Remove the dark sand vein from the center back of each shrimp and wash meat in cold water. Bring salted water to boil and add shrimp. Boil approximately 6 minutes or until shrimp turn pink in color. Shrimp may be eaten hot or cold. Dip shrimp in Cocktail Sauce. Serve with fresh steamed vegetables and rice. Serves 4

Fat: None
Oil: None

SHRIMP KABOBS

1/2 pound large shrimp
Teriyaki Sauce
1 15 1/2-ounce can new potatoes
8–10 fresh mushrooms
1 15 1/2-ounce can large pineapple chunks
1 10-ounce package frozen small onions
1 bell pepper, cut in 1/2-inch squares
1 package wooden skewers (approximately 12)

Marinate shrimp for 2 hours in Teriyaki Sauce. On wooden skewers alternately thread shrimp, vegetables, and pineapple. Broil until shrimp is tender, brushing frequently with Teriyaki Sauce and turning kabobs. Serve with rice. Serves 4

Fat: None
Oil: None

SWEET AND SOUR SHRIMP

1/4 cup packed brown sugar
2 tablespoons cornstarch
1 teaspoon salt
1/8 teaspoon black pepper
1/4 teaspoon dry mustard
1/4 cup lemon juice
1 tablespoon soy sauce
Few drops of hot pepper sauce
1 cup orange juice
2 oranges, cut in bite-size pieces
1 green pepper, cut in thin strips
1 medium onion, chopped
3/4 pound shrimp, shelled, or 2 5-ounce cans shrimp, drained
2 cups cooked rice
Orange slices

Blend brown sugar, cornstarch, salt, pepper, and mustard in large frying pan. Slowly stir in lemon juice, soy sauce, hot pepper sauce, and orange juice. Cook over medium heat until thickened, stirring constantly. Stir in oranges, green pepper, onion, and shrimp. Cover and simmer until vegetables are tender but still crisp, 8–10 minutes, and shrimp is done. Serve over rice. Garnish with orange slices. Serves 4

Fat: None
Oil: None

SHRIMP IN GARLIC SAUCE

2 tablespoons vegetable oil
1 small onion, chopped
1 teaspoon grated gingerroot
4 garlic cloves, sliced
5–6 Chinese dried black mushrooms, soaked 30 minutes
1 cup fresh or frozen peas, shelled or defrosted
1 pound cooked and cleaned shrimp
1/2 cup chicken broth or water
2 teaspoons soy sauce
1 tablespoon cornstarch in 2 tablespoons water

Heat oil in wok until sizzling. Stir-fry onion, ginger, and garlic for 1–2 minutes. Add mushrooms and peas and stir-fry 1–3 minutes. Add shrimp and continue to stir-fry 1–2 minutes. Combine broth, soy sauce, and cornstarch mixture. Add to wok and heat until sauce boils and has thickened. Serve immediately with boiled rice. Serves 4

Fat: None
Oil: Total—6 teaspoons; per serving—1 1/2 teaspoons

PRAWNS WITH GARLIC AND OREGANO

2 pounds prawns or jumbo shrimp in shells
3/4 cup olive oil
1/2 cup Marsala wine
1/2 cup lemon juice
4 garlic cloves, finely chopped
4 green onions, finely chopped
Salt and freshly ground pepper
2 teaspoons crumbled dried oregano
Fresh mint sprigs

Preheat oven to 375° F. Cut prawns down back and devein; do not remove shell. Transfer to shallow baking dish. Add all remaining ingredients except oregano and mint. Bake 10 minutes, basting prawns occasionally. Mix in oregano and baste again. Continue baking until prawns just turn bright pink, about 2 more minutes. Garnish with mint and serve. Serves 8

Fat: None
Oil: Total—36 teaspoons; per serving—4 1/2 teaspoons

BAKED SCALLOPS

1 pound scallops
1 tablespoon oil
2 tablespoons minced onion
1 tablespoon lemon juice
1/4 teaspoon salt
1/8 teaspoon marjoram
1/4 teaspoon paprika
3/4 cup dry white wine
1 1/2 cups chopped mushrooms
3/4 cup skim milk enriched with 2 tablespoons nonfat dry milk powder
1 1/2 tablespoons all-purpose flour
1/4 teaspoon salt
2 tablespoons mayonnaise
1/4 cup cracker crumbs

Preheat oven to 375° F. If scallops are large, cut in half. Heat oil in skillet, add onion, and stir until tender. Add scallops, lemon juice, seasonings, and wine; simmer 10 minutes, stirring occasionally. Add mushrooms and simmer another 2 minutes. Drain liquid from scallops and place scallops in individual baking dishes. Blend 1/4 cup of the milk with the flour; set to one side. Combine the liquid from the scallops with the remaining milk and heat until steaming. Add the flour mixture and salt; stir until thickened. Beat in the mayonnaise until well blended. Pour over the scallops and cover with crumbs. Bake until bubbly, about 10–15 minutes. Serves 4

Fat: None
Oil: Total—6 teaspoons; per serving—1 1/2 teaspoons

SKEWERED SCALLOPS

1 pound scallops
2 large green peppers, cut in 1-inch squares
1 pint cherry tomatoes
1/3 cup lemon juice
3 tablespoons honey
2 tablespoons prepared mustard
1 1/2 teaspoons curry powder
1 tablespoon oil
1 package wooden skewers

Preheat broiler. Rinse and clean scallops. Slice large scallops across grain in half; leave small scallops whole. Alternate scallops, peppers, and tomatoes on skewer. Place on aluminum-foil-lined broiler pan. Combine remaining ingredients to make a sauce. Brush kabobs with this sauce. Broil approximately 4 inches from heat for 5–7 minutes. Turn and brush with sauce. Broil 5–7 minutes longer, basting once. Serves 4

Fat: None
Oil: Total—3 teaspoons; per serving—3/4 teaspoon

GAZPACHO WITH SCALLOPS

6 ounces scallops
1 tablespoon oil
1 green onion, chopped
1 teaspoon lemon juice
4 large tomatoes, peeled
2 12-ounce cans tomato juice
1 tablespoon red wine vinegar
Pinch of sugar
1/4–1/2 cup hot or mild salsa
1/2 medium cucumber, peeled and shredded
1/3 cup diced green bell pepper
1/2 cup Garlic Croutons

Slice large scallops across grain 1/4 inch thick; leave small scallops whole. Heat oil in a medium skillet. Add green onion, lemon juice, and scallops. Sauté until scallops are just firm and opaque, 3–5 minutes. Remove from heat. Cut peeled tomatoes in half crosswise. Dice tomatoes. In a large bowl or plastic storage container, stir together diced tomatoes, tomato juice, vinegar, and sugar to taste. Stir in choice of *salsa* to taste. Stir in cucumber, bell pepper, and sautéed scallops. Cover and refrigerate at least 4 hours. Serve chilled gazpacho with Garlic Croutons sprinkled on each serving. Serves 6

Fat: None
Oil: Total—3 teaspoons; per serving—1/2 teaspoon

OYSTERS ROCKEFELLER

1/2 10-ounce package frozen chopped spinach
1/2 cup finely chopped green onion
2 tablespoons oil
1/4 teaspoon powdered thyme
1/4 teaspoon garlic powder
2 teaspoons dehydrated parsley
1/8 teaspoon cayenne pepper or 1/2 teaspoon Worcestershire sauce
31/2 tablespoons all-purpose flour
1 teaspoon salt (none if you use oyster juice)
1/2 cup skim milk
1/2 cup clam juice or oyster juice (if you shuck your oysters)
2 tablespoons mayonnaise
1 tablespoon lemon juice and/or dry sherry
1–2 dozen oysters, depending upon size, cleaned and shucked, or 1 pint small oysters

Cook frozen spinach as directed on package, drain, and set aside. Sauté onion in oil, then add seasonings. Blend in flour and salt and make a very light brown roux. Add skim milk and clam juice gradually and stir until thick. Blend in the cooked, drained spinach. Remove from heat and whip in the mayonnaise and lemon juice. Place oyster shells on 1/2-inch-thick bed of rock salt (or sand). This is very important as it is a heat conductor and is necessary to cook the oysters evenly. Put an oyster in each shell and cover with the spinach mixture, approximately 2–3 teaspoons per oyster. Preheat broiler for 1–2 minutes, then place oysters 4–5 inches under the broiling element until lightly browned. Serve hot. Serves 4

Fat: None
Oil: Total—9 teaspoons; per serving—21/4 teaspoons

SCALLOPED OYSTERS

1 pint oysters
1/4 cup diced celery
2 tablespoons minced parsley
1/2 teaspoon salt
1/4 teaspoon pepper
2/3 cup liquid (oyster liquid and skim milk)
1 1/2 cups bread crumbs, toasted
1 tablespoon oil

Preheat oven to 350° F. Combine all ingredients except the crumbs and oil. Mix together crumbs and oil; spread 1/3 of the mixture in a 10″ × 6″ × 1 1/2″ baking dish. Arrange the oyster combination and crumbs alternately in the baking dish, ending with crumbs. Bake 30 minutes. Serves 4

Fat: None
Oil: Total—3 teaspoons; per serving—3/4 teaspoon

MINCED BAKED CLAMS

4 teaspoons oil
4 teaspoons all-purpose flour
1/4 cup dry white wine or sherry
1 teaspoon salt
1/8 teaspoon pepper
2 tablespoons minced green onion
2 cups minced clams
1 4-ounce can sliced mushrooms
Crumb Topping Mix

Preheat oven to 350° F. Heat oil; stir in flour and wine. Cook, stirring constantly until thick. Add salt, pepper, onion, and minced clams. Spoon into clam shells. Add sliced mushrooms and sprinkle with Crumb Topping Mix. Bake 20 minutes. Serves 6

Fat: None
Oil: Total—4 teaspoons; per serving—2/3 teaspoon

CLAM FRITTERS

1 can drained clams, minced
1 egg or 2 egg whites
1/2 cup bread crumbs
1/2 teaspoon salt
1/8 teaspoon pepper
1–2 tablespoons all-purpose flour
3 tablespoons skim milk

Drain clams. Combine remaining ingredients and add clams. Form into patties. Fry at 375° until patties are lightly browned and warm through.

Fat: Total—1 teaspoon using complete egg; per serving—1/4 teaspoon
Oil: Trace from frying

CLAM SCRAMBLE

4 eggs
1/2 cup skim milk enriched with 2 tablespoons nonfat dry milk powder
1/4 teaspoon salt
1 6 1/2-ounce can minced clams, drained
2 tablespoons cracker crumbs

Preheat oven to 350° F. Mix eggs with milk and salt. Pour mixture into nonstick skillet and cook slowly, stirring until thick. Add clams. Spoon into baking dish or individual baking dishes, cover with crumbs. Bake until lightly browned, about 10 minutes. Serves 4

Fat: Total—4 teaspoons; per serving—1 teaspoon
Oil: None

DEVILED CRAB

1 tablespoon oil
2 tablespoons all-purpose flour
1 cup skim milk, heated
Dash of cayenne pepper
1 teaspoon salt
1 teaspoon Worcestershire sauce
2 egg yolks, slightly beaten
2 cups crabmeat or flaked white fish
1/4 teaspoon lemon juice
1/4 cup dry sherry
2/3 cup toasted bread crumbs
6 slices lemon
Paprika

Preheat oven to 450° F. Heat oil; stir in flour and heated skim milk. Season with cayenne, salt, and Worcestershire sauce; cook, stirring constantly, until thick. Add egg yolks and crab; cook for 3 minutes. Stir in lemon juice and sherry. Spoon into baking shells or ramekins; cover with crumbs. Bake about 20–25 minutes until brown. Top with a lemon slice and a sprinkling of paprika. Serves 6

Fat: Total—2 teaspoons; per serving—1/3 teaspoon
Oil: Total—3 teaspoons; per serving—1/2 teaspoon

CRAB CAKES

1 pound crabmeat
1 pound flaked cooked fish (sole, halibut, etc.)
2 eggs
8 water chestnuts, finely chopped or 1/2 cup celery, finely chopped
6–8 green onions, finely chopped
2 tablespoons oil
Parsley

Thoroughly blend together all ingredients except oil. Form into patties 3 inches in diameter and 1 inch thick. Cook slowly in oil, turning once, until patties are a deep golden brown. Drain on absorbent paper, add parsley, and serve hot. Serves 8

Fat: Total—2 teaspoons; per serving—1/4 teaspoon
Oil: Total—6 teaspoons; per serving—3/4 teaspoon

QUICK-BROILED SHELLFISH

12–13 ounces crabmeat or shrimp or combination
1/4 cup mayonnaise
1/4 cup nonfat yogurt
2 teaspoons instant minced onion or 1/8 teaspoon onion powder
1/4 teaspoon curry powder
2 tablespoons minced parsley
1/2 teaspoon Angostura bitters
1/2 teaspoon salt
1/4 teaspoon ground white pepper
3 tablespoons bread crumbs

Preheat broiler. Combine all ingredients except the bread crumbs and mix lightly. Divide mixture into four individual serving dishes and sprinkle with crumbs. Broil 4–5 inches from heat, approximately 5 minutes or until mixture bubbles and crumbs are brown. Serves 4

Fat: None
Oil: Total—6 teaspoons; per serving—1 1/2 teaspoons

CHAPTER 19

Poultry

With the elimination of red meat from your diet, you will rely more on poultry and fish as your main source of protein unless you are a vegetarian. Chicken can be substituted in most recipes calling for beef. Because of its mild flavor, it blends well with sauces, in soups, salads, and adapts well in most any type of cuisine.

Always skin the chicken and turkey before cooking. Trim off all visible fat. If you are baking chicken in the oven, cover with foil or place in a clay pot to retain moisture. It is permissible to fry chicken with skin removed in pure vegetable oil.

The dark meat of chicken or turkey contains saturated fat and must be avoided during the first year on the diet. Following the first year, 3 ounces can be eaten once a week in place of red meat. The only part of the chicken or turkey considered as white meat is the breast.

TERIYAKI CHICKEN

3 large chicken breasts, skinned and boned
3/4 cup soy sauce
1/4 cup packed brown sugar
1/4 cup dry sherry or white rice wine
2 tablespoons grated gingerroot
1 small garlic clove, minced

Preheat oven to 450° F. Skin and trim all fat from chicken. Cut breasts in half. Place cut chicken in shallow bowl. Combine remaining ingredients and pour over chicken. Cover and refrigerate for 1–2 hours. Drain chicken, saving sauce. Place chicken in an oiled baking dish. Bake in oven for 10 minutes. Turn chicken and bake for 10 additional minutes. Reduce oven temperature to 350° F. Pour off and discard liquid in pan. Continue cooking for 30 minutes longer or until tender, brushing frequently with sauce. Turn oven to Broil and broil for 2 minutes or until chicken is brown. Serve with rice and fresh vegetables. Serves 4–6

Fat: None
Oil: None

TANGY CHICKEN

1/2 cup bottled steak sauce
1/2 cup water
2 chicken breasts, skinned and boned

Combine steak sauce and water. Trim any visible fat from chicken. Place chicken in a nonstick or lightly oiled pan. Pour sauce over chicken. Brown chicken, and cover and cook until tender. Serves 2–4

Fat: None
Oil: None

HONEY MUSTARD CHICKEN

2 chicken breasts, skinned and boned
6 tablespoons honey
1/4 cup prepared mustard
Salt
1/4 teaspoon curry powder

Preheat oven to 325° F. Remove all visible fat from chicken. Combine honey, mustard, salt, and curry powder. Mix well. Brush chicken evenly with sauce. Place chicken in covered baking dish and bake 45 minutes. Yields 2–4 servings

Fat: None
Oil: None

EASY OVEN CHICKEN

2 chicken breasts, skinned
Aluminum foil for baking
1 teaspoon basil
1/2 teaspoon pepper
Sprinkling of paprika
1 teaspoon Worcestershire sauce
2 tablespoons instant rice
1 large potato, cubed
1 tomato, chopped
2 green pepper rings
1 small can mushrooms

Preheat oven to 350° F. Arrange chicken in foil. Season with spices and sprinkle on Worcestershire sauce. Cover chicken with rice and vegetables. Close foil tightly and bake 1 1/2 hours. Serves 2–4

Fat: None
Oil: None

PINEAPPLE CHICKEN

1 20-ounce can sliced pineapple in syrup
2 chicken breasts, split and skinned
2 tablespoons oil
1 large onion, chopped
1 large garlic clove, pressed
2 tablespoons plum jam
1/4 cup chopped parsley
1 teaspoon salt
1 teaspoon crumbled tarragon
2 teaspoons cornstarch
Hot rice

Drain pineapple, reserving syrup. Brown chicken in oil. Remove. Drain excess oil from skillet, leaving one tablespoon. Sauté onion and garlic until soft. Stir in jam until melted; stir in pineapple syrup, parsley, salt, and tarragon. Return chicken to skillet. Cover, simmer 30 minutes. Remove chicken to warmed serving platter. Combine small amount of pan juices with cornstarch. Mix well and add back to pan juices, cooking until mixture is clear and thickened. Serve over rice. Serves 2–4

Fat: None
Oil: Total—6 teaspoons; per serving—1 1/2 teaspoons

CRANBERRY CHICKEN

1 16-ounce can whole cranberries
1 package dry onion soup mix
1 8-ounce jar creamy French dressing
3 chicken breasts, skinned and boned

Preheat oven to 400° F. Mix cranberries, onion soup, and dressing in mixing bowl. Add chicken and coat well. Cover and marinate at least 1 hour. Place chicken in uncovered baking dish and bake for 30–45 minutes, basting occasionally. Serves 3–6

Fat: None
Oil: None

dressing

Preheat oven to 400° F. Mix cranberries, onion soup, and dressing in mixing bowl. Add chicken and coat well. Cover and marinate at least 1 hour. Place chicken in uncovered baking dish and bake for 30–45

2 cups finely chopped or ground cooked white meat of poultry
1 egg, slightly beaten
1/2 cup mayonnaise
1/4 teaspoon salt
1/4 teaspoon pepper
2 tablespoons grated onion
1/4 cup fine dry bread crumbs

Preheat oven to 375° F. In medium-sized bowl mix poultry with the remaining ingredients except bread crumbs. Chill thoroughly, then shape into patties. Roll in bread crumbs. Place on baking sheet and bake 20–25 minutes or until brown. Yields approximately 18 croquettes, which freeze very well. Serves 6

Fat: 1 teaspoon; per croquette—negligible
Oil: Total—12 teaspoons; per croquette—2/3 teaspoon

CHICKEN BREASTS WITH PASTA AND OLIVES

1/4 cup olive oil
1 medium onion, chopped
1–2 garlic cloves, minced
1 teaspoon salt
1 teaspoon turmeric
1 teaspoon cumin
1/4 teaspoon cayenne (less if too hot)
2 whole chicken breasts, skinned and boned
1 8 1/4-ounce can whole tomatoes, cut into quarters, liquid reserved
3 mushrooms, sliced
1 2.2-ounce can sliced black olives
1/4–1/2 cup dry white wine
Freshly cooked spaghettini

Heat oil in medium skillet over medium-high heat. Add onion and garlic, and sauté until translucent, about 5 minutes. Stir in salt, turmeric, cumin, and cayenne. Add chicken and cook until light golden,

1 teaspoon turmeric
1 teaspoon cumin
1/4 teaspoon cayenne (less if too hot)
2 whole chicken breasts, skinned
1 2.2-ounce can sliced black olives
1/4–1/2 cup dry white wine
Freshly cooked spaghettini

pasta. Serves 4

Fat: None
Oil: Total—16 teaspoons; per serving—4 teaspoons

CHICKEN CELESTE

4–6 chicken breasts, skinned
1/3 cup all-purpose flour
1 teaspoon salt
1/8 teaspoon pepper
1/4 teaspoon paprika
2 tablespoons oil
1 medium onion, chopped
1/2 cup dry sherry
1/4 cup water
1/4 cup mayonnaise
1/2 cup nonfat yogurt
2 tablespoons minced parsley

Clean and skin chicken; dust with flour that has been seasoned with salt, pepper, and paprika. Pour oil in heavy skillet or Dutch oven; brown chicken on both sides. Add onion, sherry, and water. Cover and simmer until tender, about 1 hour. Remove chicken to hot platter and keep warm. Add mayonnaise and yogurt to liquid in skillet, blending until smooth; add parsley and additional seasoning if desired. Pour over chicken. Serves 6

Fat: None
Oil: Total—12 teaspoons; per serving—2 teaspoons

CHICKEN-RICE CASSEROLE

3 tablespoons oil
1/3 cup all-purpose flour
1 1/2 teaspoons salt
1/8 teaspoon pepper
1 cup chicken broth
1 1/2 cups skim milk
1 1/2 cups cooked long grain or wild rice
2 cups cubed cooked chicken or turkey (white meat only)
1 4-ounce can mushroom stems and pieces, drained
1/3 cup chopped green pepper
2 tablespoons chopped pimiento
1/4 cup slivered almonds

Preheat oven to 350° F. Heat oil in 2-quart saucepan. Blend in flour, salt, and pepper. Cook over low heat, stirring constantly, until bubbly; remove from heat. Stir in broth and milk. Heat to boiling, stirring constantly. Boil and stir 1 minute. Stir in remaining ingredients. Pour into ungreased 2-quart casserole. Bake uncovered until bubbly, 40–45 minutes. Serves 6

Fat: None
Oil: Total—14 teaspoons; per serving—2 1/3 teaspoons

LEMON FRIED CHICKEN

1 2–2 1/2-pound chicken, skinned and cut into serving pieces
2 tablespoons lemon juice
2 tablespoons oil
1/4 teaspoon garlic powder
3/4 teaspoon salt
1 teaspoon soy sauce
1/4 teaspoon ground thyme
1/4 teaspoon ground marjoram
1/3 teaspoon pepper
1/2 teaspoon grated lemon rind
1/2 cup all-purpose flour
1/2 teaspoon paprika

Preheat oven to 400° F. Wash and skin chicken; dry well and place in large shallow dish. Mix together lemon juice, oil, garlic powder, salt, soy sauce, thyme, marjoram, pepper, and lemon rind. Pour over chicken and marinate in refrigerator at least 3 hours, turning occasionally. Drain chicken on absorbent paper. Mix flour and paprika. Coat chicken pieces with mixture; shake off excess. Place in baking dish. Bake for 30 minutes; turn and bake about 30 minutes longer or until chicken is tender. Serves 4–6

Fat: 2 ounces dark meat—1 teaspoon
White meat—None
Oil: Total—6 teaspoons; per serving—1 1/2 teaspoons

CHICKEN HUNGARIAN GOULASH

2 chicken breasts, skinned, boned, and cut into strips
Salt
Pepper
All-purpose flour
1/2 cup oil
1 large onion, sliced
1 garlic clove, finely chopped
1 1/2 cups tomato juice
1 16-ounce can stewed tomatoes
1 tablespoon or 3 cubes chicken bouillon
2 teaspoons paprika
1/2 teaspoon thyme leaves
1/4 teaspoon pepper
1 cup plain nonfat yogurt
1/2 16-ounce package wide egg noodles

Sprinkle chicken lightly with salt and pepper; coat with flour. In large skillet brown chicken in oil. Pour off all but 3 tablespoons drippings. Add onion and garlic; cook until tender. Add remaining ingredients except yogurt and noodles. Cover and simmer 20–25 minutes. Uncover, remove from heat, and cool 5 minutes. Stir 1/4 cup sauce into yogurt; add slowly to mixture in skillet, stirring constantly until yogurt is blended. Heat through (do not boil). Serve over hot cooked noodles. Serves 4

Fat: None
Oil: Total—24 teaspoons; per serving—6 teaspoons

CHICKEN AND RICE

2 pounds chicken breasts, skinned and boned
2 tablespoons oil
3/4 cup uncooked rice
1 tablespoon grated onion or 1 teaspoon dry onion flakes
Salt
Pepper
1 3-ounce can sliced mushrooms
1 3/4 cups water
2 chicken bouillon cubes

Preheat oven to 350° F. Brown chicken in oil. Put rice, onion, salt, and pepper in oiled casserole dish. Add mushrooms and juice. Arrange chicken on top. Pour water and dissolved bouillon over the top. Cover and bake for 1 hour. Serves 4

Fat: None
Oil: Total—6 teaspoons; per serving—1 1/2 teaspoons

CHICKEN PICANTE

1/2 cup medium-chunky salsa *or taco sauce*
1/4 cup Dijon mustard
2 tablespoons lime juice
6 chicken breast halves, skinned and boned
2 tablespoons vegetable oil
6 tablespoons plain nonfat yogurt
1 lime, peeled and sliced into 6 segments, membrane removed
Cilantro

In a large bowl, make marinade by mixing *salsa,* mustard, and lime juice. Add chicken, turning to coat. Marinate for at least 30 minutes. In large skillet heat oil over medium heat. Remove chicken from marinade and place in skillet. Cook until brown on all sides. Add marinade and cook about 5 minutes more, until fork can be inserted in chicken with ease and marinade is slightly reduced and beginning to glaze. Remove chicken to warmed serving platter. Increase heat to High and boil marinade 1 minute; pour over chicken. Place 1 tablespoon yogurt on each breast half and top each with a lime segment. Garnish with cilantro. Serves 6

Fat: None
Oil: Total—6 teaspoons; per serving—1 teaspoon

SESAME CHICKEN

1/4 cup soy sauce
1 tablespoon sugar
1 tablespoon dry sherry
1 tablespoon grated fresh ginger
1–2 garlic cloves, pressed or minced
3 large chicken breasts, split, skinned, and boned (3 pounds total)
2 eggs
1/2 cup all-purpose flour
1/2 cup sesame seeds
4 tablespoons vegetable oil

Preheat oven to 500° F. Stir together soy sauce, sugar, sherry, ginger, and garlic. Place chicken in shallow pan and marinate in sauce 1–2 hours. Heat a 10″ × 15″ pan in oven. Lift chicken from marinade. In a rimmed plate, blend eggs with 2 tablespoons of the marinade. On a piece of waxed paper mix flour and sesame seeds. Dip the chicken in egg, then coat in sesame mixture and set aside in a single layer. When pan is hot, add oil. Put chicken in pan and turn to coat with oil. Bake, uncovered, 5 minutes; turn chicken and continue cooking until no longer pink in thickest part (cut to test), about 5 minutes. Serves 6

Fat: Total—2 teaspoons; per serving—1/3 teaspoon
Oil: Total—20 teaspoons; per serving—3 1/3 teaspoons

CHICKEN AND PASTA SALAD

2 chicken breasts, skinned and boned
1 cup salted chicken stock or bouillon
1/4 cup dry white wine
3/4 pound pasta bows or medium-sized conchiglie
Garlic Mayonnaise
1 cup coarsely chopped cooked green beans
1 cup cherry tomatoes
1 cup coarsely chopped celery
4 green onions, coarsely chopped
1/2 cup coarsely chopped pitted black olives
1/4 cup toasted pine nuts or blanched almonds
Salt to taste

Prepare chicken. Gently cook chicken breasts in stock and wine until tender. Chop coarsely. Cook pasta in rapidly boiling salted water. Drain and cool.

GARLIC MAYONNAISE

In blender or food processor mix 2 egg yolks, 4 garlic cloves, 1/4 cup lemon juice, 2 teaspoons Dijon mustard, and a pinch each of salt and pepper. With motor running *slowly,* drizzle 1 1/2 cups oil to make a thin sauce. Yields 1 pint

Two cups commercial mayonnaise may be used with just garlic and Dijon mustard added to it. This will reduce amount of oil in recipe by half.

Set aside 1 tablespoon of each vegetable for garnish. Mix all remaining ingredients in a large bowl with chicken and pasta. Add mayonnaise to taste and toss gently. (There will be extra mayonnaise. Add as necessary if salad is kept for several days). Salt to taste. Serves 6

Fat: None
Oil: Total—13 teaspoons; per serving—2 1/5 teaspoons

Fat: Total from mayonnaise—2 teaspoons; per serving—negligible
Oil: Total from mayonnaise—72 teaspoons; 1 teaspoon mayonnaise—1 teaspoon oil

CHILI WITH CHICKEN

1/4 cup olive oil
1 cup minced onion
2 garlic cloves
1 pound cubed chicken or ground turkey breasts
1 tablespoon cumin
2 tablespoons chili powder
2 teaspoons oregano
2 teaspoons salt
1 teaspoon pepper
1 tablespoon sugar
3 8-ounce cans tomato sauce
1 12-ounce can tomatoes, cut in pieces
1 8-ounce can kidney beans (optional)

In olive oil sauté onion and garlic until clear. Remove from heat. In large skillet fry chicken or turkey until brown, then add to onion and garlic. Add remaining ingredients and simmer for 30 minutes. Serves 6

Fat: None
Oil: Total—12 teaspoons; per serving—1 1/2 teaspoons

CHICKEN AND NOODLES

1 pound chicken breasts, skinned and boned
2 bay leaves
1 teaspoon or more salt
1 1/2 pints water
Chopped onion or onion powder to taste
3 tablespoons cornstarch mixed with 3 tablespoons water
1 10 3/4-ounce can condensed chicken broth, chilled and with fat removed
4 cups noodles

Preheat oven to 350° F. In large saucepan combine chicken breasts, bay leaves, salt, water, and onion, and cook 45 minutes to 1 hour. Remove breasts and cut into small pieces. Add cornstarch to sauce and mix with whisk. Add chicken broth and cook until thickened. In 1 quart of water cook 4 cups noodles until tender. Drain and rinse. In a large baking dish combine noodles and diced chicken. Cover with sauce and bake 1/2 hour. Serves 4–6

Fat: None
Oil: None

CHICKEN AND SAUERKRAUT

2 chicken breasts, skinned, boned and cut in 2-inch chunks
3 tablespoons oil
3 tablespoons all-purpose flour
1 cup lukewarm water
1 16-ounce can sauerkraut, rinsed once
Pepper to taste

Prepare chicken. Heat 1 tablespoon oil in large skillet. Add chicken and fry until golden brown. Remove chicken. Add 2 tablespoons oil. Heat on Medium to Medium-high. Add flour and stir with a fork, browning lightly. Add 1 cup lukewarm water. Stir quickly and work lumps out with fork or wire whisk. Cook until thickened. Add sauerkraut and chicken and continue cooking 10–15 minutes. Season with pepper if desired. Serve over boiled potatoes. Serves 2–4

Fat: None
Oil: Total—9 teaspoons; per serving—4 1/2 teaspoons

BLANQUETTE DE POULET

2 large chicken breasts, skinned and boned
2 tablespoons oil
1/2 pound medium mushrooms
2 medium carrots, chopped
1 medium onion, cut into quarters
1 1/2 teaspoons salt
1 teaspoon chicken bouillon
1/4 teaspoon thyme
1/2 teaspoon pepper
1 cup water
1 tablespoon all-purpose flour or 1 1/2 teaspoons cornstarch
2 teaspoons lemon juice
2 egg yolks, slightly beaten
1 tablespoon chopped parsley (optional)

Cut chicken breasts into bite-size pieces. Heat 1 tablespoon oil in 12-inch skillet over medium-high heat and cook chicken until tender, about 3–5 minutes, stirring frequently. With slotted spoon remove chicken to bowl.

Cut mushrooms in half. In same skillet over medium heat, in 1 tablespoon oil, cook mushrooms, carrots, onion, salt, bouillon, thyme, and pepper until vegetables are tender, about 15 minutes, stirring occasionally.

In cup, stir water and flour until smooth. Gradually stir flour mixture into mixture in skillet; cook over medium heat until mixture is slightly thickened and boils, stirring constantly. Return chicken to skillet.

In small bowl, mix lemon juice and egg yolks until blended; stir in small amount of hot liquid from skillet. Slowly pour egg mixture back into simmering liquid, stirring rapidly to prevent lumping. Cook over medium-low heat, stirring constantly, until mixture is slightly thickened. (DO NOT BOIL, or mixture will curdle.) Serve over rice. Serves 4

Fat: Total—2 teaspoons; per serving—1 1/2 teaspoons
Oil: Total—6 teaspoons; per serving—1 1/2 teaspoons

CURRY CHICKEN

2 large onions, chopped (1 1/2–2

1 garlic clove, finely chopped

Serves 4

Fat: Total—2 teaspoons; per serving—1 1/2 teaspoons
Oil: Total—6 teaspoons; per serving—1 1/2 teaspoons

1 16-ounce can whole or stewed tomatoes, drained
1 cube chicken bouillon dissolved in 3/4 cup warm water
1/2 cup chopped parsley or parsley flakes

2–3 tablespoons all-purpose flour
2 tablespoons oil
1/3 cup toasted slivered almonds

In medium skillet sauté onion in oil until lightly browned, about 5 minutes. Add green pepper; cook 5 minutes. Stir in curry powder; cook 1 minute, stirring constantly. Add tomatoes, bouillon, parsley, garlic, salt, and mace. Bring to boiling. Lower heat; simmer, covered, 5 minutes. Remove from heat; add raisins. Set aside.

Preheat oven to 375° F. Dust chicken with flour. Brown in 2 tablespoons oil in large (second) skillet, adding more oil if necessary. Place sauce and chicken in large baking dish. Bake covered, for 15 minutes or until bubbling. Serve over rice. Sprinkle with almonds before serving.

To make ahead: Prepare a day ahead, but omit raisins, almonds, and baking until before serving. After baking add raisins and almonds. Serves 4

Fat: None
Oil: Total—26 teaspoons; per serving—4 1/3 teaspoons

CHICKEN CASHEW

3 chicken breasts, skinned and boned (6 halves)
2 tablespoons oil
1/2 pound fresh pea pods (snow peas) or 2 10-ounce packages frozen peas
1 cup sliced mushrooms
1/2 cup sliced green onion
1 6-ounce can bamboo shoots, drained
1/2 cup sliced water chestnuts
1 teaspoon chicken bouillon granules or 1 cube
1/4 cup soy sauce
2 tablespoons cornstarch
1/2 teaspoon sugar
Dash of pepper
1/2 teaspoon salt
4 ounces salted cashew nuts

Cut chicken into small bite-size pieces. In large skillet or wok cook chicken in 2 tablespoons oil until tender. Toss chicken frequently

1/2 pound fresh pea pods (snow peas) or 2 10-ounce packages frozen peas
1 cup sliced mushrooms
1/2 cup sliced green onion
1/4 cup soy sauce
2 tablespoons cornstarch
1/2 teaspoon sugar
Dash of pepper
1/2 teaspoon salt

sugar, pepper, and salt, and add to chicken mixture. Toss. Cover and cook until the sauce has thickened. Stir in cashew nuts. Serve with rice. Yields 6 servings

Fat: None
Oil: Total—10 teaspoons; per serving—1 2/3 teaspoons

CHICKEN AND BROCCOLI CRÊPES

6 tablespoons olive oil
6 tablespoons all-purpose flour
Dash of salt
3 cups skim milk
1/2 cup nonfat yogurt
1/4 cup dry white wine
1 2 1/2-ounce can sliced mushrooms
1 10-ounce package frozen broccoli
2 cups cooked chicken, finely chopped
12 main-dish Crêpes

SAUCE

In medium saucepan blend oil, flour, and salt. Add milk all at once. Cook, stirring constantly, until thickened and bubbly. Stir in yogurt and wine. Cook 1 minute. Remove 1/2 cup of the sauce; set aside. Stir mushrooms into remaining sauce.

FILLING

Cook broccoli; drain. Combine with chicken and the reserved 1/2 cup sauce.

To assemble: Spread 1/4 cup filling over unbrowned side of crêpe, leaving 1/4-inch rim around edge. Roll up crêpe. Place seam side down in skillet or chafing dish. Repeat with remaining crêpes. Drizzle sauce over crêpes. Cook covered over low heat until bubbly. Serves 6

Fat: None
Oil: Total—18 teaspoons; per serving—3 teaspoons

CHICKEN TACO MEAT

8 ounces uncooked chicken breast, skinned and boned
1/2 package commercial taco seasoning
1/2 cup water

Grind chicken breast. In medium skillet mix together chicken, taco seasoning, and water. Cover and cook slowly for 1/2 hour. Remove lid and cook down. Use this recipe in place of red meat in tacos and enchiladas. Serves 4

Fat: None
Oil: None

TURKEY LOAF I

1 pound ground skinned turkey breast
1 1/2 tablespoons sage
3 tablespoons prepared mustard
2 tablespoons ketchup
1 egg
3 slices dried bread, crumbled
1/2 cup skim milk
1 teaspoon salt
1/2 teaspoon coarsely ground pepper

Preheat oven to 350° F. Oil a 9-inch loaf pan. Combine all ingredients and shape into a loaf. Place in 9″ × 5″ × 3″ loaf pan and smooth out top. Bake 45–55 minutes. Pour 1 small can tomato sauce over the top during the last 20 minutes if desired. Serves 4

Variations:

Add to mixture

1. 1 large garlic clove, minced
2. 2 teaspoons garlic salt and 1 small onion, diced
3. 2 tablespoons Worcestershire sauce

Fat: Total—1 teaspoon; per serving—1/4 teaspoon
Oil: None

TURKEY LOAF II

1 cup bread crumbs
1/4 cup wheat germ
2 pounds ground or finely diced skinned turkey breast
1/2 cup chopped onion
1/2 cup grated carrot
1/2 cup chopped celery
Dash of hot pepper sauce
1 egg
1 8-ounce can tomato sauce or evaporated skim milk
1 1/2 teaspoons salt
1 teaspoon oregano
1 teaspoon Worcestershire sauce
1 teaspoon dried parsley

Preheat oven to 350° F. Mix all ingredients and bake in 9″ × 5″ × 3″ loaf pan for 1 hour. Serves 6

Fat: Total—1 teaspoon; per serving—1/6 teaspoon
Oil: None

CHAPTER 20

Beef

The largest single source of fat in the Western diet is meat. This is particularly true of corn-fattened beef, which is the source of marbled steaks and other high-grade meat cuts. For this reason we are recommending that the meat intake be sharply reduced and confined to lean portions. In accordance, we have limited the recipes in this section to discourage the use of red meat in your diet.

During the first year red meat intake will be restricted completely. Patients generally lose the desire for red meat at the end of this time. Following the first year you will be allowed 3 ounces once a week. We strongly suggest, however, that your red meat allowance be used only on special occasions.

A small food scale showing graduated measurements in ounces is necessary to accurately determine serving size. Weigh all meat after cooking. The recipes will indicate the amount of fat after cooking. Although we have included a few oven-baked recipes, it is always best to broil or cook so fat drains easily from the meat.

The oven-baked recipes will be slightly higher in fat than will the broiled meats.

When considering cuts of meat, always buy the leanest and least marbled. All visible fat must be discarded before cooking.

Meat Preparation

Remove meat from wrapper as soon as possible and place in refrigerator. When ready to cook, do not wash meat or pierce while cooking or valuable juices will be lost.

For best results sear the surface of the meat as soon as possible. This locks in juices. Cooking should be slow to develop the flavor. Tougher cuts should be cooked slowly for best results.

Gravy

It is important that all gravy containing fat be eliminated. This is possible by the simple expedient of defatting the gravy.

1. When you wish to defat meat juices in a hurry, pour the juices into a deep bowl or jar, add a few ice cubes, and place the bowl in the freezing compartment of the refrigerator for about 15 minutes. You can also pour off the meat juices when the roast is three quarters done and allow them to congeal in the refrigerator. The hardened fat can then be easily removed and the remainder can be made into a fat-free gravy.

2. Cook or fry the meat well in advance of mealtime or even the day before. Remove the meat from the pan, place the juice in a bowl or jar, and refrigerate until completely cold. The fat will have risen to the top and hardened, thus making it easy to remove. The meat juice can now be used for cooking without concern for the small traces of fat that may still remain. The meat can then be rewarmed quickly without loss of taste.

Two cups of liquid (meat juice) will make 1 1/2 to 2 cups of gravy. Use 1 1/2 tablespoons of flour for each cup of gravy desired. Mix flour with a small amount of cold water; add slowly to liquid in pan; cook, stirring constantly, until thick and smooth. Season to taste.

MEAT LOAF

2 pounds lean ground beef
1/4 cup finely chopped onion
2 teaspoons salt
1/4 teaspoon pepper
1/4 teaspoon sage
1/4 teaspoon poultry seasoning
1 tablespoon Worcestershire sauce
3 egg whites, lightly beaten
1 cup tomato sauce
4 slices whole grain bread

Preheat oven to 350° F. Combine meat with onion and seasonings. Beat egg whites and add tomato sauce. Cube bread and soak in the liquid mixture. Mix well. Add to meat and mix lightly. Pack into 5″ × 9″ meat loaf pan with rack in bottom for fat to drain. Bake for 1 1/4 hours. Let loaf stand for 20 minutes. Remove from pan and spread with ketchup or hot tomato sauce. Serves 10

Fat: Total—14 teaspoons; per serving—1 1/2 teaspoons
2 ounces cooked beef—1 teaspoon
Oil: None

BEEF AND EGGPLANT CASSEROLE

1 medium-sized eggplant
1 pound lean ground beef
1 tablespoon oil
1 medium onion, chopped
1/4 cup blanched chopped green pepper
3/4 teaspoon salt
1/4 teaspoon oregano
1 cup chopped, peeled tomatoes (canned or fresh)
1 tablespoon all-purpose flour

Preheat oven to 350° F. Peel and slice eggplant. Cook in boiling water until tender but not soft. Drain. In large skillet cook beef until free of fat. Drain beef and pat between paper towels to remove fat. Set aside. In 1 tablespoon oil brown onion and green pepper with seasonings. Add beef, tomatoes, and flour. Cook until thickened. Arrange in casserole dish in layers with eggplant. Bake 30 minutes. Serves 6

Fat: Total—6 teaspoons; per serving—1 teaspoon
2 ounces cooked beef—1 teaspoon
Oil: Total—3 teaspoons; per serving—1/2 teaspoon

SALISBURY STEAK

2 pounds ground round steak
1 medium onion, minced
2 tablespoons minced green pepper
1 tablespoon chopped parsley
1 teaspoon salt
1 teaspoon pepper
1 teaspoon Worcestershire sauce

Preheat broiler. Mix all ingredients lightly. Shape into patties. Place 3 inches under broiler heat. Broil 12 minutes, turning once. Yields 10 patties

Fat: Total—14 teaspoons; per serving—1 1/2 teaspoons
2 ounces cooked beef—1 teaspoon
Oil: None

VINEYARD BEEF ROAST

1 5-pound beef roast
2 cups Burgundy
1 garlic clove, minced
1 large onion, quartered
1 tablespoon oregano
1/2 teaspoon black pepper
Salt

Preheat oven to 350° F. Prick roast deeply with ice pick on all sides, reaching to the center. Combine remaining ingredients in a glass or plastic bowl capable of holding the roast plus about 1 1/2 quarts liquid. Mix well. Place roast in mixture. Add more red wine if necessary to bring level to within 2 inches from top of roast. Cover and refrigerate overnight. Turn meat several times. Place meat on rack in baking dish, pour marinade over, and cover. Bake about 2 1/2 hours. If you wish to use the marinade, defat first. Serves 10–12

Fat: 2 ounces cooked beef—1 teaspoon
Oil: None

ROAST LAMB WITH WINE

1 5–6-pound leg of lamb
1 garlic clove, crushed
3 tablespoons lemon juice
1/4 teaspoon curry powder
1/4 teaspoon ground ginger
1/4 teaspoon dry mustard
Salt and pepper
3 tablespoons tart jelly
1 cup dry red wine

Preheat oven to 325° F. Wipe leg of lamb with damp cloth; do not remove fell. Rub meat with crushed garlic; spread lemon juice over evenly. Mix curry powder, ginger, and mustard; rub evenly over meat. Cover lamb and refrigerate several hours or overnight. Uncover and place in roasting pan; season with salt and pepper. Bake uncovered 20–35 minutes per pound or until meat thermometer registers 140° F for rare or 165° F for well done. Mix jelly and wine together. About 45 minutes before lamb is done, remove from pan; pour off fat or place lamb in clean roaster. Glaze with jelly-wine mixture and baste at least 3 times during last cooking period. Serves 10–12

Fat: 3 ounces cooked lamb—1 teaspoon
Oil: None

VEAL SCALLOPINI WITH MUSHROOMS

6 shoulder veal steaks
1/2 cup all-purpose flour
3 tablespoons oil
1 4-ounce can mushrooms or mushroom stems and pieces (reserve liquid)
2 garlic cloves, finely chopped, or 1/2 teaspoon garlic powder
1 cup dry white wine or sherry
1/2 cup cut-up tomatoes
1 teaspoon salt
1/4 teaspoon pepper
Chopped parsley

Dredge veal with flour. Heat oil in large heavy skillet and cook meat until brown. Drain mushrooms and save liquid. Add mushrooms and garlic to meat. Let simmer 5 minutes, covered. Add wine, tomatoes, and mushroom liquid. Season to taste with salt and pepper, cover, and let simmer for about 15 minutes until meat is tender. Sprinkle steaks with chopped parsley and serve. If you use gravy, it must be defatted. Serves 6

Fat: 2 ounces cooked veal—1 teaspoon
Oil: Total—9 teaspoons; per serving—1 1/2 teaspoons

VENISON SWISS STEAK

1 1/2 pound venison steak, cut in half
All-purpose flour
1 tablespoon oil
1 1 3/8-ounce package dry onion soup mix
2 teaspoons spaghetti sauce seasoning
2 small bay leaves
Salt and pepper
1 cup dry red wine
1 8-ounce can tomato sauce

Dredge meat in flour. Heat oil in heavy skillet; brown meat over medium heat. Add soup mix, spaghetti sauce seasoning, bay leaves, salt, and pepper. Add wine and tomato sauce. Simmer, covered, 30–45 minutes until meat is tender. If sauce seems too thick, add more wine or water. Serves 6

Fat: Total—8 teaspoons; per serving—1 1/3 teaspoons
Oil: Total—3 teaspoons; per serving—3/4 teaspoon

TACO SALAD

1 pound lean ground beef
1 head lettuce, chopped
3 medium tomatoes, chopped
1 15 1/2-ounce can sliced olives
1/2 cup grated Count Down Cheese
Taco Sauce
Sour Cream Substitute
1 15 1/2-ounce can red kidney beans, drained and rinsed
3 cups oven-baked Tortilla Chips

In medium skillet cook ground beef until well done. Drain off fat and pat meat with paper towel to absorb any remaining fat. Let cool. Combine remaining ingredients and add enough Taco Sauce to flavor. Add cooked ground beef. Toss. Top with Sour Cream Substitute. Serves 6

Fat: Total—6 teaspoons; per serving—1 teaspoon
Oil: Total—8 teaspoons; per serving—1 1/3 teaspoons

CHAPTER 21

Oriental Cuisine

Methods of cooking used by the Chinese and Japanese are particularly well suited to the low-fat diet and can add a whole new dimension to one's enjoyment of food and the pleasures of interesting cuisine. The dairy products that we have eliminated in this diet such as butter, cream, whole milk, and cheese, as well as margarine, were unknown to the Chinese and Japanese before the nineteenth century and vegetable oils were used extensively. Their methods of preparing a variety of foods are low in fat as well as being an economical way to "stretch" the use of these ingredients. To understand this form of cooking, a glimpse into their past is interesting and informative.

The Chinese with their great cultural history extending back some four thousand years considered cooking a form of art. Their enjoyment of food is revealed in ancient silk screens and literature. Before the revolutionary period of the twentieth century, they believed that food was health as well as life and that it nourished both mind and body. It is interesting to note that in the sixth century A.D., the Imperial Court dietitian said, "A true doctor finds out the cause of the disease; and having found that out, he tries to cure it first by food. When food fails, then he prescribes medicine."

This great cuisine was developed over many centuries in a country that was frequently devastated by flood, droughts, and wars. The Chinese cooks were forced to utilize all possible sources of food as well as to develop techniques for cooking food quickly. Thus cooking in China evolved partly in response to the scarcity of fuel and partly to China's agricultural limitations. While China is comparable to the United States in size, it is very mountainous, its climate has a far greater range of temperature, and only 11 percent of its land is available for agriculture. Consequently, the Chinese found that they could feed more people by utilizing the land to raise grain than by using the land to feed cattle. Their sources of meat were limited to pigs and poultry, with lamb and mutton popular in the north, because these animals did not affect their agriculture. However, they preferred fish to meat, which was readily available in the saltwater areas, rivers, and lakes, and great quantities were sun-dried as a method of preserving them for shipment to the inland areas.

Rice was grown in southern China, with its warm climate and rain, but wheat predominated in the northern provinces where it was made into flour for noodles, steamed buns, and pancakes. The inland provinces utilized spices, vinegar, lemons, garlic, chives, scallions, and leeks to replace salt, which was almost impossible for them to obtain. However, it was the soybean that was the most well-developed product in China, and next to rice the most important. Soybeans were made into milk, bean curds, and sauces; they were cooked whole or sprouted as a vegetable. Eggs were not only a sign of good luck and happiness, but also were an important part of the diet. The Chinese were as versatile in their use of eggs as they were with soybeans and vegetables. Tea was first cultivated for medicinal purposes in the fifth century but gradually developed into a beverage because it was believed that those who drank boiled water were healthier than those who did not. Today China still has the problem of feeding its people beyond the basic foods; consequently they enjoy few of the Western delicacies. Meat is a luxury and the Chinese prefer having it cut into small pieces and mixed with vegetables. Stir frying is also popular as an efficient, economical, and healthful method of cooking.

Until the sixth century, when the Japanese first became aware of their sophisticated neighbor, China, their diet was limited to rice, fruit, vegetables, and fish, which were found in abundance in the waters surrounding the islands. During the open-door period when the Chinese influence was at its peak, the Japanese were introduced to soybeans and tea. Soybeans soon became as important to the Japanese as they were to the Chinese and were developed into a wide variety of products. Also, as in China, tea was used for medicinal purposes or as a special beverage for aristocrats and priests and did not become a popular beverage until later. Deep-fat frying was introduced to the Japanese by Portuguese traders in the midsixteenth century and this method of cooking was modified into their own technique of deep frying with oil called tempura. Eggs were never an important part of the Japanese diet, but now they have been adopted enthusiastically along with other Western foods such as steak, hamburgers, and ice cream. As a result, the urban Japanese are beginning to suffer from such Western maladies as obesity and vascular disease previously not experienced by them.

Chinese cuisine has influenced all of Asia and there are few cities in the world that do not have at least one Chinese restaurant. Most importantly, it is a healthful cuisine, low in fat content and low in calories. The Chinese method of cooking vegetables is one of their greatest contributions to the Western culture. Their skill is unlimited and the variety unbelievable. Unlike their Western counterparts, Oriental cooks never boil vegetables in water, never overcook them or butter them, thereby ensuring that the vegetables retain their natural crispness, full flavor, and bright color. Traditionally, vegetables were rarely eaten raw for hygienic reasons. Harmony, contrast, and accent are the three principles of their culinary art.

For the beginner there are some basic and simple recipes included in this book. We will attempt to acquaint you with only a few methods of Chinese and Japanese cooking. For the most part the ingredients will be easily found in your local supermarket and the recipes can be cooked in an ordinary pan with ordinary utensils. If you find that you enjoy this method of cooking, then you may want to make a small investment in some basic utensils. For Chinese cooking you will want a wok and a spatula, which can be found in specialty or department stores, a cleaver for chopping and slicing, and some extra-long chopsticks. With these utensils you can do just about everything. Most large cities have Oriental markets where a variety of canned, dried, and fresh foods can be found. For those interested in Oriental cooking, there are many excellent recipe books available.

Selecting Your Vegetables and Meats

Quality ingredients are essential to delicious meals in any type of cuisine. Quality is even more important in Oriental dishes for many reasons. Old vegetables do not have time to soften with this quick method of cooking and tough meat does not have time to tenderize. Select your vegetables and meats carefully. Learn to look for signs of freshness.

When buying seafood, if it's frozen make certain it has not been partially thawed and refrozen. If frozen too long it will appear grayish in color. Buy fish that have not been frozen, if possible. The eyes of the fish should be firm, clear, and bright. The gills should be reddish inside. The whole fish should be firm with no trace of sliminess. If the fish has been cut, the pieces should be moist and bright in color.

Stir Frying

This is a method of quick cooking at a high temperature in very hot oil to seal in the juices and preserve the texture, color, and taste. It demands the cook's constant attention and food prepared in this manner must be served immediately. Therefore it is necessary to become well acquainted with the method, know what you are going to do, prepare and organize all of the ingredients (chopping, slicing, dicing) before you begin. Read your recipe thoroughly before beginning to cook; you will not have time to consult it once you have started.

Heat a heavy skillet or wok to a hot temperature (375° F), or until a drop of water sizzles in it, then add oil and heat until bubbling. Add the seasonings directly to the oil as instructed in the recipes. If garlic is whole, it can be removed for a delicate flavor, or minced if a stronger flavor is desired. Meat is usually stir-fried by itself in very hot oil while you toss it vigorously. Vegetables are added after the meat is partially cooked; however, this depends upon the recipe. The coarse vegetables need a longer time and go in the pan before the more tender ones. Add the vegetables a fistful at a time instead of all at once. This allows the vegetables to be coated with oil at the high temperature without reducing the temperature. An experienced cook can determine by the color of the vegetables when they are done. Unfortunately, there is no set timetable because the age and degree of freshness influences the cooking time, but cooking time is never more than a few minutes.

After you have tried a few of these basic recipes, you can experiment with your own combinations of vegetables and meats or whatever you have on hand.

Sukiyaki or "saucepan" food is the Japanese method of preparing meat or fish and various vegetables, dried foods, and seasonings in one saucepan. The Japanese sit around the saucepan while it is cooking and eat directly from it, taking what they want with their chopsticks and putting it into small dishes.

Tempura is a method of frying in plenty of oil food that has been dipped in a batter of egg, water, and flour. It is delicious using either fish, meat, or vegetables.

STIR-FRY MEDLEY

1/2 pound of one of the following, skinless, boneless chicken breast, fish fillets, small shrimp, bay or sea scallops
1 teaspoon vegetable oil
2 tablespoons olive oil
1 tablespoon minced fresh parsley
1 tablespoon minced onion
2 medium garlic cloves, minced
Pinch of crushed hot red pepper
1 1/4 cups cut vegetables such as asparagus, broccoli, cauliflower, celery, bell pepper, cucumber, or zucchini
1/4 teaspoon salt
Pinch of sugar
1/4 cup brightly colored vegetables such as carrot, bell pepper, or butternut squash
Salt and pepper to taste

MARINADE

1/2 egg white
1 1/2 teaspoons dry vermouth
1 1/2 teaspoons cornstarch
1/2 teaspoon salt

Cut chicken or fish into 1-inch pieces. For the marinade in a medium bowl whisk together the egg white, vermouth, cornstarch, and salt. Add the chicken or fish and mix well. Cover and refrigerate for 1 hour.

Heat a large pot of water and 1 teaspoon of vegetable oil. Add chicken or fish and cook, stirring gently for approximately 30 seconds for fish and 1 minute for chicken. Drain and rinse to remove any excess cornstarch.

Warm wok or heavy skillet over high heat until a drop of water evaporates on contact. Pour olive oil in a thin stream around edge.

Add parsley, onion, garlic, and hot red pepper all at once to wok. Cook, stirring until fragrant, about 10 seconds; do not let garlic brown.

Add first set of vegetables to wok, tossing to coat with oil. Sprinkle with salt and sugar, and toss until the vegetables are almost crisp, 1 1/2–2 minutes.

Add the precooked fish or chicken and toss to coat with oil. Cook, tossing to blend the flavors, until warmed through, about 30 seconds.

Add remaining colored vegetables. Cook, tossing to blend flavors, about 20 seconds.

Remove from heat and season well with salt and pepper. Serves 2

Fat: None
Oil: Total—7 teaspoons; per serving—3 1/2 teaspoons

CHICKEN AND VEGETABLES

2 teaspoons salt, divided
1 teaspoon sugar
1/4 teaspoon ground ginger
1/4 teaspoon cayenne pepper
2 1/4 tablespoons soy sauce
2 garlic cloves, minced
2 whole chicken breasts, skinned, boned, and cut into 1-inch cubes
1/3 cup oil
2 cups diagonally sliced fresh broccoli
2 cups sliced mushrooms
1 medium onion, thinly sliced
4 cups hot cooked rice
1/2 cup water

Combine 1 teaspoon of salt, sugar, ginger, cayenne pepper, soy sauce, and garlic. Add chicken. Marinate 25 minutes. Heat 3 tablespoons of oil to sizzling in pan over medium heat. Add chicken mixture. Stir-fry 5 minutes or until chicken loses all pinkness and fork can be inserted with ease. Remove from pan. Add remaining oil and heat to sizzling. Add broccoli and remaining 1 teaspoon salt. Stir-fry 5 minutes. Add mushrooms and onion. Stir-fry until mixture is tender-crisp. Return chicken to pan. Add rice and water. Heat thoroughly. Serves 4

Fat: None
Oil: Total—16 teaspoons; per serving—4 teaspoons

STIR-FRIED CHICKEN AND VEGETABLES

2 tablespoons vegetable oil
1 cup coarsely chopped onion
1 teaspoon minced garlic
1 pound boneless and skinless chicken breasts, cut into 3/4-inch pieces
1/2 cup cold water
1 teaspoon cornstarch
3/4 teaspoon ground ginger
1 1/2 teaspoons Worcestershire sauce
2 medium-sized tomatoes, cut into wedges (3 cups)
1 cup diced green pepper

Heat oil in a 10-inch skillet. Add onion and garlic; sauté until barely tender. Remove to a bowl, leaving as much oil as possible in skillet. Add chicken to sizzling oil in skillet and stir-fry until chicken is almost cooked through, about 2 minutes; remove skillet from heat.

In a measuring cup combine water, cornstarch, ginger, and Worcestershire sauce; mix well and set aside. Return onion and garlic to skillet. Add tomatoes and green pepper. Stir in Worcestershire mixture. Cook and stir, uncovered, until sauce is thickened and green pepper is barely tender, about 2 minutes. Serves 4

Fat: None
Oil: Total—6 teaspoons; per serving—1 1/2 teaspoons

STIR-FRIED CHICKEN

1 whole chicken breast, skinned and boned
1/2 cup snow peas
1/2 cup soy sauce
1/2 cup chicken stock
2 tablespoons cornstarch
3 tablespoons oil
1 teaspoon salt
1 tablespoon grated fresh ginger
1/2 cup thinly sliced celery
1/2 cup sliced green onion
1/2 cup sliced water chestnuts
1/2 cup sliced mushrooms

Slice chicken into very thin strips. Wash snow peas and remove ends. Heat wok or skillet to approximately 375° F. While wok is heating, mix soy sauce, chicken stock, and cornstarch, and set to one side. Add oil to wok and heat until sizzling. Then add salt and stir; add ginger and stir. Add chicken pieces and stir constantly until they lose their pinkness, about 2 minutes. Add snow peas, celery, and green onion, and stir for 2 minutes. Cover and steam for 2 minutes. Add water chestnuts and mushrooms and stir for 2 additional minutes. Add cornstarch mixture and cook until sauce is clear and thick, stirring constantly. Serves 4

Fat: None
Oil: Total—9 teaspoons; per serving—2 1/4 teaspoons

CHICKEN ALMOND

3 tablespoons cornstarch
2 cups chicken broth
2 tablespoons soy sauce
4 tablespoons oil
Salt to taste
2 cups thinly sliced chicken breast, skinned and boned
2 cups diced bamboo shoots
2 cups diced celery
1 cup sliced bok choy (Chinese chard)
1 cup sliced water chestnuts
1/2 cup blanched almonds

Mix cornstarch with chicken broth and soy sauce, and set to one side. Heat heavy skillet or wok; add oil and salt. When oil is sizzling, add chicken, stirring constantly for 2–3 minutes. Add vegetables and half the almonds; mix thoroughly. Cover and steam 5 minutes. Remove lid and add cornstarch mixture, stirring constantly until sauce is clear and thick. Garnish with remaining almonds. Serve immediately. Serves 6

Fat: None
Oil: Total—22 teaspoons; per serving—3 2/3 teaspoons

STIR-FRIED SHRIMP

1 teaspoon cornstarch
1/4 teaspoon ground ginger
2 tablespoons soy sauce
2 tablespoons dry sherry
1/2 cup chicken broth
3/4 pound snow peas
3 tablespoons oil
1 garlic clove, minced
1 pound shrimp, shelled and deveined
1/2 cup sliced water chestnuts

Mix cornstarch and ginger; blend in soy sauce, sherry, and chicken broth; set to one side. Wash snow peas and nip the ends. Heat 2 tablespoons of oil in wok or skillet until sizzling. Add garlic and shrimp. Cook, stirring until shrimp becomes pink and firm, 2–3 minutes, then remove to serving dish. Reheat wok; add additional tablespoon of oil, then peas and water chestnuts. Stir and cook 1–2 minutes. Add cornstarch mixture and return shrimp to pan. Stir until sauce becomes clear and thickens, about 1 minute. Serves 4

Fat: None
Oil: Total—9 teaspoons; per serving—2 1/4 teaspoons

STIR-FRIED SWEET-AND-SOUR SHRIMP

2 tablespoons oil
1 tablespoon soy sauce
2 tablespoons cornstarch
1 pound shrimp, shelled and deveined
1 8-ounce can pineapple chunks, drained, or 1 cup fresh pineapple chunks
1 cup thinly sliced celery
1/2 cup diced green pepper
1/4 cup vinegar
1/4 cup packed brown sugar
1 tablespoon slivered fresh or crystallized ginger
1 cup pineapple juice

Preheat heavy skillet or wok to 375° F. Add oil. Combine soy sauce and cornstarch and put to one side. When oil is sizzling add shrimp, pineapple, celery, and green pepper, stirring continuously for 2–3 minutes. Add vinegar, brown sugar, ginger, and pineapple juice and bring to a boil. Add soy sauce and cornstarch mixture and cook until thick and clear, stirring constantly. Serve with rice. Serves 6

Fat: None
Oil: Total—6 teaspoons; per serving—1 teaspoon

CANTONESE SHRIMP AND PEA PODS

1 1/2 teaspoons chicken stock base
1 cup boiling water
1 tablespoon oil
1/4 cup thinly sliced green onion
1 garlic clove, crushed
1 1/2 pounds shrimp, shelled and deveined
1 teaspoon salt
1 teaspoon ginger, grated fresh or ground
1 9-ounce package frozen snow peas
1 tablespoon cornstarch
1 tablespoon cold water

Fifteen minutes before cooking preheat electric skillet or wok to 375° F. Dissolve chicken stock base in boiling water and set to one side. Add oil to wok and heat to sizzling. Add onion, garlic, and shrimp, stirring frequently. If necessary, add small amount of broth to prevent sticking. Stir in salt, ginger, and snow peas. Add broth. Cover and simmer 5–7 minutes until snow peas are cooked but still slightly crisp. Combine cornstarch and water. Add to shrimp and cook until thick and clear, stirring constantly. Serves 6

Fat: None
Oil: Total—3 teaspoons; per serving—1/2 teaspoon

SKILLET SCALLOPS

1 1/2 pounds scallops
3 tablespoons oil
1 7-ounce package frozen snow peas or 1 cup fresh snow peas
2 tomatoes, cubed
2 tablespoons dry sherry or soy sauce
1/2 teaspoon salt
1 1/2 tablespoons cornstarch
1/4 cup chicken broth or water
1 1/2 teaspoons lemon juice
3 tablespoons parsley

Cut large scallops crosswise. Heat oil in skillet or wok. Add scallops and cook over low heat, 3–4 minutes, stirring frequently, until translucent. Add snow peas and tomatoes, stirring frequently. Blend sherry, salt, cornstarch, broth, and lemon juice. Add to scallops and vegetables, and cook until thick, stirring constantly. Garnish with parsley. Serve with rice. Serves 6

Fat: None
Oil: Total—9 teaspoons; per serving—1 1/2 teaspoons

TOMATO FRIED RICE

4 tablespoons oil
1 small onion, finely chopped
3 cups cold cooked rice
1 tablespoon soy sauce
Dash of pepper
1 2-ounce can pimiento, drained
2 tablespoons dry sherry or dry white wine or water
2 medium-sized tomatoes, peeled and chopped
Chopped parsley or *sliced green onion tops (for garnish)*

Heat skillet or wok over medium-high heat. Add oil. When sizzling, add onion and stir-fry until golden, about 2 minutes. Add rice; continue stir-frying until golden brown, about 3 minutes. Add soy sauce, pepper, pimiento, and wine. Stir-fry about 1 minute, adding liquid if needed. Add tomatoes, toss, and cook 1–2 minutes. Turn onto warm serving dish and garnish with parsley or green onions. Serves 6

Fat: None
Oil: Total—12 teaspoons; per serving—2 teaspoons

TEMPURA

BATTER

1 cup all-purpose flour
1 medium egg
1 cup ice water

Blend flour, egg, and ice water together mixing lightly. Surround the bowl with ice to keep the batter as cold as possible.

Prepare meat, vegetables, and fish:

water chestnut slices
carrot strips
asparagus tips
eggplant slices
mushroom slices
green beans
green pepper rings
broccoli flowerets
onion rings
raw beef strips
scallops
raw fish (any white fish), cut in small pieces
raw shrimp, shelled and deveined

Pour enough oil into a deep pan or wok to measure about 2 inches deep and heat to 375° F.

Coat vegetables and meat lightly, and quickly drop into the hot oil a few pieces at a time. Fry in the order given—mild-flavored vegetables first, fish last. Fry until golden brown on both sides. Drain well on absorbent paper and serve very hot. Each food should be served as it is cooked. Serve with individual dishes of Tempura Sauce. Serves 4

Fat: 2 ounces beef—1 teaspoon
Tempura batter—Negligible
Oil: For frying—approximately 2 teaspoons per average serving

TEMPURA SAUCE

1/3 cup soy sauce
1/2 cup chicken stock
1/3 cup dry sherry
1/4 teaspoon powdered ginger

Combine all ingredients and mix well. Yields approximately 1 cup

Fat: None
Oil: None

BEEF SUKIYAKI

1 1/2 pounds sirloin steak
2 tablespoons oil
1/2 cup soy sauce
2/3 cup water
3 tablespoons sugar
1 5-ounce can bamboo shoots (3/4 cup)
1 cup 1-inch pieces green onion
2 medium onions, thinly sliced
2 cups bean sprouts
1 5-ounce can sliced water chestnuts (2/3 cup)
1 cup sliced fresh or canned mushrooms

Fifteen minutes before cooking preheat heavy skillet or wok to 375° F.

Cut meat into paper-thin slices across the grain, then into strips about 1 inch wide. Brown strips in hot oil in skillet or wok, 2–3 minutes. Combine soy sauce, water, and sugar, and pour over meat. Push meat to one side of the skillet or wok. Keeping the ingredients separate, add bamboo shoots, green onion, and onion slices. Cook 3–5 minutes, turning vegetables. Push vegetables to one side. Add bean sprouts, water chestnuts, and mushrooms. Cook 2 minutes until hot. Serve with rice. Serves 6

Fat: Total—9 teaspoons; 2 ounces beef—1 teaspoon
Oil: Total—6 teaspoons; per serving—1 teaspoon

SUKIYAKI

2 tablespoons oil
1 1/2 pounds lean meat, cut crosswise into thin slices
1/2 cup sliced mushrooms
1/2 cup sliced bamboo shoots
2 medium onions, sliced
1/2 cup dry sherry or sake or dry white wine
1/2 cup soy sauce
1/2 pound firm Chinese bean curd, cut into cubes (optional)
1/2 cup 1-inch pieces green onion
2 cups cooked rice

Heat skillet or wok. Add oil. When oil begins to sizzle, drop in meat and brown, cooking 2–3 minutes. Add mushrooms, bamboo shoots, and onion. Stir-fry for 5 minutes, turning vegetables frequently. Add sherry and soy sauce. Bean curd and green onion require very little cooking so they should be added last, just before serving. Serve over rice. Serves 6

Fat: Total—9 teaspoons; 2 ounces beef—1 teaspoon
Oil: Total—6 teaspoons; per serving—1 teaspoon

EGG FOO YUNG

2 tablespoons oil
6 eggs
1/2 cup sliced water chestnuts
1/4 cup sliced green onion
1/2 cup bean sprouts
1/2 cup chopped cooked shrimp
1 teaspoon salt

Heat oil in skillet. Beat eggs lightly and add remaining ingredients. Drop by spoonfuls into skillet. Brown on each side. Serve with sauce. Yields 12 pancakes

Fat: Total—6 teaspoons; per pancake—1/2 teaspoon
Oil: Total—6 teaspoons; per pancake—1/2 teaspoon

EGG FOO YUNG SAUCE

1 tablespoon cornstarch
2 tablespoons vinegar
2 tablespoons soy sauce
1 cup water
1 tablespoon brown sugar
1/2 teaspoon salt

Combine cornstarch, vinegar, and soy sauce. Blend. Add remaining ingredients and cook until thick and clear, stirring constantly. Yields 1 1/4 cups

Fat: None
Oil: None

SPICY FRIED TOFU

3–5 tablespoons oil
1 pound firm Chinese bean curd (tofu), cut into 1/2-inch cubes and patted dry
2 garlic cloves, minced
1/2 teaspoon curry powder
1/2 teaspoon crumbled dried dillweed
1/4 teaspoon turmeric
1/4 teaspoon crumbled dried basil
1/4 teaspoon crumbled dried thyme
1/4 teaspoon cumin
2 tablespoons soy sauce
1/2 cup Count Down cheese

Heat 3 tablespoons oil in large skillet or wok over high heat. Add bean curd and sauté 3 minutes. (If excess water drains from bean curd, carefully tip skillet and remove with bulb baster or spoon.)

Reduce heat to Medium, add garlic, curry powder, dillweed, turmeric, basil, thyme, and cumin, and stir well, adding remaining 2 tablespoons oil to prevent sticking if necessary. Increase heat to medium-high, add soy sauce, and stir until thoroughly heated, about 1 minute. Transfer bean curd to serving dish, using slotted spoon. Sprinkle with Count Down cheese and toss until cheese melts. Serve immediately. Serves 4–6

Fat: None
Oil: Total—15 teaspoons; per serving of 4—3 1/2 teaspoons; per serving of 6—2 1/2 teaspoons

STIR-FRIED ASPARAGUS

1 pound fresh asparagus
1/2 teaspoon salt
2 tablespoons oil

Clean and trim asparagus and cut into diagonal slices. Place in a colander or porous steamer and cook in boiling water for 2 minutes. Remove and drain. Heat a large skillet or wok, add salt and oil, then asparagus. Stir and toss for several minutes until asparagus is bright green. Remove before it is overcooked and a dark green. Serves 4

Fat: None
Oil: Total—6 teaspoons; per serving—1 1/2 teaspoons

STIR-FRIED CABBAGE

2 pounds Chinese cabbage
3 tablespoons oil
1/2 teaspoon salt
3/4 cup water

Cut cabbage crosswise into 1/2-inch strips. Heat oil in skillet or wok. Add the white stems of the cabbage. Stir for 1 minute. Add salt and water. Cover and cook over medium heat for 3 minutes. Add the green leaves, cover, and cook 2–3 minutes longer. Serve juice that remains with the cabbage. Serves 4

Fat: None
Oil: Total—9 teaspoons; per serving—2 1/4 teaspoons

STIR-FRIED FROZEN VEGETABLES

1 9–10-ounce package frozen broccoli or cauliflower or Brussels sprouts
1 tablespoon oil
1/2 teaspoon salt
1 garlic clove

Thaw vegetable. Cut into small pieces. Heat skillet or wok; add oil, salt, and garlic. Add vegetables and stir for 30 seconds. Cover and cook for 2 minutes, stirring occasionally. The vegetables should be crisp yet tender and the color bright. Serves 4

Fat: None
Oil: Total—3 teaspoons; per serving—3/4 teaspoon

STIR-FRIED SPINACH OR LEAFY VEGETABLES

1 pound spinach
1 tablespoon oil
1/2 teaspoon salt
1 garlic clove

Wash spinach thoroughly, trim stems, and pat leaves dry. Heat skillet or wok; add oil and salt, then garlic. Toss in spinach and stir thoroughly. Cover and cook for 45 seconds. Uncover and stir for 3 minutes. Serves 4

Fat: None
Oil: Total—3 teaspoons; per serving—3/4 teaspoon

TERIYAKI SAUCE

BASIC MARINADE

1/2 cup soy sauce
Freshly grated gingerroot to taste
1/3 cup sugar
1 or more garlic cloves, sliced or minced, to taste

OTHER ADDITIONS TO THE MARINADE

Chopped green onion
1–2 tablespoons sesame oil
2 tablespoons sesame seeds
Red pepper flakes
Minced onion
Sherry or white wine or sake

Mix ingredients together. Marinate meat, chicken, or fish for at least 30 minutes. Meat and chicken can be marinated overnight. Cook under broiler or over charcoal grill. Yields approximately 2/3 cup

Fat: None
Oil: Total—6 teaspoons if using sesame oil
Total—2 teaspoons if using sesame seeds

SWEET-AND-SOUR SAUCE

1 tablespoon oil
1 8-ounce can pineapple tidbits, drained
1 tablespoon chopped green onion
1 1/2 tablespoons sugar
1 1/2 tablespoons cornstarch
1 1/2 tablespoons soy sauce
1/2 teaspoon salt
1 1/2 tablespoons tomato juice
2 tablespoons vinegar
1 cup pineapple juice
1 tablespoon brandy

Heat oil in medium-sized skillet. Sauté pineapple and green onion in oil. Combine sugar, cornstarch, soy sauce, salt, tomato juice, vinegar, and pineapple juice. Add to the pineapple and simmer for 5 minutes, stirring constantly. Just before serving add the brandy. Yields 1 3/4 cups

Fat: None
Oil: Total—3 teaspoons; per 1 tablespoon sauce—1/10 teaspoon

MISO SOUP

BASIC SOUP

5 cups water
1 packet fish stock powder (.35 ounces)*
1/4 cup miso†
1 or 2 eggs, beaten

Bring water to a boil. Add fish stock powder. Make a thin paste by mixing the miso with 2 tablespoons water. Add miso paste to fish stock. Bring to a boil. Turn off heat. Add beaten egg while stirring. Serve hot. Serves 4

* Fish stock powder is available in Oriental grocery stores.
† Miso is available in Oriental grocery stores or natural food stores.

ADDITIONS TO MISO SOUP

cubed tofu
green onion slices
canned clams (whole baby clams or chopped clams)
thin slices of daikon (white Japanese radish)
fresh spinach
udon noodles (wide Japanese noodles)
fishcake slices

Fat: Total—2 teaspoons; per serving—1/2 teaspoon
Oil: None

CHAPTER 22

Meatless Cooking

Vegetarianism or meatless cooking has become popular in the last several years. For many reasons people are converting to vegetable-grain-fruit diets and eliminating meat.

Before trying a meatless diet it is necessary to have a good working knowledge of the diet. Because of the high concentration of cheese and other dairy products in most vegetarian diets, it is important to understand what foods can be substituted for these dairy products to ensure an adequate protein balance and at the same time maintain a low-fat diet.

It is important not to rely on one or even two plant foods. Legumes are an excellent source of protein, B vitamins, and trace minerals. Nuts supply the diet with oils and additional protein, B vitamins, and iron. Dark leafy vegetables are valuable sources of calcium and other minerals, riboflavin, and carotene; they are a general source of other vitamins.

Tofu, also known as Chinese bean curd, is high in protein, low in calories, fats, and carbohydrates. One-fourth pound contains eighty-six calories, 9.4 g protein, 5 g unsaturated fat, 2.9 g carbohydrates, 154 mg calcium, 151 mg iron, 8 mg sodium, 50 mg potassium, and small amounts of niacin, riboflavin, and thiamine. It is a very versatile protein. It serves well as an alternative to meat dishes. It is also economical. Tofu can be purchased in most markets or can always be found in a natural food store.

Because of its mild flavor, it can be added to meatless sauces and chiles to improve the protein content.

It can be added to main dishes, salads, desserts, soups, and party dips. It is frequently used in Oriental cooking.

We have included a few tofu recipes to help introduce you to this versatile protein food. It is not our goal to make this a vegetarian cookbook; however, for variety in your diet, we have included a number of meatless recipes.

BROWN RICE VEGGIE CASSEROLE WITH *SALSA*

2 1/2 cups water
2 vegetable bouillon cubes
1 cup long grain brown rice
1 pound broccoli
1 small head cauliflower (1 pound)
2 medium crookneck or zucchini squash
1/4 cup sliced celery
1/4 pound mushrooms, sliced
1/4 cup shredded carrots
1/4 cup chopped green onion
1/4 teaspoon soy sauce
1 7-ounce can mild green chili salsa
20 cherry tomatoes
1/2 cup Count Down cheese
3 tablespoons salted, roasted sunflower seeds (optional)

Preheat oven to 350° F. In a 2-quart saucepan, bring water and bouillon cubes to a boil. Add rice, cover, and simmer for 45 minutes. Remove from heat and uncover. Break broccoli into bite-size flowerets, leaving about 2 inches of stem; break cauliflower into bite-size flowerets; cut squash into 1/2-inch-thick slices. Combine broccoli, cauliflower, squash, and celery in a large steamer. Cover and steam for 8–10 minutes, or until vegetables are almost tender. Add mushrooms, cover, and steam for 2 minutes. Remove vegetables from heat. Add carrots, green onion, and soy sauce to rice; toss lightly with a fork. Spread rice mixture evenly in a greased shallow 2-quart casserole or baking pan. Spoon *salsa* evenly over rice and top with vegetables and tomatoes. Cover with Count Down cheese. Bake, uncovered, at 350° F for 15–20 minutes or until heated. Sprinkle with sunflower seeds and serve. Serves 6

Fat: None
Oil: Total—1 teaspoon; per serving—negligible

HOLIDAY NUT LOAF

1/2 cup water containing 1 tablespoon nutritional yeast
1 cup seasoned bread crumbs
1/2 cup toasted wheat germ
1/2 cup chopped peanuts
2 cups grated carrots (1 pound)
1 cup finely chopped onion
1/2 cup finely chopped celery
1 4-ounce can mushroom pieces, drained
1/2 teaspoon sage
1/2 teaspoon thyme
2 tablespoons dried parsley or 1/4 cup chopped fresh parsley

Mix all ingredients. Turn into oiled 8″ × 4″ loaf pan and bake at 350° F for 30 minutes. Serves 4

Fat: None
Oil: Total—10 teaspoons; per serving—2 1/2 teaspoons

SUNDAY STEW

3 thin-skinned white potatoes, washed and cubed
4 carrots, peeled and sliced 1 inch thick
1 large onion, peeled and quartered
1 rutabaga, peeled and cubed (optional)
2 parsnips, peeled and cubed (optional)
1 turnip, peeled and cubed (optional)
5 vegetable bouillon cubes
1 tablespoon dry onion
Gravy browning sauce
3 tablespoons flour
1/4 cup water

Add the following:

1 cup frozen peas, thawed
1 17-ounce can whole kernel corn, drained

Cook vegetables in boiling water to cover. Drain them into a bowl. Save the cooking water.

Gravy: Return 4 cups of the vegetable cooking water to the cooking pan. Add 5 vegetable bouillon cubes and 1 tablespoon dry onion. Add gravy browning sauce until liquid is a pleasant brown color. Prepare a paste of 3 tablespoons flour and 1/4 cup water. Mix well. Add to mixture and cook until gravy thickens.

Return well-drained vegetables to gravy and reheat. Serve in casserole dish with hot biscuits on top. Serves 4–6

Note: Vegetable bouillon cubes are available from natural food stores and many supermarkets; they are good for brown gravy and for soup stock. Gravy browning sauce is available in most supermarkets.

Fat: None
Oil: None

TOFU PATTIES

1 pound tofu (firm soybean curd)
2 cups rolled oats
1 tablespoon ketchup
1 tablespoon Worcestershire sauce
1 small onion, finely diced
1 teaspoon prepared mustard
1 teaspoon salt
1/4 teaspoon pepper

Break up soybean curd in glass bowl with wooden spoon. Add remaining ingredients and mix with wooden spoon until consistency for making patties. Wet hands and form thin patties. Brown on both sides in lightly oiled frying pan for about 5 minutes. Serve on a bun with ketchup, relish, tomato, and lettuce. Serves 4–6

Fat: None
Oil: None

TOFU SLOPPY JOES

1 large onion, diced
2 medium green peppers, seeded and diced
6 tablespoons oil
2 15-ounce cans Spanish-style tomato sauce
1 1/2 tablespoons chili powder
3/4 teaspoon salt
1/8 teaspoon pepper
1/2 teaspoon dried or 1 1/2 teaspoons chopped fresh oregano
1 tablespoon soy sauce
1 tablespoon prepared mustard (Dijon)
1 tablespoon sugar
1–1 1/2 pounds tofu (firm soybean curd), squeezed and crumbled
1 tablespoon Worcestershire sauce

In large skillet, sauté onion and pepper in 3 tablespoons oil until just tender. Add tomato sauce, chili powder, salt, pepper, oregano, soy sauce, mustard, and sugar. Stir and simmer 20–25 minutes. Heat remaining 3 tablespoons oil in another skillet. Add tofu and Worcestershire sauce. Stir until browned and sauce is absorbed. Add to tomato sauce mixture and simmer 5 minutes. Serve over toasted whole wheat bun and with green salad. Serves 6

Fat: None
Oil: Total—18 teaspoons; per serving—3 teaspoons

TOFU LOAF

1 1/2 pounds tofu (Chinese soybean curd), mashed
1/3 cup ketchup
1/3 cup soy sauce
2 tablespoons Dijon mustard
1/2 cup chopped parsley
1/4 teaspoon black pepper
1 medium onion, finely chopped
1/4 teaspoon garlic or onion powder
1 cup whole grain bread crumbs or rolled oats

Preheat oven to 350° F. Mix all ingredients together. Oil a 5″ × 7″ loaf pan. Press the mixture into the pan. Bake for 1 hour. Let cool 10–15 minutes before removing from the pan. Garnish with ketchup and parsley. May be sliced and fried and used for sandwiches the next day. Serves 4–6

Fat: None
Oil: None

POTATO-TOFU CASSEROLE

3 cups mashed potatoes
1 1/2 pounds tofu (Chinese soybean curd), mashed
1 1/4 teaspoons salt
1/4 teaspoon black pepper
1/4 teaspoon garlic powder or onion powder
1/4 cup chopped fresh parsley
1 medium onion, chopped
1 tablespoon oil
Paprika for garnish

Preheat oven to 325° F. In a medium-sized bowl mix together potatoes, tofu, salt, pepper, garlic powder, and parsley. Sauté onion in oil until translucent and add to potato mixture. Oil an 8″ × 8″ × 2″ baking dish, spread mixture into the dish, and sprinkle with paprika. Bake for 35 minutes. Serves 6

Fat: None
Oil: Total—3 teaspoons; per serving—1/2 teaspoon

HERBED LENTILS AND RICE

2 2/3 cups vegetable broth
3/4 cup chopped onion
1/4 cup dry white wine
1/4 teaspoon salt
1/4 teaspoon thyme
1/8 teaspoon pepper
3/4 cup dry lentils
1/2 cup uncooked brown rice
1/2 teaspoon dry basil
1/4 teaspoon dry oregano
1/8 teaspoon garlic powder

Preheat oven to 350° F. Mix all ingredients, stirring well. Turn into 1 1/2-quart covered casserole.

Bake covered for 90 minutes–2 hours, until rice and lentils are cooked. Stir twice during baking. Serves 4

Fat: None
Oil: None

COTTAGE CHEESE PATTIES

1 1/2 cups cottage cheese, low-fat, rinsed, or dry-curd
1 cup rolled oats, quick or old-fashioned
1 cup crushed cracker or cereal crumbs
1 medium onion, diced
2 eggs
1 cup chopped walnuts or other nuts
2 tablespoons oil

Mix all ingredients and form into patties. Fry in oil until brown. For casserole, bake at 350° F for 30 minutes and serve with mushroom or onion gravy. Serves 6

Fat: Total—2 teaspoons; per serving—1/3 teaspoon
Oil: Total—30 teaspoons; per serving—5 teaspoons

CHAPTER 23

Sauces

Sauces, especially in a gourmet dinner, are frequently an important addition to a meal, but they are a "double-edged sword," with one edge giving delight to the palate while the other adds unwanted calories, too often due to the inclusion of large amounts of fat. Because they add substantially to the pleasure of eating, we have included many sauces in this book. We have, however, reduced calories and the high-fat content by substituting mayonnaise or oil for butter and meat fats, or by using tasty ingredients that contain neither fats nor oils.

These sauces have been added to the diet over the years after being tested, altered, and then retested. They have been accepted surprisingly well by our patients, most of whom now prefer them to the fatty sauces they formerly used. It is interesting to note that patients who have been on the Swank low-fat diet for several years can recognize the presence in food of saturated fats such as meat fat and butter. These fats adhere to their hard palates, causing the mouth to feel unclean. Since fats are relatively insoluble in the saliva, this sensation may remain for several minutes. It is a reminder to patients on the low-fat diet that they have just eaten too much forbidden fat.

GOURMET CREAM SAUCE

1 cup skim milk enriched with 4 tablespoons nonfat dry milk powder
1 1/2 tablespoons all-purpose flour
1/4 teaspoon salt
2 tablespoons mayonnaise

Mix skim milk and nonfat dry milk powder together and reserve enough to mix with flour. In a medium saucepan bring milk mixture to a scald. Add flour that has been mixed with reserved milk, and stir until thickened. Add salt and beat in mayonnaise until well blended. Yields 1/4 cup

Fat: None
Oil: Total—3 teaspoons; per 1/4 cup serving—3/5 teaspoon

EASY WHITE SAUCE

THIN

1 tablespoon oil
1 tablespoon all-purpose flour
1 cup skim milk
1/4 teaspoon salt

Heat oil on low temperature. Blend in flour thoroughly, keeping heat low. Add milk slowly, increasing heat slightly. Stir constantly until mixture thickens. Add salt. Yields approximately 1 cup

Fat: None
Oil: Total—3 teaspoons; per 1/3 cup—1 teaspoon

MEDIUM

2 tablespoons oil
2 tablespoons all-purpose flour
1 cup skim milk
1/4 teaspoon salt

Follow procedure for thin Easy White Sauce. Yields approximately 1 cup

Fat: None
Oil: Total—6 teaspoons; per 1/3 cup—2 teaspoons

THICK

3 tablespoons oil
3 tablespoons all-purpose flour
1 cup skim milk
1/4 teaspoon salt

Follow procedure for thin Easy White Sauce. Yields approximately 1 cup

Fat: None
Oil: Total—9 teaspoons; per 1/3 cup—3 teaspoons

Note: For a slightly richer sauce, buttermilk can be substituted for skim milk. If preparing larger amounts of white sauce, use the same method, but add hot milk and finish cooking in a double boiler to save time and energy required for stirring.

MUSHROOM SAUCE

Following recipe for Gourmet Cream Sauce, adding 1–2 cups either canned or fresh sliced mushrooms.

HOT MAYONNAISE

Prepare the medium Easy White Sauce and add 1 cup mayonnaise. Use as a sauce for green beans and asparagus. Yields approximately 2 cups

Fat: None
Oil: Total—30 teaspoons; per 1/3 cup—5 teaspoons

MOCK HOLLANDAISE SAUCE I

1 cup thick Easy White Sauce
2 egg yolks
3 tablespoons lemon juice
Dash of cayenne pepper

In medium saucepan prepare Easy White Sauce. Add beaten yolks to the hot sauce and mix well. Bring slowly to the boiling point, stirring constantly until smooth. Remove from heat; add lemon juice and cayenne pepper. Yields 1 cup

Fat: Total—2 teaspoons; per 1/4 cup serving—1/2 teaspoon
Oil: Total—9 teaspoons; per 1/4 cup serving—2 1/4 teaspoons

MOCK HOLLANDAISE SAUCE II

1 tablespoon cornstarch
1/2 cup water
2 tablespoons lemon juice
3 tablespoons oil
1/4 teaspoon salt
1 packet Butter Buds
3 egg yolks

In medium saucepan mix cornstarch with small amount of water until a smooth paste is formed. Add remaining water and bring to a boil. Remove from heat and add remaining ingredients. Mix until smooth, using a wire whisk. Reheat very slowly for a short period of time until mixture is thickened. Yields 1 cup

Fat: Total—3 teaspoons; per 1/4 cup serving—3/4 teaspoon
Oil: Total—9 teaspoons; per 1/4 cup serving—2 1/4 teaspoons

MARINARA SAUCE

1 garlic clove, minced
3 tablespoons olive oil
3 8-ounce cans tomato sauce
1 teaspoon oregano
1 teaspoon thyme
2 tablespoons chopped fresh parsley
1 teaspoon dried onion flakes
1/4 cup red wine
1 teaspoon brown sugar

Sauté garlic lightly in olive oil. Add tomato sauce. Stir in oregano, thyme, parsley, and onion. Add wine and brown sugar. Simmer for 1 hour or longer. This sauce can be used as a basic tomato sauce or a pizza sauce. Yields approximately 4 cups

Variations: Chopped zucchini, chopped mushrooms, chopped olives, chopped green pepper.

Fat: None
Oil: Total—9 teaspoons; per 1/2 cup—1 1/8 teaspoons

EASY BARBECUE SAUCE

2 tablespoons brown sugar
2 tablespoons lemon juice or vinegar
1 tablespoon prepared mustard or 1 teaspoon dry mustard
2 teaspoons horseradish
1 tablespoon Worcestershire sauce
1 teaspoon onion juice
1 teaspoon salt
3/4 cup ketchup

Combine all ingredients, mixing well. Sufficient for 1 pound of meat. Yields approximately 1 cup

Fat: None
Oil: None

PIQUANT BARBECUE SAUCE

1/2 cup beer
1/2 cup ketchup
2 tablespoons vinegar
2 tablespoons brown sugar
2 tablespoons Worcestershire sauce
Salt and pepper to taste

Combine all ingredients, mixing well. Sauce is sufficient for about 1 1/2–2 pounds of meat.

Fat: None
Oil: None

HORSERADISH SAUCE

1/2 cup mayonnaise
4 tablespoons horseradish
2 tablespoons currant jelly
1 tablespoon tarragon vinegar
1 teaspoon dry mustard
1/8 teaspoon salt
1/4 cup nonfat yogurt
Dash of hot pepper sauce (optional)
1 tablespoon dry sherry

Mix mayonnaise and horseradish. Beat jelly to soften; add to mayonnaise mixture. Stir in vinegar, mustard, and salt. Fold in yogurt. Add hot pepper sauce if desired. Add sherry just before serving. Yields 1 3/4 cups

Fat: None
Oil: Total—12 teaspoons; per 2 teaspoons—1/4 teaspoon

TANGY TOMATO SAUCE

1 16-ounce can whole tomatoes
1/4 cup diced celery
2 tablespoons diced green pepper (optional)
1 tablespoon minced onion
1 tablespoon vinegar
1 teaspoon Worcestershire sauce
1/2 teaspoon sugar
1/2 teaspoon salt

Dice tomatoes. In medium saucepan combine diced tomatoes with remaining ingredients. Simmer 10 minutes. Yields 2 cups

Fat: None
Oil: None

TARTAR SAUCE

1 cup mayonnaise
1 teaspoon grated onion
1 tablespoon minced dill pickle
1 teaspoon dill
1/8 teaspoon salt
1 tablespoon minced parsley
1 tablespoon chopped pimiento
1 tablespoon chopped olives
1/2 teaspoon Worcestershire sauce
1/8 teaspoon mustard

Combine all ingredients and mix well. Yields 1 1/4 cups

Fat: None
Oil: Total—25 teaspoons; per tablespoon—1 1/4 teaspoons

CREOLE SAUCE

1/3 cup minced onion
1 garlic clove, minced
2 tablespoons olive oil
2 1/2 cups canned tomatoes
1 teaspoon celery seed
1 teaspoon chili powder
1/4 cup chopped green pepper
1 bay leaf
2 teaspoons salt
2 teaspoons sugar
2 sprigs parsley
8 whole cloves
1/2 teaspoon basil

Sauté onion and garlic in oil until onion turns yellow, about 5 minutes. Add remaining ingredients and simmer over low heat until mixture thickens. May be used over fish, shrimp, crab, or chicken. Yields 2 cups

Fat: None
Oil: Total—6 teaspoons; per 1/4 cup—3/4 teaspoon

CRANBERRY CUMBERLAND SAUCE

2 medium oranges
1 cup red currant jelly
1 cup light port wine
3 cups sugar
4 sticks cinnamon
1/2 teaspoon whole allspice
4 cups fresh cranberries

Juice oranges and reserve liquid. Cut peel into fine strips; simmer in water 10 minutes until tender. Drain. Combine orange juice, jelly, wine, and sugar. Place spices in a cheesecloth and secure ends. Add to juice mixture. Bring mixture to a boil, reduce temperature, and simmer for 5 minutes. Remove spices. Add cranberries and orange peel. Bring to a full boil until berries pop. Yields 3 pints

Fat: None
Oil: None

CUMBERLAND SAUCE

1/3 cup red currant jelly
1/4 cup port wine
1/4 cup orange juice
2 tablespoons lemon juice
2 tablespoons dry mustard
1 teaspoon paprika
1/2 teaspoon ground ginger
1 teaspoon cornstarch
2 tablespoons grated orange peel

In medium saucepan stir jelly over low heat until melted. Combine remaining ingredients; add to jelly. Bring to boiling point; reduce heat and simmer, stirring constantly, for 5 minutes. Let stand an hour or longer before serving. Best with game, cold turkey, or chicken. Yields approximately 1 cup

Fat: None
Oil: None

MEATLESS SPAGHETTI SAUCE

1 cup chopped onion
3 garlic cloves, crushed
2 tablespoons olive oil
1 teaspoon salt
Pepper to taste
1 teaspoon oregano
1 teaspoon basil
1/8 teaspoon cayenne pepper or chili powder to taste
1/2 green pepper, chopped
2 6-ounce cans tomato paste
3–4 8-ounce cans tomato sauce
1/2 cup dry red wine
1 tablespoon brown sugar
8–10 fresh mushrooms
1 16-ounce can ripe sliced olives

In a 4-quart saucepan sauté onion and garlic in olive oil until the onion is transparent but not brown. Thoroughly stir in the spices and green pepper. Add tomato paste and tomato sauce. Add wine and brown sugar. Add mushrooms and olives, and simmer 3–4 hours. Taste improves when served the following day. Serves 10

Fat: None
Oil: Total—22 teaspoons; per serving—2 1/3 teaspoons

CLAM SAUCE

1 large garlic clove, chopped
2 tablespoons oil
2 tablespoons all-purpose flour
2 8-ounce bottles clam broth (2 cups)
Salt and pepper to taste
1 1/2 teaspoons dried thyme leaves
1/2 cup sliced mushrooms
2 10 1/2-ounce cans clams, minced
1/4 cup dry sherry or white wine
1/4 cup chopped fresh parsley

In medium saucepan sauté garlic in oil. Stir in flour, then gradually add clam broth, salt, pepper, and thyme, and stir until slightly thickened. Add the mushrooms and clams. Just before serving, add the sherry and garnish with parsley. Serves 4

Fat: None
Oil: Total—6 teaspoons; per serving—1 1/2 teaspoons

RED CLAM SAUCE

3 garlic cloves, chopped
2 tablespoons olive oil
1 8-ounce can tomato paste
1 27-ounce can Italian-style tomatoes
1/2 teaspoon chopped parsley
1 teaspoon salt
1/4 teaspoon pepper
1/2 teaspoon oregano
Pinch of sugar (optional)
2 10-ounce cans whole baby clams with juice or 2 8-ounce cans minced clams with juice

In large saucepan sauté garlic in olive oil until lightly browned. Slowly stir in tomato paste and whole tomatoes. Add parsley, salt, pepper, oregano, and sugar. Simmer 1/2 hour. Add clams and simmer an additional 15 minutes. Serve over spaghetti. Serves 6

Fat: None
Oil: Total—6 teaspoons; per serving—1 teaspoon

SEAFOOD COCKTAIL SAUCE

2 teaspoons prepared horseradish
3 tablespoons tomato ketchup
1 teaspoon salt
2 tablespoons vinegar
4 tablespoons lemon juice (optional)
1/4 teaspoon hot pepper sauce

Combine all ingredients and mix well. Store in refrigerator until needed. Yields approximately 1/2 cup

Fat: None
Oil: None

SWEET-AND-SOUR SAUCE

6 tablespoons sugar
2 tablespoons soy sauce
1 tablespoon dry white wine
3 tablespoons vinegar
1/2 cup pineapple juice
3 tablespoons ketchup
2 tablespoons cornstarch
1/2 cup water

In small saucepan over medium heat, combine sugar, soy sauce, wine, vinegar, pineapple juice, and ketchup; bring to a boil. Mix together cornstarch and water until smooth. Add to sauce; stir until thickened. Yields approximately 2 cups

Fat: None
Oil: None

CURRY SAUCE

1 tablespoon oil
1 tablespoon curry powder
2 tablespoons all-purpose flour
1 cup buttermilk or skim milk
1 teaspoon onion flakes
1/2 teaspoon salt
1/2 teaspoon pepper

Heat oil. Combine curry powder and flour, and add to oil. Stir until smooth. Add milk and stir until thickened and smooth. Add onion flakes, salt, and pepper. Yields approximately 1 cup

Fat: None
Oil: Total—3 teaspoons; per 1/2 cup—1 1/2 teaspoons

BROWN MUSHROOM SAUCE

2 tablespoons chopped onion
1 cup sliced fresh or canned mushrooms
4 tablespoons oil
4 tablespoons all-purpose flour
2 cups bouillon or beef stock
1 teaspoon salt
1 teaspoon pepper

In medium saucepan sauté onions and mushrooms in oil. Add flour and stir until well mixed. Add liquid and stir constantly until thickened. Add salt and pepper. Yields approximately 2 cups

Fat: None
Oil: Total—12 teaspoons; per 1/4 cup—3 teaspoons

CHEESE SAUCE

2 tablespoons mayonnaise
1 1/2 tablespoons all-purpose flour
1 cup buttermilk
1/2 cup grated Count Down cheese
1/4 teaspoon salt

In medium saucepan stir mayonnaise and flour over medium heat until smooth. Add buttermilk slowly and stir until thickened. Add cheese and salt, and cook over low heat until melted. Yields approximately 1 cup

Fat: None
Oil: Total—3 teaspoons; per 1/4 cup—3/4 teaspoon

TARRAGON SAUCE

12 slices white bread, crusts removed, cut into 1-inch squares
1 cup chicken stock or double strength bouillon
1/4 cup sherry vinegar
4–5 garlic cloves, minced
4 fresh parsley sprigs without stems
1 tablespoon crumbled dried tarragon
3/4 teaspoon coarsely ground pepper
Salt to taste

Place all ingredients in blender. Purée until smooth. Can be made a day ahead. If refrigerated, bring to room temperature before serving. Serve with chicken. Yields 2 cups

Fat: None
Oil: None

VINAIGRETTE

Grated peel of 1/2 orange
5 tablespoons oil
3/4 teaspoon sugar
1/4 teaspoon salt (optional)
2 tablespoons cilantro leaves
4 teaspoons red wine vinegar
1/2 teaspoon Dijon mustard
Freshly ground pepper

Combine all ingredients in blender. Blend well. Will keep in refrigerator about 3 weeks. Good on fruit as well as green salads. Serves 6

Fat: None
Oil: Total—15 teaspoons; per serving—2 1/2 teaspoons

ROUILLE

1/2 cup parsley leaves
4 large garlic cloves, minced
1 4-ounce jar pimientos, undrained
1/2 teaspoon crushed dried basil
1/4 teaspoon cayenne pepper
1 1/2 slices white bread, crusts trimmed, cut in 1-inch pieces
1 teaspoon dried red pepper flakes
1/2 teaspoon salt
1/3 cup oil

Place all ingredients in blender except oil, and purée until smooth. Add oil with machine running and blend 15 seconds. Can be refrigerated for 2 weeks. Bring to room temperature and stir well before serving. Serve with seafood. Yields 1 cup

Fat: None
Oil: Total—16 teaspoons; per 1/4 cup—4 teaspoons

TERIYAKI SAUCE

1/2 cup soy sauce
4 teaspoons brown sugar
3 garlic cloves, minced
2 tablespoons sherry
1/4 teaspoon salt
1 inch fresh gingerroot, crushed

Combine all ingredients. Use as a basic sauce for chicken and fish. Yields 1 cup

Fat: None
Oil: None

CHAPTER 24

Vegetables

Vegetables are an important part of the American diet. Proper cooking is especially important since the low-fat diet does not allow seasoning with rich sauces or butter. Fresh vegetables should be cooked in small amounts of water, steamed or microwaved for the briefest time, and served immediately. It is possible to cook them so that they retain their natural flavor, nutrients, and appearance. Consommé, a bouillon cube, or basic stock can be added to the cooking water. We also encourage you to try your hand at the Chinese method of stir frying. Directions with a few recipes can be found in Chapter 21.

To assist you in the art of seasoning vegetables, we would like to suggest some accompaniments for each.

ASPARAGUS: Lemon juice with a dash of nutmeg, chives, or chervil
BEETS: Lemon juice, caraway seeds, dill, tarragon, thyme, yogurt with grated orange rind and dash of allspice
BROCCOLI: Curried mayonnaise, poppy seeds, tarragon, marjoram, yogurt-horseradish mixture
BRUSSELS SPROUTS: Caraway seeds, sage, nutmeg
CABBAGE: Lemon juice and curry, horseradish or mustard-flavored yogurt, caraway, dill, or celery seeds
CARROTS: Fresh mint, dill, chives, parsley, ginger, nutmeg, poppy seeds
CORN: Garlic salt, curry
GREEN BEANS: Diced water chestnuts, mushrooms, scallions or green onions, dill, rosemary, mint

ONIONS: Soy sauce, caraway seeds, curry
PEAS: Onions, water chestnuts, curry, savory, marjoram, scallions, chives
SAUERKRAUT: Dill, celery and caraway seeds, onion powder
SPINACH AND OTHER GREENS: Lemon juice, oil, onion salt, Worcestershire sauce, tarragon vinegar with caraway, poppy or sesame seeds
SQUASH, ACORN: Minced onion, honey and orange juice, nutmeg
SQUASH, SUMMER: Fresh dill, oregano, chives, parsley, scallions or green onions
TOMATOES: Dill, basil, sage, marjoram, thyme, rosemary
ZUCCHINI: Soy sauce, basil, marjoram, okra, tomatoes, and minced onion

Try poaching your vegetables in consommé or chicken broth, dry white wine, a mixture of one of the recommended herbs, and salt and pepper. Add enough water barely to cover. Bring to a boil very slowly, then reduce the heat and poach until just crisply tender. Remove from the heat, taste the liquid for seasoning. Serve hot or let the vegetables cool in the liquid for use in salads. Be sure that your poached vegetables are not overcooked. They should still have a slight crisp bite to them and be well marinated in the poaching liquid or dressing so that the flavors mingle with and enhance the natural goodness of the vegetables.

BAKED BEANS

1 pound dry navy beans
6 cups water
1/2 cup chopped onion
Salt to taste
1 teaspoon dry mustard
1/2 cup ketchup
1/2 cup packed brown sugar
1/4 cup molasses
1 cup beer

Soak beans overnight in enough water to cover. Drain. In large kettle simmer beans in 6 cups water until beans are tender, about 1 1/2 hours. Preheat oven to 325° F. Mix cooked beans with remaining ingredients. Cover and bake for 1 1/2 hours, stirring twice during cooking. Uncover and cook 15 minutes longer. Serves 6

Fat: None
Oil: None

REFRIED BEANS

1/2 pound small red pinto beans (dried)
5 cups water
1 1/2 teaspoons salt
1/4 cup finely minced onion
6 tablespoons oil
1 teaspoon cumin
1 garlic clove, minced

Combine beans with water in large saucepan and bring to a boil over medium-high heat. Reduce heat, cover, and simmer without stirring until beans are tender but not completely soft, 1 1/2–2 hours. Add 1 1/2 teaspoons salt and simmer for another 30 minutes. In large skillet over medium heat cook onion in oil until soft but not brown. Increase heat to High. Add 1 cup beans with small amount of liquid and mash well. (A wooden mallet works best.) Add remaining beans and liquid 1 cup at a time. Mash and mix until coarse paste is formed. Add cumin and garlic. Continue cooking, stirring and swirling mixture until beans begin to dry out and start coming away from skillet, 15–20 minutes. Turn onto hot dish to serve. Serves 6

Fat: None
Oil: Total—18 teaspoons; per serving—3 teaspoons

STRING BEANS WITH MUSHROOMS AND ALMONDS

2 16-ounce cans French-cut green beans
1/2 cup chicken stock base
1 teaspoon salt
2 teaspoons instant minced onion
1/2 pound mushrooms, sliced
1/4 cup sliced blanched almonds
2 tablespoons oil

Drain liquid from beans. In medium saucepan combine beans, chicken stock base, salt, and onion. Bring to a boil. Sauté mushrooms and almonds in oil until lightly browned. Pour over the beans and mix lightly. Serve at once. Serves 6

Fat: None
Oil: Total—11 teaspoons; per serving—1 4/5 teaspoons

GERMAN-STYLE BRUSSELS SPROUTS

2 cups or 2 10-ounce packages Brussels sprouts
2 tablespoons vinegar
2 tablespoons honey
1 teaspoon prepared mustard

Cook or steam Brussels sprouts until tender. Drain. Combine vinegar, honey, and mustard, and stir into sprouts. Serves 4

Fat: None
Oil: None

SWEET-AND-SOUR RED CABBAGE

2 tablespoons chopped onion
2 tablespoons oil
6 tablespoons brown sugar
3 tablespoons vinegar or dry white wine
6 cups shredded red cabbage

In large skillet sauté the onion lightly in oil; add brown sugar and vinegar. Add cabbage, stirring thoroughly, and cook for 25 minutes. Serves 4

Fat: None
Oil: Total—6 teaspoons; per serving—1 1/2 teaspoons

GOLDEN VEGETABLE BAKE

2 tablespoons oil
2 tablespoons all-purpose flour
1 cup skim milk, scalded
1 teaspoon salt
1/8 teaspoon pepper
3/4 teaspoon paprika
2 eggs, beaten
1 1/2 cups shredded carrots
1 16 1/2-ounce can cream-style corn (1 3/4 cups)
1/3 cup chopped green pepper
2 tablespoons chopped onion

Preheat oven to 350° F. In medium saucepan heat oil and gradually add flour. Slowly add milk, stirring constantly, and cook until thickened. Add seasonings. Stir 1/4 cup sauce into eggs. Add egg mixture to remaining sauce. Stir in vegetables. Pour into an oiled 1 1/2-quart casserole. Bake for 50–55 minutes. Serves 6

Fat: Total—2 teaspoons; per serving—1/3 teaspoon
Oil: Total—6 teaspoons; per serving—1 teaspoon

GINGERED CARROTS

1 pound carrots, cut in julienne strips
1/2 cup chicken stock
1/2 teaspoon sugar
1/2 teaspoon ground ginger
1 tablespoon oil
1/2 teaspoon salt

In medium saucepan cook carrots in chicken stock until tender. Add sugar, ground ginger, oil, and salt. Continue cooking 3–4 minutes, tossing gently. Serves 6

Fat: None
Oil: Total—3 teaspoons; per serving—1/2 teaspoon

GOLDEN HONEYED CARROTS

2 cups sliced carrots
2 tablespoons honey
3 tablespoons orange juice
1 1/2 tablespoons golden raisins
2 tablespoons coarsely chopped walnuts
1/8 teaspoon cinnamon

Cook or steam carrots until tender. Drain. In small saucepan heat remaining ingredients; toss with carrots. Serves 4

Fat: None
Oil: Total—2 1/2 teaspoons; per serving—2/3 teaspoon

MUSHROOM–WILD RICE CASSEROLE

1 cup wild rice
1/2 green pepper, diced
1/2 pound fresh button mushrooms or 1 4 1/2-ounce can mushrooms
3 tablespoons oil
2 tablespoons all-purpose flour
1/2 teaspoon salt
1/8 teaspoon pepper
1/2 cup chicken bouillon
1/2 cup dry white wine

Preheat oven to 325° F. Cook rice following package directions. In a skillet sauté green pepper and mushrooms in oil until mushrooms are lightly browned. Add flour, salt, and pepper. Gradually stir in bouillon and wine. Cook over low heat, stirring constantly, until slightly thickened. Add rice. Place in 1-quart casserole. Bake about 30 minutes. Serves 4

Fat: None
Oil: Total—9 teaspoons; per serving—2 1/4 teaspoons

HARVARD BEETS

1/2 cup sugar
1 tablespoon cornstarch
1/4 cup vinegar
1/4 cup water
12 small beets, peeled and cooked
2 tablespoons oil

In medium saucepan combine sugar and cornstarch. Add vinegar and water, bring to a boil, and boil 5 minutes. Add beets and let stand 30 minutes. Before serving, bring to a boil and add oil. Serves 4

Fat: None
Oil: Total—6 teaspoons; per serving—1 1/2 teaspoons

PEAS SAVORY

1 10-ounce package frozen peas
2/3 cup sliced fresh or canned mushrooms
1 tablespoon oil
2 tablespoons chopped onion
2 tablespoons water
3/4 teaspoon salt
1/4 teaspoon ground savory
Dash of pepper

Place all ingredients in a saucepan. Bring to a full boil over medium-high heat, separating peas with fork. Cover, reduce heat, and simmer 2–3 minutes or until just tender. Serves 4

Fat: None
Oil: Total—3 teaspoons; per serving—3/4 teaspoon

CREAMED PEAS AND NEW POTATOES

2 cups medium Easy White Sauce
1 16-ounce can new potatoes, cut in medium-sized pieces
1 10-ounce package tiny frozen peas
1 teaspoon parsley
1 teaspoon salt
1 teaspoon pepper

Add potatoes and peas to sauce. Season to taste. Cook until potatoes are warm. Yields approximately 2 cups

Fat: None
Oil: Total—6 teaspoons; per serving—1 1/2 teaspoons

MODESTO POTATOES

2 tablespoons oil
1 tablespoon all-purpose flour
4 medium-sized potatoes, peeled and sliced
1 medium-sized onion, sliced
1 garlic clove, minced
Salt and pepper to taste
1/3 cup dry white wine
1/2 cup bouillon
1/2 teaspoon minced thyme and/or marjoram
1 tablespoon minced parsley

Heat oil in heavy skillet; mix in flour and brown quickly. Add potatoes, onion, garlic, salt, and pepper. Fry, turning often, until potatoes are slightly browned. Add wine, bouillon, and thyme. Cover tightly. Simmer until potatoes are tender and liquid is absorbed. Add parsley; mix well. Good with a baked fish dinner. Serves 6

Fat: None
Oil: Total—6 teaspoons; per serving—1 teaspoon

LEMON-STUFFED POTATOES

3 medium potatoes
1/4 cup skim milk
1 1/2 teaspoons grated lemon peel
2 tablespoons chopped parsley
Salt and pepper to taste

Preheat oven to 375° F. Wash potatoes. Bake for 1 hour or until soft. Cut each potato in half lengthwise. Scoop out the pulp, leaving a thin shell of potato. Add milk to the pulp and mash with a fork. Season with remaining ingredients and divide among potato shells. Return to oven and heat for 5–10 minutes. Serves 6

Fat: None
Oil: None

POTATO PUFFS

1 cup mashed potatoes
1/3 cup skim milk
1 cup all-purpose flour
2 teaspoons baking powder
1 teaspoon salt
2 teaspoons caraway seeds
Oil for frying

Combine all ingredients and mix well. Heat heavy skillet to 325° F with oil to depth of 2 inches. Drop potato mixture by spoonfuls into hot oil. When brown on one side, turn and cook until brown on other side. Discard oil. Yields 15–20 small puffs

Fat: None
Oil: Approximately 1 teaspoon per puff from frying

BAKED POTATO WITH AVOCADO PURÉE AND CHIVES

1 large baking potato
1/2 teaspoon oil
1/2 teaspoon salt
1/4 teaspoon black pepper
1/2 avocado, mashed to a purée
2 teaspoons snipped fresh chives

Preheat oven to 350° F. Rub the potato with the oil and bake until soft, approximately 1 hour, or cook in microwave. Split the potato lengthwise in half. Scoop out the pulp, leaving a thin shell of potato. Mash the pulp with a fork and season with the salt and pepper. Mix in the avocado purée until blended. Divide among potato shells and sprinkle with chives. Yields 2 servings

Fat: None
Oil: Total—4 1/2 teaspoons; per 1/2 potato—2 1/4 teaspoons oil

OVEN FRENCH FRIES

2 medium raw potatoes, peeled
1 tablespoon oil
Salt to taste

Preheat oven to 425° F. Wash and cut raw potatoes into desired-sized strips. Place on baking sheet and brush with oil. Bake 45 minutes or until brown. Salt lightly and serve. Serves 2

Fat: None
Oil: Total—3 teaspoons; per serving—1 1/2 teaspoons

PILAF

1 cup uncooked rice
2 tablespoons oil
1/2 cup vermicelli
2 cups chicken stock
1/4 cup chopped almonds

Preheat oven to 375° F. In medium-sized skillet brown rice in oil for 10 minutes, stirring to prevent burning. Add vermicelli, stock, and almonds. Bake in a covered baking dish for 30 minutes. Remove lid, stir, and bake for another 10 minutes. Serves 4

Fat: None
Oil: Total—11 teaspoons; per serving—2 3/4 teaspoons

STUFFED TOMATOES PARISIENNE

6 medium even-sized tomatoes
2 teaspoons oil
1/2 pound mushrooms, chopped
1 small onion, chopped
1 teaspoon salt
1/8 teaspoon pepper
1 teaspoon chopped parsley
1/4 cup chicken bouillon

Preheat oven to 375° F. Wash tomatoes. Cut 1-inch pieces from stem ends of tomatoes. Scoop out pulp and discard. Heat oil in medium-sized skillet. Add mushrooms and onion, and sauté 5 minutes. Season with salt, pepper, and parsley. Stuff tomatoes with mixture. Pour bouillon into shallow baking dish. Arrange tomatoes in dish. Bake 30 minutes until brown and tender. Serves 6

Fat: None
Oil: Total—2 teaspoons; per serving—1/3 teaspoon

FRIED TOMATOES

6 medium firm ripe tomatoes
1/2 cup sifted all-purpose flour
1 teaspoon garlic salt
1/2 teaspoon rosemary or thyme
1 tablespoon oil
2 teaspoons brown sugar
2/3 cup dry red wine

Core tomatoes; remove skin if desired. Cut each tomato in half. Combine flour and seasonings, and dredge tomatoes. In medium skillet sauté tomatoes in oil. Add sugar and wine; continue cooking until tomatoes are tender, about 5 minutes. Serve with any remaining liquid. Serves 6

Fat: None
Oil: Total—3 teaspoons; per serving—1/2 teaspoon

FESTIVAL SWEET POTATOES

3 large sweet potatoes or yams
1 teaspoon salt
1/2 cup packed brown sugar
1 8-ounce can sliced pineapple (6 slices)
1/3 cup rum or brandy or dry sherry or water

Preheat oven to 350° F. In medium saucepan boil sweet potatoes in their skins 20–30 minutes or until tender. Peel and put through ricer or mash. Season with salt and 1/4 cup brown sugar or to taste. Form into balls, using an ice-cream scoop, and place a mound on top of each slice of pineapple. Heat remaining brown sugar and liquid together until sugar is dissolved; pour over potatoes and pineapple. Bake 30 minutes, basting often with syrup in pan. Serves 6

Variation: Omit sauce and place half a marshmallow on top of each potato mound about 2 minutes before removing from oven.

Fat: None
Oil: None

BARLEY PILAF

2 tablespoons oil
2 medium onions, chopped
1/2 pound mushrooms, sliced
13/4 cups barley or part barley, bulgar wheat, and rice
1 quart chicken broth
Salt and pepper to taste

Preheat oven to 350° F. Heat 1 tablespoon oil in heavy skillet and cook onion and mushrooms until tender. Add remaining oil and barley. Cook very slowly, turning mixture until browned. Add 13/4 cups chicken broth. Pour into a casserole dish and cover. Bake 30 minutes, remove lid, season to taste, and add remaining broth. Cover and cook 30 minutes longer. If barley appears dry, add slightly more stock. Cook until tender but not mushy. Serves 8

Fat: None
Oil: Total—6 teaspoons; per serving—3/4 teaspoon

BAKED SOYBEANS

1 cup dried large soybeans
4 quarts water
2 tablespoons oil
2 tablespoons molasses
1 onion, thinly sliced
11/4 teaspoons salt
1 teaspoon lemon juice

Soak soybeans in 1 quart water for 24 hours in refrigerator. Change water 4 times during the 24 hours to prevent souring. When soaking, 1 quart of water should be used to every cup of soybeans. After soybeans have soaked, bring to a boil in 1 quart water and cook slowly, keeping the beans covered. Simmer for 3–4 hours until the beans are light tan. Transfer to a covered baking dish and add the oil, molasses, onion, and salt. Bake in a moderate oven, 325° F, for 1–2 hours, until beans are brown and well done. Stir occasionally during the baking and keep the beans covered and moist. Remove cover the last half hour of cooking, add the lemon juice, and continue cooking until the top is brown. Serves 4

Fat: None
Oil: Total—6 teaspoons; per serving—11/2 teaspoons

SOYBEAN CASSEROLE

4 cups soybeans, cooked
1 onion, grated
1/2 green bell pepper, chopped
1 carrot, grated
1/2 cup chopped celery and tops
3 tablespoons molasses
3 tablespoons minced parsley
1/4 teaspoon thyme
1/4 teaspoon savory
1/2 teaspoon garlic powder
Tomato juice as needed

Preheat oven to 350° F. Combine all ingredients except tomato juice. Turn into covered casserole dish. Bake for 2 hours, adding tomato juice as needed. Uncover for last 30 minutes of baking. Serves 6

Fat: None
Oil: None

CREAMED SPINACH

2 teaspoons all-purpose flour
1 cup skim milk
2 10-ounce packages frozen chopped spinach
1/4 teaspoon garlic powder
1/4 teaspoon ground nutmeg (or to taste)
Salt and pepper to taste

Brown flour in dry pan, stirring constantly. Cool pan and flour. Reheat and add milk slowly, stirring until thickened. Add spinach and seasonings. Simmer 5–10 minutes. Serves 8

Fat: None
Oil: None

CHAPTER 25

Muffins and Breads

Breads generally contain a relatively small amount of fat even though there is a wide variation in the amount of fat or oil that commercial bakeries use. Some of the quick loaf breads may contain as much as a teaspoon of oil per slice, but this is not true of breads made with yeast where a slice contains only a trace of fat or oil. No restrictions have been placed on eating yeast breads unless obesity is a problem. Homemade bread is delicious and worth the time and effort to make. Several bread recipes using whole grain products and high-protein supplements are included. These breads will provide maximum nutrition as well as delicious sandwiches and toast. Also included are recipes for biscuits, muffins, and quick loaf breads to illustrate how easy it is to use oil instead of butter or shortening.

Bread Rising

If you find it difficult to find a warm, moist place, free from drafts for bread rising, try this simple no-fail solution.

Place both oven racks as low as possible. Place a shallow pan on the bottom rack. Pour 1 quart of boiling water in the pan and immediately place the covered bread dough on the upper rack. Close the oven door and set timer for desired rising time. Do not open door. Do not turn oven on during this part of process.

For the second rising do not refill the water. Place the bread back in oven and set timer. Remove the water when baking the bread or the oven will be too moist.

TIME-SAVING MIXES

The following mixes can be prepared ahead of time and stored for several weeks or months. You will find them convenient, easy, and economical.

CORNMEAL MIX

4 cups all-purpose flour
1 tablespoon salt
3/4 cup sugar
1/4 cup baking powder
3/4 cup vegetable oil
4 1/2 cups cornmeal

In a large bowl combine flour, salt, sugar, and baking powder. Stir to blend well. With a pastry blender, cut in oil until evenly distributed. Add cornmeal and mix well. Put in airtight container. Store in refrigerator. Use within 10–12 weeks. Yields 10 1/2 cups

Fat: None
Oil: Total—36 teaspoons; per 1 cup serving—3 1/2 teaspoons

Use this mix for the following cornmeal recipes:

CORNMEAL MUFFINS

2 1/2 cups Cornmeal Mix
1 egg
1 1/4 cups skim milk

Preheat oven to 425° F. Oil and flour muffin pans. Put Cornmeal Mix in medium bowl. Combine egg and milk in small bowl. Add to mix. Blend. Bake 15–20 minutes until golden brown. Yields 1 dozen muffins

Fat: Total—1 teaspoon; per serving—negligible
Oil: Total—8 3/4 teaspoons; per muffin—3/4 teaspoon

CORNBREAD

Prepare same recipe for cornmeal muffins. Oil an 8-inch-square pan. Spread batter in pan and bake for 25 minutes until golden brown. Yields 1 8-inch-square loaf

HOT ROLL MIX

5 pounds all-purpose flour
1 1/2 cups sugar
4 teaspoons salt
1 cup instant nonfat dry milk powder

Combine all ingredients in large bowl. Store in airtight container. Use within 6–8 months. Yields 22 cups

Fat: None
Oil: None

This mix can be used for Pan Rolls and Basic Bread.

PAN ROLLS

1 package active dry yeast
1 1/2 cups lukewarm water
2 eggs, beaten
1/2 cup oil
5–6 cups Hot Roll Mix

In a large bowl dissolve yeast in lukewarm water. Blend in eggs and oil. Add 5 cups Hot Roll Mix. Blend well. Add additional mix to make a soft, but not too sticky dough. Knead about 5 minutes until dough is smooth. Lightly oil bowl and let rise in a warm place until doubled in size, approximately 1 hour. Oil a 13″ × 9″ pan. Punch down dough. Divide into 24–30 balls of equal size. Place balls in pan. Cover and let rise again until double in size, approximately 30 minutes. Preheat oven to 375° F. Bake 20–25 minutes until golden brown. Yields 2 dozen rolls

Fat: Total—2 teaspoons; per serving—negligible
Oil: Total—24 teaspoons; per roll—1 teaspoon

BASIC BREAD

2 packages active dry yeast
1 cup lukewarm water
2 eggs, beaten
1 cup water
1/4 cup vegetable oil
1/4 cup packed brown sugar
2/3 cup wheat germ
6 1/2–7 cups Hot Roll Mix

In a large bowl dissolve yeast in lukewarm water. When yeast begins to bubble, add eggs, water, and oil. Blend well. Add sugar and wheat germ. Blend well. Add Hot Roll Mix 1 cup at a time until dough is stiff. On a lightly floured surface knead dough 5–7 minutes until smooth. Oil bowl and add dough. Cover with damp towel and let rise in a warm place until double in size, approximately 60 minutes. Punch down dough. Let stand 10 minutes. Shape into 2 loaves. Oil two 9″ × 5″ loaf pans. Place dough in pans. Cover and let rise until slightly rounded above top of pan, approximately 30 minutes. Preheat oven to 375° F. Bake 45–55 minutes until golden brown. Remove from pans and cool on a wire rack. Yields 2 loaves (16 slices per loaf)

Fat: Total—2 teaspoons; per slice—negligible
Oil: Total—12 teaspoons; per slice—1/3 teaspoon

MUFFIN MIX

8 cups all-purpose flour
2/3 cup sugar
1/3 cup baking powder
1 tablespoon salt
3/4 cup oil

In a large bowl combine flour, sugar, baking powder, and salt. Mix well. With a pastry blender cut oil into dry ingredients. Store in airtight container in refrigerator. Use within 10–12 weeks. Yields 10 cups

Fat: None
Oil: Total—36 teaspoons; per 1 cup—3 3/5 teaspoons

Use this recipe for some easy tasty muffins:

BASIC MUFFINS

2 1/3 cups Muffin Mix
1 egg, beaten
1 cup skim milk

Preheat oven to 400° F. Oil muffin pans. Pour Muffin Mix in medium bowl. Combine egg and milk, and add to mix. Stir until just moistened. Batter should be lumpy. Fill muffin pans 2/3 full. Bake 15–20 minutes until golden brown. Yields 1 dozen muffins

Fat: Total—Negligible
Oil: Total—8 1/3 teaspoons; per muffin—2/3 teaspoon

APPLE MUFFINS

2 1/3 cups Muffin Mix
1/2 cup chopped nuts
1/4 teaspoon cloves
1 cup sweet applesauce
1/4 cup skim milk
1 egg, beaten

Preheat oven to 400° F. Oil muffin pans. In a medium bowl combine Muffin Mix, nuts, and cloves. Combine applesauce, milk, and egg, and add to dry ingredients. Stir until just moistened; batter should be lumpy. Fill muffin pans 2/3 full. Bake 15–20 minutes until golden brown. Yields 1 dozen large muffins

Fat: Total—1 teaspoon; per muffin—negligible
Oil: Total—20 1/3 teaspoons; per muffin—1 2/3 teaspoons

APPLE BRAN MUFFINS

1 cup all-purpose flour
1 teaspoon baking powder
1/2 teaspoon salt
1/4 teaspoon baking soda
1/4 teaspoon cinnamon
1/8 teaspoon nutmeg
1 egg
1/2 cup buttermilk
1/3 cup packed brown sugar
3 tablespoons oil
1/2 cup grated raw apple
1/2 cup raw bran
2 tablespoons chopped nuts

Preheat oven to 400° F. Oil muffin pans. Mix together the flour, baking powder, salt, baking soda, cinnamon, and nutmeg, and put to one side. Beat egg, buttermilk, brown sugar, and oil. Add grated apple, then dry ingredients, bran, and nuts. Stir. Fill muffin pans 2/3 full. Bake 15–20 minutes. Yields 1 dozen muffins

Fat: Total—1 teaspoon; per muffin—negligible
Oil: Total—12 teaspoons; per muffin—1 teaspoon

BRAN MUFFINS

1 cup all-purpose flour
3/4 teaspoon salt
1 teaspoon baking powder
1/2 teaspoon baking soda
1/4 teaspoon cinnamon
1 cup raw bran
1/4 cup water
1 cup buttermilk
2 tablespoons oil
1 egg, beaten
1/4 cup packed brown sugar
1/2 cup raisins or dates

Preheat oven to 400° F. Oil muffin pans. Mix flour with salt, baking powder, baking soda, and cinnamon. Stir in bran. Combine water, buttermilk, oil, and egg. Add brown sugar. Quickly stir into dry ingredients. Add raisins. Fill muffin pans 2/3 full. Bake 15–20 minutes. Yields 1 dozen muffins

Fat: Total—1 teaspoon; per muffin—negligible
Oil: Total—6 teaspoons; per muffin—1/2 teaspoon

MOLASSES-BRAN MUFFINS

1 cup bran cereal
3/4 cup skim milk
2 tablespoons molasses
1 egg
1 1/4 cups Muffin Mix

Preheat oven to 400° F. Oil muffin pans. In small bowl combine bran and milk. Combine molasses and egg, and add to bran mixture. Add bran molasses mixture to Muffin Mix. Stir until moistened; batter should be lumpy. Fill muffin pans 2/3 full. Bake 15–20 minutes. Yields 1 dozen muffins

Fat: Total—1 teaspoon; per muffin—negligible
Oil: Total—4 1/2 teaspoons; per muffin—1/3 teaspoon

ZUCCHINI BRAN MUFFINS

1 1/4 cups bran flakes cereal
1 cup skim milk
1 1/3 cups all-purpose flour
1 tablespoon baking powder
1/2 teaspoon salt
1/2 cup sugar
1/4 teaspoon coriander
1/8 teaspoon nutmeg
1/8 teaspoon cinnamon
1/4 cup oil
1 egg
1 cup grated zucchini

Preheat oven to 425° F. Oil muffin pans. Soak bran in milk 6–7 minutes. Mix dry ingredients and spices together. Beat together oil and egg. Add to bran-milk mixture. Fold zucchini into flour mixture and gradually add liquid. Stir until just wet (mixture should remain lumpy). Fill muffin pans 2/3 full. Bake 30–35 minutes or until done. Yields 1 dozen muffins

Fat: Total—1 teaspoon; per muffin—negligible
Oil: Total—12 teaspoons; per muffin—1 teaspoon

REFRIGERATOR BRAN MUFFINS

1 cup boiling water
1 cup 100% raw bran flakes cereal
2 eggs
1/2 cup oil
3/4 cup packed brown sugar
2 teaspoons salt
3 teaspoons baking soda
2 cups buttermilk
2 1/2 cups all-purpose flour
2 cups all-bran cereal

Preheat oven to 350° F. Oil muffin pans. Pour boiling water over raw bran flakes cereal and set to one side to cool. Beat eggs; add oil, sugar, and salt. Stir the baking soda into the buttermilk, stirring until foamy, then add to the egg mixture alternately with flour. Add bran mixture and All-Bran cereal bran. Fill muffin pans 2/3 full. Bake for 20 minutes or until done. Batter may be stored in covered container in refrigerator for 1 month. Yields approximately 3 dozen muffins

Fat: Total—2 teaspoons; per muffin—negligible
Oil: Total—24 teaspoons; per muffin—2/3 teaspoon

NUTTY LEMON YOGURT MUFFINS

3/4 cup whole wheat flour
1 cup all-purpose flour
1 1/2 teaspoons baking powder
1/2 teaspoon baking soda
1 cup chopped walnuts
1 teaspoon grated lemon peel
1 egg
2/3 cup lightly packed brown sugar
2/3 cup buttermilk
1/3 cup oil
1/4 cup plain nonfat yogurt
1/2 teaspoon vanilla extract

Preheat oven to 375° F. Oil muffin pans. Set aside. In medium bowl combine flours, baking powder, baking soda, walnuts, and lemon peel. Mix well. In a large bowl beat egg lightly. Stir in brown sugar, buttermilk, oil, yogurt, and vanilla. Blend well. Add flour mixture and gently fold together until dry ingredients are moistened. Fill muffin cups 3/4 full. If desired, place a walnut half on top of each muffin. Bake 20–25 minutes or until toothpick inserted in center comes out clean. Serve warm. Yields 1 dozen muffins

Fat: Total—1 teaspoon; per muffin—negligible
Oil: Total—40 teaspoons; per muffin—3 1/3 teaspoons

CORNELL BREAD

2 packages active dry yeast
3 cups warm water
2 tablespoons sugar
6 cups unbleached flour plus 1/2 cup all-purpose flour
3 tablespoons wheat germ
1/2 cup stirred soy flour
3/4 cup nonfat dry milk powder
4 teaspoons salt
3 tablespoons oil

In a large bowl soften yeast in warm water with sugar. Let stand for 5 minutes. Mix together 3 cups flour, wheat germ, soy flour, and nonfat dry milk powder. Stir salt and the remaining 3 cups of flour into the yeast mixture. Add 2 tablespoons oil and remaining dry ingredients. Turn out on a lightly floured board. Knead vigorously, about 5 minutes, using remaining 1/2 cup flour. Put in a large bowl and brush lightly with remaining oil. Cover and let rise in a warm place until double in bulk, about 35 minutes. Punch down dough, fold over edges, and turn upside down in bowl to rise another 20 minutes. Turn onto board and divide into 3 equal portions. Shape 3 loaves or 2 loaves and a pan of rolls. Place in oiled 8 1/2″ × 4 1/2″ × 2 1/2″ loaf pans or 9-inch round layer cake pans for rolls. Brush lightly with oil. Cover.

Let rise in a warm place until double in bulk, about 30–45 minutes. Preheat oven to 350° F. Bake about 50 minutes. Substitute whole wheat flour for half the regular flour for a half-and-half loaf. Yields 3 loaves (approximately 16 slices per loaf)

Fat: None
Oil: Total—9 teaspoons; per slice—1/3 teaspoon

OATMEAL CORNELL BREAD

2 packages active dry yeast
3/4 cup warm skim milk
1/3 cup packed brown sugar
2 cups regular or quick oats
21/2 cups boiling water
1/4 cup oil
4 teaspoons salt
51/2 cups unbleached flour plus 1/2 cup for kneading
2 tablespoons wheat germ
1/2 cup stirred soy flour
3/4 cup nonfat dry milk powder

Soften yeast in warm milk with brown sugar. Let stand 5 minutes. In a large bowl mix together uncooked oats, boiling water, oil, and salt. Cool to lukewarm. Mix together flour, wheat germ, soy flour, and nonfat dry milk powder. Stir the yeast and sugar into the lukewarm oatmeal mixture. Add half the dry ingredients. Beat until smooth. Stir in remaining dry ingredients. Turn out on a lightly floured board. Knead well, about 5 minutes, using about 1/2 cup more flour. Put in a large oiled bowl. Brush lightly with oil. Let rise in a warm place until double in bulk, about 35 minutes. Punch down dough, fold over edges, and turn upside down in bowl to rise another 20 minutes. Turn onto floured board and divide into two portions. Shape into loaves. Place in oiled 81/2" × 41/2" × 21/2" loaf pans. Brush lightly with oil. Cover. Let rise in a warm place until dough is almost double in bulk, about 30 minutes. Preheat oven to 350° F. Bake for about 50 minutes. Yields 2 loaves (approximately 16 slices per loaf)

Fat: None
Oil: Total—12 teaspoons; per slice—3/8 teaspoon

QUICK WHOLE WHEAT CORNELL BREAD

2 packages active dry yeast
3 cups warm water
1/4 cup molasses
1/4 cup packed brown sugar
6 cups whole wheat flour
1/2 cup stirred soy flour
3/4 cup nonfat dry milk powder
3 tablespoons wheat germ
2 tablespoons nutritional yeast
4 teaspoons salt
1/4 cup oil

Dissolve yeast in warm water in large bowl. Add molasses and brown sugar. Let stand 5 minutes. Mix together flours, dry milk powder, wheat germ, nutritional yeast, and salt. Stir the yeast mixture and add half the flour and the oil. Beat vigorously, adding as much flour mixture as can be beaten. Stir and work in remaining flour. Turn into two oiled 8 1/2″ × 4 1/2″ × 2 1/2″ loaf pans. Brush with oil. Let rise 30 minutes or until double in bulk. Preheat oven to 375° F. Bake 50 minutes. Yields 2 loaves (approximately 16 slices per loaf)

Fat: None
Oil: Total—12 teaspoons; per slice—3/8 teaspoon

WHOLE GRAIN BREAD

1 package active dry yeast
1/2 cup warm water
1 teaspoon granulated sugar
1/2 cup potato water
1/2 cup scalded skim milk
1 1/2 cups all-purpose flour plus 1/2 cup for kneading
2 teaspoons salt
1/4 cup molasses
1 tablespoon brown sugar or honey
2 tablespoons oil plus 2 teaspoons to oil bowl
1 cup graham flour
3/4 cup whole wheat flour
2 tablespoons raw bran
2 tablespoons rye flour
2 tablespoons wheat germ
2 tablespoons nonfat dry milk powder

Dissolve yeast in warm water with sugar and let stand 10 minutes. Combine potato water and milk, add to the yeast mixture, then stir in the flour and salt. Beat well for 5 minutes with an electric mixer. Let rise in a warm place until full of bubbles, approximately 30–35 minutes. Add molasses, brown sugar, and 2 tablespoons oil to the risen sponge. Blend together the graham flour, whole wheat flour, bran, rye flour, wheat germ, and nonfat dry milk powder, and add to sponge. Mix thoroughly. Turn onto a floured board and let rest for 10 minutes covered. Knead, adding all-purpose flour to keep from sticking until dough is springy in hands, about 10 minutes. Turn into oiled bowl, rolling to coat underside, and let rise until double in bulk, about 1 hour. Punch down. Turn into two oiled 8 1/2″ × 4 1/2″ × 2 1/2″ loaf pans. Cover and let rise again until double in bulk, about 1–1 1/2 hours. Preheat oven to 375° F. Bake 45 minutes. Yields 2 loaves (approximately 16 slices per loaf)

Fat: None
Oil: Total—8 teaspoons; per slice—1/4 teaspoon

GRAHAM BREAD

1 cup graham flour
1/2 cup all-purpose flour
1/4 cup wheat germ
1 teaspoon baking soda
1/2 teaspoon salt
2 tablespoons oil
1/3 cup packed brown sugar
2 tablespoons molasses
1 cup buttermilk
1/2 cup raisins (optional)

Preheat oven to 350° F. Mix together the graham flour, all-purpose flour, wheat germ, baking soda, and salt; put to one side. Mix oil, brown sugar, molasses, and buttermilk until well blended. Add the dry ingredients. Beat until smooth. Add the raisins if desired. Turn into one oiled 8 1/2″ × 4 1/2″ × 2 1/2″ loaf pan. Bake 1 hour 10 minutes. Yields 1 loaf (approximately 16 slices per loaf)

Fat: None
Oil: Total—6 teaspoons; per slice—3/8 teaspoon

SWEDISH RYE BREAD

1 package active dry yeast
1/4 cup warm water
1/4 cup packed brown sugar
1/4 cup light molasses
1 tablespoon salt
2 tablespoons oil
1 1/2 cups hot water
2 1/2 cups medium rye flour
3 tablespoons caraway seeds or 2 tablespoons grated orange peel
3 1/2–4 cups all-purpose flour
1/2 cup stirred soy flour
1/4 cup nonfat dry milk

Soften yeast in water. In a large bowl combine the brown sugar, molasses, salt, and oil. Add the hot water to this mixture and stir until sugar is dissolved. Cool to lukewarm. Stir in rye flour and beat well. Add softened yeast and caraway seeds or orange peel. Mix well. Stir in the all-purpose flour, soy flour, and nonfat milk. Cover and let rest for 10 minutes. Knead on a well-floured board until smooth and satiny, about 10 minutes. Place dough in lightly oiled bowl, turning over once to oil surface. Cover, let rise in warm place until double in bulk, about 1 1/2 hours. Punch down. Turn out on a lightly floured board and divide into 2 portions. Round each piece into a ball and let rest, covered, for 10 minutes. Pat ball of dough into 2 round loaves. Place on nonstick or oiled baking sheet or shape into 2 loaves and place in two nonstick or oiled 8 1/2″ × 4 1/2″ × 2 1/2″ loaf pans. Cover and let rise until double in bulk, about 1 1/2 hours. Preheat oven to 375° F. Bake 25–35 minutes. For soft crust, brush with oil. Yields 2 loaves (approximately 16 slices per loaf)

Fat: None
Oil: Total—6 teaspoons; per slice—3/8 teaspoon

ORANGE BREAD

Peelings from 2 oranges
1/4 cup water
3/4 cup sugar
2 3/4 cups all-purpose flour
2 1/2 teaspoons baking powder
1/2 teaspoon salt
1 egg
1 cup skim milk
1/2 cup chopped nuts

Preheat oven to 350° F. Place orange peelings in a saucepan and cover with water. Bring to a boil and simmer for 2–3 minutes. Drain. Again cover with water and bring to a boil, then simmer for 7–10 minutes or until peeling is tender but not mushy. Drain. Trim pith from inside peeling and cut into narrow strips 1 inch long. Return the cut peeling to the saucepan and add 1/4 cup water and the sugar. Boil until the consistency of corn syrup. While the syrup cools, mix flour, baking powder, and salt. Combine the egg and milk. Gradually add the dry ingredients, beating until smooth. Add the syrup, peel, and the chopped nuts. Spread dough in an oiled 8 1/2″ × 4 1/2″ × 2 1/2″ pan and permit to stand for 10 minutes before baking. Bake about 1 hour. Yields one 1-pound loaf (16 slices per loaf)

Fat: Total—1 teaspoon; per slice—negligible
Oil: Total—12 teaspoons; per slice—3/4 teaspoon

PUMPKIN BREAD

2 1/2 cups all-purpose flour
2 teaspoons baking soda
1/2 teaspoon salt
1/2 teaspoon cinnamon
1/2 teaspoon ground cloves
2 cups sugar
1 16-ounce can puréed pumpkin (2 cups)
1/4 cup oil
1/2 cup chopped nuts (optional)
1/2 cup chopped dates

Preheat oven to 350° F. Mix together flour, baking soda, and salt. Add spices. Combine sugar, pumpkin, and oil; beat well. Add dry ingredients, nuts, and dates. Pour batter into two oiled 8 1/2″ × 4 1/2″ × 2 1/2″ loaf pans. Bake 1 hour or until done when tested with a toothpick. Yields 2 loaves (approximately 12 slices per loaf)

Fat: None
Oil: Total—12 teaspoons (24 teaspoons if nuts are used); per slice—1/2 teaspoon (1 teaspoon if nuts are used)

DATE NUT BREAD

1 teaspoon baking soda
1 cup boiling water
1 cup chopped pitted dates
2 cups all-purpose flour
1 cup chopped walnuts (optional)
1 tablespoon oil
1 cup packed brown sugar
1 egg, beaten
1/2 teaspoon salt
1/2 teaspoon vanilla

Preheat oven to 350° F. Dissolve the baking soda in the boiling water and mix with dates. Set aside to cool. Mix 1/3 of the flour with the walnuts and reserve. Gradually add oil and brown sugar to the egg, then the salt. Add date mixture and flour alternately. Add floured nuts and vanilla. Bake in an 8 1/2″ × 4 1/2″ × 2 1/2″ oiled loaf pan for 1 hour. Yields 1 loaf (16 slices per loaf)

Fat: Total—1 teaspoon; per slice—1/16 teaspoon
Oil: Total—3 teaspoons (27 teaspoons if nuts are used); per slice—3/16 teaspoon (1 11/16 teaspoons if nuts are used)

BANANA TEA BREAD

1 1/2 cups all-purpose flour
1 teaspoon baking soda
1/2 teaspoon salt
2 large—or 2 1/2 medium—bananas (1 cup when mashed)
1/2 cup nonfat yogurt
1 cup sugar
2 eggs
1 teaspoon vanilla or 1/2 teaspoon lemon extract
1/2 cup oil
1/2 cup chopped nuts (optional)

Preheat oven to 350° F. Mix together flour, baking soda, and salt in large mixing bowl. Break peeled bananas in chunks and place in blender. Push down with rubber scraper. Cover and blend on Low a few seconds, then on High until mashed. Add yogurt, sugar, eggs, flavoring, and oil. Cover; blend on High for 1/2 minute. Add nuts and blend on High briefly until nuts are coarsely chopped. Pour over flour mixture. Beat with mixer at low speed for 1/2 minute, scraping bowl, or mix by hand. Turn into an oiled 8 1/2″ × 4 1/2″ × 2 1/2″ loaf pan. Bake for 1 hour, or until done when tested with a toothpick. Yields 1 loaf (16 slices per loaf)

Fat: Total—2 teaspoons; per slice—scant 1/6 teaspoon
Oil: Total—24 teaspoons (36 teaspoons if nuts are used); per slice—1 1/2 teaspoons (2 1/4 teaspoons if nuts are used)

POPPY SEED BREAD

3 cups all-purpose flour
2 3/4 cups sugar
1 1/2 teaspoons baking powder
1 1/2 teaspoons salt
3 eggs
1 1/2 cups oil
1 1/2 cups skim milk
1 teaspoon vanilla extract
1 teaspoon almond extract
1 teaspoon butter extract
3 tablespoons poppy seeds

Preheat oven to 350° F. Combine dry ingredients. Set aside. Beat eggs and oil together. Add milk. Add this to dry ingredients. Add vanilla, almond, and butter extracts. Add poppy seeds. Mix well. Turn into two 8 1/2″ × 4 1/2″ × 2 1/2″ oiled loaf pans. Bake for 1 hour. Yields 2 loaves (16 slices per loaf)

Fat: Total—3 teaspoons; per slice—negligible
Oil: Total—72 teaspoons; per slice—2 1/4 teaspoons

HOLIDAY CRANBERRY NUT BREAD

2 cups all-purpose flour
1 1/2 teaspoons baking powder
1/2 teaspoon baking soda
1 teaspoon salt
1 cup sugar
3 tablespoons oil
1 egg, unbeaten
3/4 cup orange juice
Peel of 1 orange, cut in strips
1 cup washed drained cranberries
1/2 cup chopped nuts (optional)

Preheat oven to 350° F. Mix together in large bowl flour, baking powder, baking soda, and salt. Combine in blender sugar, oil, egg, and orange juice. Cover; blend on high speed briefly. Add orange peel and cranberries. Cover; blend on low speed briefly, then high speed briefly. Add nuts. Cover; blend on high speed only until nuts are coarsely chopped. Pour over flour mixture. Mix by hand. Turn into an oiled 8 1/2″ × 4 1/2″ × 2 1/2″ loaf pan. Bake 1 hour 15 minutes or until toothpick inserted in center comes out clean. Yields 1 loaf (16 slices per loaf)

Fat: Total—1 teaspoon; per slice—1/16 teaspoon
Oil: Total—9 teaspoons (21 teaspoons if nuts are used); per slice—9/16 teaspoon (1 5/16 teaspoons if nuts are used)

SUNSHINE ROLLS

1 package active dry yeast, softened in 1/2 cup warm water
1 cup cooked cubed squash or yams
1/2 cup sugar
3/4 teaspoon salt
1 egg, beaten
1/3 cup oil plus 4 teaspoons for brushing
3 cups all-purpose flour plus 1/4–1/2 cup for kneading

Preheat oven to 375° F. Dissolve dry yeast in warm water. Let stand 5 minutes. Put squash through food mill and then sieve to remove fiber. In a large bowl combine the squash, sugar, salt, egg, yeast mixture, 1/3 cup oil, and 1 cup flour, and mix thoroughly. Let rise until full of bubbles, approximately 45 minutes. Add 2 cups of flour and beat well. Turn onto a floured board and let rest for 10 minutes covered. Knead well, adding 1/4–1/2 cup additional flour. Turn into oiled bowl, rolling to coat all sides, and let rise until double in bulk, about 1 hour. Turn out onto floured board and cut as desired to make rolls. Brush rolls with oil. Let rise until double in bulk, about 1 1/2–2 hours. Bake for 20 minutes. Yields 2 dozen cloverleaf rolls

Fat: Total—1 teaspoon; per roll—negligible
Oil: Total—20 teaspoons; per roll—5/6 teaspoon

ZUCCHINI LOAVES

3 eggs
1 cup oil
2 cups sugar
1 teaspoon vanilla
2 cups finely shredded zucchini, well packed
1 1/2 cups cake flour
1 cup whole wheat flour
1/2 cup wheat germ
1 teaspoon salt
2 teaspoons nutmeg
1 teaspoon baking soda
1/2 teaspoon baking powder
2 tablespoons grated orange peel
1/2 cup chopped nuts

Preheat oven to 325° F. In a mixing bowl beat eggs, oil, sugar, vanilla, and zucchini. Reduce speed to Low and begin adding all remaining ingredients as you measure them. Stir in nuts last. Batter is quite thin. Line two 8 1/2″ × 4 1/2″ × 2 1/2″ loaf pans with oiled double waxed paper. Fill loaf pans 2/3 full. Bake 1 hour. Yields 2 loaves (16 slices per loaf)

Fat: Total—3 teaspoons; per slice—negligible
Oil: Total—60 teaspoons; per slice—1 3/4 teaspoons

BUTTERMILK BISCUITS

2 cups all-purpose flour
2 teaspoons baking powder
1/4 teaspoon baking soda
1 teaspoon salt
1/3 cup oil
2/3 cup buttermilk

Preheat oven to 475° F. Mix together flour, baking powder, baking soda, and salt. Pour oil and buttermilk into one measuring cup; do not stir. Then pour all at once into flour. Stir with a fork until mixture cleans sides of bowl and rounds up into a ball. For drop biscuits, drop dough onto ungreased cookie sheet. For rolled or patted biscuits, smooth by kneading dough about 10 times without additional flour. With the dough on waxed paper, press about 1/4 inch thick with hands, or roll out between waxed papers. For higher biscuits, roll dough 1/2 inch thick. Cut with unfloured biscuit cutter. Bake 10–12 minutes on ungreased cookie sheet. Yields 16 2-inch biscuits

Note: For sweet milk biscuits, omit baking soda and use 3 teaspoons baking powder.

Fat: None
Oil: Total—16 teaspoons; per biscuit—1 teaspoon

QUICK BUTTERMILK ROLLS

1 envelope active dry yeast
1/4 cup warm water
3/4 cup lukewarm buttermilk or nonfat yogurt
1/4 teaspoon baking soda
1 teaspoon sugar
1 teaspoon salt
3 tablespoons oil
21/2 cups all-purpose flour

Dissolve yeast in warm water in medium-sized bowl of mixer. Let stand 5 minutes. Add buttermilk, baking soda, sugar, salt, oil, and 1 cup flour. Beat 2 minutes on Medium or 200 strokes with spoon. Stir in remaining flour. Turn onto lightly floured board. Knead until smooth and elastic, 4–5 minutes. Roll out and shape into crescents, rolling up a triangle from the wide end, or any shape you like. Place on lightly oiled sheet and let rise until double in bulk, 11/2 hours. Preheat oven to 400° F. Bake for 15 minutes or until golden brown. Because there is only one rising time, these could be made for a dinner. Yields 11/2 dozen rolls

Fat: None
Oil: Total—9 teaspoons; per roll—1/2 teaspoon

PIZZA CRUST

1 package active dry yeast
3/4 cup warm water
4 cups all-purpose flour
1 tablespoon sugar
1 teaspoon salt
1 egg, beaten
2 tablespoons oil

Dissolve yeast in warm water. Let stand 5 minutes. Mix flour with sugar and salt. Add dissolved yeast, beaten egg, and oil. Blend until flour is moistened and dough becomes tacky. Turn out on floured board and knead until elastic and pliable. Turn into well-greased bowl. Let rise once about 45 minutes and punch down. Flip over and let rise a second time, approximately 1 hour. Preheat oven to 425° F. Divide dough into 4 pieces and roll out to fit pizza pans. Bake 20 minutes. Yields 4 pizza crusts (8 slices each)

For topping, see Meatless Spaghetti Sauce.

Fat: Total—1 teaspoon; per slice—negligible
Oil: Total—6 teaspoons; per slice—3/16 teaspoon

CHAPTER 26

Pies and Cakes

Butter, margarine, or vegetable shortening is a standard ingredient in recipes for cakes, cookies, pies, and pastries. Since these fats are forbidden, you will have to learn to adapt your recipes to the use of oil. A table for substituting oil for fat is found on p. 121.

It will take a little experimenting to learn the best way to combine oil with the other ingredients when making adjustments in your own recipes. There are two methods that we have found to be the most satisfactory when the recipe calls for eggs. You can gradually add the oil to the beaten eggs, thus emulsifying the oil (as in making mayonnaise), then beat in the sugar before adding the dry ingredients. Or you can gradually add the sugar to the beaten eggs, then gradually add the oil, beating well before adding the dry ingredients. Sometimes the oil can be mixed with the liquid in the recipe. Do not become discouraged if your first attempt does not turn out to suit you. Analyze what you think you might have done wrong and try again. You will soon learn that proper mixing is very important.

As we stated previously, 1 tablespoon of chocolate syrup a day is allowed in this diet. We have included many recipes made with chocolate syrup in this section, but you must be careful that an individual serving does not exceed this allowed amount.

Carob has become quite popular as a chocolate substitute. Carob has many advantages over chocolate. It contains more fiber and has its own natural built-in sweetening. It does not contain caffeine or theobromine. It has less sodium and more calcium and potassium.

Although it is not a perfect substitute, it might be worthwhile trying. Carob is the fruit of the carob tree and bears a close resemblance to an overgrown lima bean pod. It is often called St. John's bread. When finely ground it can be used as a substitute for cocoa, chocolate, and to some extent sugar. Carob powder can be found in specialty food stores. A general rule to remember is to use 3 level tablespoons of carob powder plus 1 tablespoon milk and 1 tablespoon water to equal 1 ounce of chocolate. You will find a recipe for carob nut brownies and a recipe for carob fudge in the candy section.

Sugar has a tendency to increase nervousness in some patients. Products containing sugar should be kept at a minimum. The content of sugar in the following recipes may appear high. It is important to remember that the bulk of salt and sugar in the diet is found in processed foods. The occasional dessert is not harmful on the low-fat diet unless you have a sensitivity to sugar. You can reduce the sugar content accordingly to suit your needs.

With experience and patience you will soon be able to judge what works best for you. Above all, DON'T BE DISCOURAGED.

A Note on Crusts

To obtain a flaky piecrust, first the oil (or mayonnaise) and water must be as cold as possible. Second, the ingredients must be mixed thoroughly and the dough rolled quickly—you must be careful not to reroll the dough more than one time. And third, the oven temperature must be sufficiently high to bake the crust quickly. Any type of crust can be made crisper if it is thoroughly chilled after it has been rolled.

MAYONNAISE PASTRY

8-INCH SINGLE CRUST

1 cup all-purpose flour
1/2 teaspoon salt
1/3 cup mayonnaise
2 tablespoons ice water

Mix flour and salt. Blend mayonnaise and water together. (This is very important.) Then add to flour, stirring until it is completely worked together in a ball. Roll out on a pastry cloth. Or, roll out gently between 2 pieces of waxed paper (wipe table with damp cloth to keep paper from slipping). Roll pastry into 12-inch circle. Peel off top paper; place loosely in pan. Mend cracks in pastry with pieces from edge. Trim 1/2 inch beyond pan edge. Fold extra pastry back and under, then build up fluted edge. Finish pie according to each recipe.

For shell: Preheat oven to 475° F. Prick pastry to prevent puffing during baking. Bake for 12–15 minutes or until light golden brown.

Fat: None
Oil: Total—8 teaspoons; 1/6 recipe—1 1/3 teaspoons

9-INCH SINGLE CRUST
(or small double crust)

1 1/2 cups all-purpose flour
1/3 teaspoon salt
1/2 cup mayonnaise
3 tablespoons ice water

Follow the procedure for the single 8-inch crust.

Fat: None
Oil: Total—12 teaspoons; 1/8 recipe—1 1/2 teaspoons

DOUBLE CRUST

2 cups all-purpose flour
1 teaspoon salt
2/3 cup mayonnaise
4 tablespoons ice water

Follow the procedure for the single 8-inch crust.

Fat: None
Oil: Total—16 teaspoons; 1/8 recipe—2 teaspoons

For two-crust pie: Preheat oven to 425° F. Divide dough in half. Use the larger portion for the bottom pastry. Fit bottom pastry into pie pan. Fill as desired; trim if necessary. Roll remaining dough in similar manner for top crust. Cut slits and place over filling. Trim 1/2 inch beyond rim of pan edge. Fold under. Seal and flute edges. Bake as directed according to each recipe.

OIL PASTRY

9-INCH DOUBLE CRUST

2 cups all-purpose flour
1 1/2 teaspoons salt
1/2 cup oil
1/4 cup skim milk

Mix flour and salt. Pour oil into measuring cup; carefully add skim milk. Pour all at once into flour. (Do not blend milk and oil.) Stir lightly until mixed. Gather into a ball. Roll out between waxed paper. Bake as directed according to each recipe.

Variations:

SPICY PASTRY

Add 1 teaspoon cinnamon or 1/2 teaspoon nutmeg to flour.

SWEET PASTRY

Add 2 tablespoons of sugar to flour.

Fat: None
Oil: Total—24 teaspoons; 1/8 recipe—3 teaspoons

CRANBERRY AND APPLE PIE

Dough for double-crust pie
2 cups cranberries
4 medium tart green apples, peeled, cored, and sliced 1/8 inch thick
*1 cup sugar**
2 tablespoons all-purpose flour
1 teaspoon freshly grated nutmeg

Preheat oven to 450° F. Roll dough out on lightly floured surface to thickness of 1/8 inch. Cut out two 11-inch rounds. Fit one round into 9-inch pie plate. Combine cranberries, apples, sugar, flour, and nutmeg. Spoon into pie plate. Cover with second round. Seal edges; crimp decoratively. Make slits in top to allow steam to escape. Bake 10 minutes. Reduce oven temperature to 375° F. Bake until crust is golden brown and fruit is tender, 35–40 minutes. Serve warm or chilled. Serves 8

Fat: None
Oil: Total—16 teaspoons; 1/8 recipe—2 teaspoons (if mayonnaise crust is used)

* Add up to 1/2 cup more sugar if sweeter flavor is desired in filling.

RHUBARB PIE

1 9-inch unbaked pie shell
2 cups diced rhubarb
1 cup nonfat yogurt
1/2 cup all-purpose flour
1 1/2 cups sugar
1 teaspoon vanilla
Pinch of salt

Preheat oven to 400° F. Prepare pie shell. Place diced rhubarb evenly in bottom of unbaked shell. Beat all remaining ingredients and pour over rhubarb. Bake 10 minutes at 400° F, reduce temperature to 375° F, and continue baking 40 minutes. Serves 8

Fat: None
Oil: Total—12 teaspoons; 1/8 recipe—1 1/2 teaspoons (if mayonnaise crust is used)

KAHLÚA PECAN PIE

1 9-inch unbaked pie shell
3 tablespoons oil
2 teaspoons butter extract
3/4 cup sugar
1 teaspoon vanilla
2 tablespoons all-purpose flour
3 eggs
1/2 cup Kahlúa
1/2 cup dark corn syrup
3/4 cup evaporated skim milk
1 cup pecan halves
Pecan halves for top (approximately 1/2 cup)

Preheat oven to 400° F. Prepare pie crust. Chill. Beat together oil, butter extract, sugar, vanilla, and flour until creamy. Mix well. Beat in eggs one at a time. Stir in Kahlúa, corn syrup, evaporated skim milk, and pecans. Mix well; pour into pie shell. Bake for 10 minutes. Reduce heat to 325° F and bake until firm, about 40 minutes. Chill. When ready to serve, garnish generously with pecan halves. Serves 8–10

Fat: Total—3 teaspoons; per serving—1/3 teaspoon
Oil: Total—57 teaspoons; per serving—7 1/8 teaspoons (including pie crust) (if mayonnaise crust is used)

BRANDIED PUMPKIN PIE

1 9-inch unbaked pie shell
1 cup canned or fresh-cooked pumpkin
1 cup evaporated skim milk, undiluted
1 cup packed light brown sugar
3 eggs, slightly beaten
1/4 cup brandy
1 teaspoon cinnamon
1 teaspoon nutmeg
1/2 teaspoon ginger
1/2 teaspoon mace
3/4 teaspoon salt

Preheat oven to 400° F. Prepare pie shell. Combine pumpkin, milk, and sugar in large bowl. Blend until well mixed. Stir in eggs, brandy, spices, and salt; mix well. Pour filling into pie shell. Bake 50–55 minutes or until tip of sharp knife comes out clean from center. Cool on racks. Serves 6

Fat: Total—3 teaspoons; per serving—1/2 teaspoon
Oil: Total (pastry)—12 teaspoons; per serving (pastry)—2 teaspoons (if mayonnaise crust is used)

LEMON CHIFFON PIE

1 9-inch baked pie shell
1 envelope unflavored gelatin
1/3 cup lemon or lime juice
2/3 cup water
2 tablespoons sugar
1/2 teaspoon grated lemon peel
3 egg whites
1/4 teaspoon salt
1/2 cup light corn syrup

Prepare pie shell. Sprinkle gelatin over lemon juice and water in small saucepan to soften. Add sugar. Stir over very low heat just until gelatin and sugar are completely dissolved. Remove from heat and stir in lemon peel. Chill about 1/2 hour or until mixture is the consistency of unbeaten egg white. Beat egg whites and salt until soft peaks form when beater is raised. Gradually add corn syrup, beating until stiff peaks form. Fold chilled gelatin mixture into beaten egg whites. Chill, stirring occasionally, until thick enough to mound, about 1/2 hour. Pile lightly into pastry shell. Chill. Serves 6

Fat: None
Oil: Total (pastry)—12 teaspoons; per serving (pastry)—2 teaspoons (if mayonnaise crust is used)

ANGEL PIE

1 9-inch baked pie shell
1 1/2 cups boiling water
4 1/2 tablespoons cornstarch
3/4 cup sugar
3 egg whites
Pinch of salt
3 tablespoons sugar
2 teaspoons vanilla
1/2 teaspoon almond extract
Whipped Cream Substitute

Prepare pie shell. Add the boiling water to the cornstarch and sugar, and cook, stirring constantly, until clear and thick. Beat the egg whites with a pinch of salt. Beat the sugar in gradually. Pour the hot mixture gradually over the egg whites, beating constantly. Add the flavorings. Cool. Pour into pie shell and chill. Garnish with Whipped Cream Substitute. Serves 6

Fat: None
Oil: Total (pastry)—12 teaspoons; per serving (pastry)—2 teaspoons (if mayonnaise crust is used)

STRAWBERRY PIE

1 9-inch baked pie shell
1 envelope unflavored gelatin
1/2 cup cold water
3 egg yolks
1/4 teaspoon salt
1 tablespoon lemon juice
1 10-ounce package frozen sliced strawberries, thawed
3 egg whites
1/4 cup sugar

Prepare pie shell. Sprinkle gelatin over cold water. Let stand 5 minutes to soften. In saucepan beat egg yolks lightly; add salt, lemon juice, and half the syrup from strawberries. Cook over low heat until thickened, stirring constantly. Add gelatin; stir until dissolved. Remove from heat. Add strawberries, including remaining syrup. Chill until mixture begins to thicken. Beat egg whites until stiff but not dry. Gradually add sugar, beating until smooth and glossy. Fold into strawberry mixture. Pile lightly into pastry shell. Chill until firm. Serves 6

Fat: Total—3 teaspoons; per serving—1/2 teaspoon
Oil: Total (pastry)—12 teaspoons; per serving (pastry)—2 teaspoons (if mayonnaise crust is used)

APRICOT CHIFFON PIE

1 9-inch baked pie shell
1 package lemon-flavored gelatin
1 1/2 cups apricot syrup (add water if not enough syrup)
1/4 cup orange juice
1/3 cup ice water
1/3 cup nonfat dry milk powder
1 teaspoon lemon juice
1 15 1/2-ounce can apricots, drained and chopped (1 cup)
Whipped Cream Substitute

Prepare pie shell. Dissolve lemon gelatin in 1 cup apricot syrup heated to boiling. Add remaining apricot syrup and orange juice. Chill mixture until it jells. Whip ice water with skim milk powder. When partially whipped, add lemon juice and continue beating until stiff. Fold whipped milk into gelatin mixture. Fold in apricots. Turn into crust and chill until firm. Garnish with Whipped Cream Substitute. Serves 6

Fat: None
Oil: Total (pastry)—12 teaspoons; per serving (pastry)—2 teaspoons (if mayonnaise crust is used)

ANGEL FOOD CAKE

1 1/2 cups egg whites
1/2 teaspoon salt
1 teaspoon cream of tartar
1 1/2 cups sugar
1 1/4 cups cake flour
1 teaspoon vanilla or almond extract
1/4 teaspoon lemon extract

Preheat oven to 350° F. Beat egg whites and salt until frothy; add cream of tartar. Continue beating until egg whites form peaks. Gradually add sugar 2 tablespoons at a time, beating thoroughly after each addition until meringue holds stiff peaks. Gently fold in the cake flour until the mixture is blended. Add flavorings. Pour into a 10-inch tube pan. Bake for 10 minutes, then increase the temperature of the oven to 400° F and continue baking for 20 minutes. Test by lightly touching middle of cake. If no imprint remains, the cake is done. Remove from oven, invert cake over bottle neck or supports, and let hang until cool. Serves 8

Fat: None
Oil: None

FRESH APPLE CAKE

1 cup sugar
1 3/4 cups coarsely chopped apples
1 1/2 cups cake flour
1 teaspoon baking soda
1/2 teaspoon salt
1 teaspoon cinnamon
1/2 teaspoon nutmeg
1/2 teaspoon allspice
1/4 cup oil
1 egg
1/2 cup raisins
1/2 cup chopped walnuts (optional)

Preheat oven to 350° F. Add sugar to apples and let stand 10 minutes. Mix flour with baking soda, salt, and spices. Blend oil and egg into apple mixture. Add cake flour, stirring just until blended. Fold in raisins and nuts. Pour into a waxed-paper-lined 9-inch square pan. Bake 50–55 minutes. Cool 10 minutes. Remove from pan. Cool and sprinkle with confectioners' sugar. Serves 12

Fat: Total—1 teaspoon; per serving—negligible
Oil: Total—12 teaspoons (24 teaspoons if nuts are used); per serving—1 teaspoon (2 teaspoons if nuts are used)

SPICED APPLESAUCE CAKE

3 cups all-purpose flour
1 16-ounce jar applesauce
1 cup sugar
1 cup mayonnaise
1/2 cup skim milk
2 teaspoons baking soda
2 teaspoons ground cinnamon
1 teaspoon vanilla
1/2 teaspoon salt
1/2 teaspoon ground nutmeg
1 cup chopped walnuts
1/2 cup raisins

Preheat oven to 350° F. Oil and flour a 13″ × 9″ × 2″ baking pan. In large bowl with mixer on low speed beat together all the ingredients except walnuts and raisins, just until blended. Increase speed to Medium and continue beating for 2 minutes. Stir in walnuts and raisins. Pour into baking pan. Bake 30–35 minutes or until cake tester inserted in center comes out clean. Cool slightly in pan. Serves 12

Fat: None
Oil: Total—48 teaspoons; per serving—4 teaspoons

CARROT CAKE

1 cup sugar
3/4 cup oil
1 teaspoon vanilla
4 eggs
2 cups all-purpose flour
2 teaspoons baking powder
1 teaspoon baking soda
1 teaspoon cinnamon
1/2 teaspoon allspice
1 8-ounce can crushed pineapple, with juice or syrup
2 cups shredded carrots
1 cup raisins
1 cup finely chopped nuts (optional)

Preheat oven to 375° F. In large bowl combine sugar, oil, and vanilla, and beat well. Add eggs one at a time while beating first ingredients. Mix together flour, baking powder, baking soda, cinnamon, and allspice, and add to egg mixture alternately with crushed pineapple and juice, mixing well. Fold in carrots, raisins, and nuts. Place mixture in an oiled 9″ × 13″ × 2″ pan. Bake 35–40 minutes. Cake is done when it pulls away from sides slightly. Cool in pan 5 minutes. Turn out on rack. When completely cool, frost with Orange Icing. Serves 16

Fat: Total—4 teaspoons; per serving—1/4 teaspoon
Oil: Total—36 teaspoons (60 teaspoons if nuts are used); per serving—2 1/4 teaspoons (3 3/4 teaspoons if nuts are used)

QUICK COFFEE CAKE

1 cup all-purpose flour
2 teaspoons baking powder
1/2 teaspoon salt
1/2 teaspoon cinnamon
1/2 cup sugar
1 egg
1/2 cup skim milk
1 tablespoon grated orange peel
2 tablespoons oil

Preheat oven to 375° F. Mix dry ingredients. Mix egg, milk, orange peel, and oil, and combine with flour mixture. Place in an 8-inch oiled square pan and bake for 25 minutes.

TOPPING

Squeeze 1 medium orange to make juice. Combine with 1/4 cup packed brown sugar, 2 tablespoons peel, and 1/2 cup chopped nuts. Spread over hot coffee cake. Serves 8

Fat: Total—1 teaspoon; per serving—1/8 teaspoon
Oil: Total—18 teaspoons; per serving—2 1/4 teaspoons

HONEY SPICE CAKE

3 1/2 cups all-purpose flour
1 cup sugar
3 teaspoons baking powder
1 teaspoon baking soda
1 teaspoon ground ginger
1 1/2 teaspoons ground cinnamon
3/4 teaspoon ground nutmeg
1/4 teaspoon ground allspice
1/8 teaspoon ground cloves
5 large eggs
1 cup honey
2 teaspoons instant coffee, dissolved in 2/3 cup boiling water and cooled
1/2 cup oil
2 teaspoons vanilla
1 1/2 teaspoons grated orange peel

Preheat oven to 325° F. In a medium bowl stir together flour, sugar, baking powder, baking soda, ginger, cinnamon, nutmeg, allspice, and cloves. In a large bowl combine eggs, honey, coffee, oil, and vanilla. Beat on low speed with an electric mixer until well blended. Gradually beat in flour mixture until smooth. Stir in orange peel. Turn into an oiled and floured 12-cup fluted tube pan. Bake until a cake tester inserted in the center comes out clean, about 1 hour 10 minutes. Cool cake in pan on a wire rack for 10 minutes; with a small narrow metal spatula loosen edges; turn out on rack and cool completely. Serves 16

Fat: Total—5 teaspoons; per serving—1/3 teaspoon
Oil: Total—24 teaspoons; per serving—1 1/2 teaspoons

ZUCCHINI CAKE

3 cups grated zucchini
3 cups sugar
1 1/2 cups oil
4 eggs
3 cups all-purpose flour
2 teaspoons baking powder
1 teaspoon baking soda
1 1/2 teaspoons cinnamon
1/2 teaspoon salt
1 cup chopped nuts

Preheat oven to 300° F. Mix zucchini, sugar, oil, and eggs. Combine dry ingredients and mix well. Add nuts. Oil and flour a 10-inch tube pan. Turn batter into pan and bake for 1 1/2 hours. Let cool in pan for 10 minutes; loosen edges; turn cake out on rack and cool completely. Serves 12

Fat: Total—4 teaspoons; per serving—1/3 teaspoon
Oil: Total—96 teaspoons; per serving—8 teaspoons

ZUCCHINI CAROB CAKE

2 cups all-purpose flour
1 teaspoon baking powder
1 teaspoon baking soda
1 teaspoon cinnamon
1/2 teaspoon nutmeg
1/2 teaspoon salt
1/4 cup carob powder
3 medium eggs
2 cups sugar
1/2 cup oil
3/4 cup buttermilk
2 cups shredded zucchini (1 or 2 medium)
1 cup coarsely chopped walnuts or pecans
1 teaspoon vanilla
1 teaspoon grated orange peel

Preheat oven to 350° F. Mix flour, baking powder, baking soda, spices, salt, and carob powder. Set aside. In large bowl beat eggs until light. Gradually beat in sugar until eggs are fluffy and pale ivory. Slowly beat in oil. Stir in flour mixture, 1/3 at a time, alternately with buttermilk and zucchini. Blend lightly but thoroughly. Stir in nuts, vanilla, and orange peel. Turn into an oiled 13″ × 9″ × 2″ pan. Bake 50–60 minutes. Cool. Serves 16

Fat: Total—3 teaspoons; per serving—1/5 teaspoon
Oil: Total—48 teaspoons; per serving—3 teaspoons

CHOCOLATE FUDGE CAKE

2 cups all-purpose flour
1 cup less 2 tablespoons sugar
2 teaspoons baking soda
1/4 cup chocolate syrup (for a moist cake, add another 1/4 cup)
1/4 teaspoon salt
1 cup mayonnaise
1 cup cold water
1 teaspoon vanilla
1 teaspoon almond extract

Preheat oven to 350° F. Combine all ingredients in large bowl. Beat with electric beater until well blended and free of lumps. Turn into an oiled 12″ × 9″ cake pan and bake 25–30 minutes until toothpick comes out clean. Serves 16

Fat: None
Oil: Total—24 teaspoons; per serving—1 1/2 teaspoons (chocolate syrup per serving—3/4–1 1/2 teaspoons)

CHOCOLATE CHIFFON CAKE I

2 1/2 cups cake flour
1 cup sugar
1 tablespoon baking powder
1 teaspoon salt
1/2 cup oil
6 egg yolks
3/4 cup chocolate syrup
1/4 cup water
1 teaspoon vanilla
1/2 teaspoon cream of tartar
6 egg whites

Preheat oven to 325° F. Mix flour, sugar, baking powder, and salt together. Make a well in the center. Add in order, oil, egg yolks, chocolate syrup, water, and vanilla. Beat with spoon until smooth. Beat cream of tartar with egg whites until very stiff. Gently fold into first mixture, blending well. Do not stir. Turn batter into an oiled 10-inch tube pan. Bake 1–1 1/2 hours until cake springs back when lightly touched with finger. Invert and let cool. Serves 12

Fat: Total—6 teaspoons; per serving—1/2 teaspoon
Oil: Total—24 teaspoons; per serving—2 teaspoons
(chocolate syrup per serving—1 tablespoon)

CHOCOLATE CHIFFON CAKE II

1 3/4 cups cake flour
1 cup sugar
1 teaspoon salt
1/3 cup oil
3/4 cup buttermilk
3/4 teaspoon baking soda
2 egg yolks
1/3 cup chocolate syrup
2 egg whites
Marshmallow Filling

Preheat oven to 350° F. Mix together flour, 1/2 cup sugar, and salt. Add oil and 1/2 cup buttermilk. Beat 1 minute. Add remaining buttermilk, baking soda, egg yolks, and chocolate syrup. Beat 1 minute. Make stiff meringue of egg whites and remaining sugar. Fold into cake batter. Pour into two 8- or 9-inch nonstick or oiled pans. Bake 25–30 minutes. Cool. Slice in two layers and fill with Marshmallow Filling. Serves 10

Fat: Total—2 teaspoons; per serving—1/5 teaspoon
Oil: Total—16 teaspoons; per serving—1 3/5 teaspoons
(chocolate syrup per serving—1/2 teaspoon)

HONEY CAKE

1 cup sugar
3 large eggs
1 cup oil
1 cup honey
2 1/2 cups all-purpose flour
1 teaspoon baking powder
1 teaspoon salt
2 teaspoons cinnamon
1/2 teaspoon allspice
1/4 cup pineapple juice
1/4 cup water
3/4 teaspoon baking soda
1 teaspoon vanilla
1/2 cup chopped pecans (optional)

Preheat oven to 325° F. Combine sugar, eggs, oil, and honey, and beat until very thick. Combine flour, baking powder, salt, and spices, and stir. Combine pineapple juice and water, bring to a boil, and add baking soda. Add juice mixture alternately with dry ingredients to egg mixture. Stir in vanilla and nuts. Pour into a 10-inch nonstick or oiled tube pan, lined with waxed paper in bottom. Bake for 1 hour 15 minutes. Let cool in pan. Serves 12

Fat: Total—3 teaspoons; per serving—1/4 teaspoon
Oil: Total—48 teaspoons (60 teaspoons if nuts are used); per serving—4 teaspoons (5 teaspoons if nuts are used)

ORANGE CHIFFON CAKE

1 1/4 cups cake flour
2 teaspoons baking powder
1/2 teaspoon salt
3/4 cup sugar
1/4 cup oil
3 egg yolks
1/3 cup orange juice
1/2 teaspoon lemon extract
1 teaspoon orange peel
1/4 teaspoon cream of tartar
3 egg whites

Preheat oven to 350° F. Blend together all ingredients except cream of tartar and egg whites. Blend until smooth. Beat egg whites with cream of tartar until very stiff. Fold into first mixture carefully. Bake in an 8-inch tube pan or an 8-inch square pan, ungreased, about 40 minutes. Invert cake in pan over bottle neck and allow to cool completely before removing. Serves 8

Fat: Total—3 teaspoons; per serving—3/8 teaspoon
Oil: Total—12 teaspoons; per serving—1 1/2 teaspoons

LEMON GOLD CAKE

2 1/4 cups cake flour
1 1/2 cups sugar
1 tablespoon baking powder
1 teaspoon salt
1/2 cup oil
6 egg yolks
3/4 cup cold water
2 teaspoons fresh lemon juice
1 teaspoon grated lemon peel
1/2 teaspoon cream of tartar
6 egg whites

Preheat oven to 325° F. Mix flour, sugar, baking powder, and salt together in bowl. Make a well and add in order, oil, egg yolks, water, lemon juice, and lemon peel. Beat with a spoon until smooth. Add cream of tartar to egg whites; beat until very stiff. Pour egg yolk mixture gradually over egg whites, carefully folding with rubber scraper just until blended. Do not stir. Pour immediately into an ungreased 10″ × 4″ tube pan. Bake approximately 1 hour or until top springs back when lightly touched. Invert cake and cool for 1 hour. Loosen sides with spatula. Serves 12

Fat: Total—6 teaspoons; per serving—1/2 teaspoon
Oil: Total—24 teaspoons; per serving—2 teaspoons

MAYONNAISE DATE AND NUT CAKE

1 cup boiling water
1 teaspoon baking soda
1 cup chopped dates
1 cup chopped nuts
1 cup mayonnaise
1 cup granulated sugar
1 cup packed brown sugar
2 tablespoons chocolate syrup
1 1/2 cups all-purpose flour
1 teaspoon vanilla

Preheat oven to 350° F. Pour the boiling water and baking soda over the chopped dates and nuts, and let stand until cool. Mix mayonnaise, sugars, and chocolate syrup. Slowly fold in flour. Add vanilla and date mixture. Bake 40–45 minutes in an 8 1/2″ × 4 1/2″ × 2 1/2″ loaf pan. Yields 1 loaf (16 slices per loaf)

Fat: None
Oil: Total—48 teaspoons; per serving—3 teaspoons
(chocolate syrup per serving—3/8 teaspoon)

DATE AND NUT CAKE

1 teaspoon baking soda
1 cup cut-up pitted dates
1 cup boiling water
1 cup packed brown sugar
2 tablespoons oil
1 egg
2 cups all-purpose flour
1/2 teaspoon baking powder
1 teaspoon vanilla
1/2 cup chopped nuts (optional)

Preheat oven to 350° F. Sprinkle baking soda over dates, add boiling water, and let stand until cool. Cream sugar and oil, add egg, and beat. Add flour, baking powder, and date mixture alternately; add vanilla; fold in nuts. Bake in a waxed-paper-lined 8 1/2″ × 4 1/2″ × 2 1/2″ loaf pan for 45 minutes. Yields 1 loaf (16 slices)

Fat: Total—1 teaspoon; per slice—negligible
Oil: Total—6 teaspoons (18 teaspoons if nuts are used); per slice—3/8 teaspoon (1 1/8 teaspoon if nuts are used)

LUSCIOUS WHITE CAKE

1 1/3 cups cake flour
3/4 cup sugar
3/4 teaspoon salt
2 teaspoons baking powder
1/3 cup oil
2 egg yolks
6 tablespoons water
1 teaspoon vanilla
1/8 teaspoon cream of tartar
3 egg whites
Lemon Filling

Preheat oven to 350° F. Mix dry ingredients together. Make a well and add in order, oil, egg yolks, water, and vanilla. Beat until smooth. Add cream of tartar to egg whites. Beat until whites form very stiff peaks. Gently fold first mixture into egg whites until well blended. Turn into a 9-inch nonstick or oiled layer cake pan. Bake in oven 35–40 minutes or until done. Cool. Split cake and add Lemon Filling. Serves 8

Fat: Total—2 teaspoons; per serving—1/4 teaspoon
Oil: Total—16 teaspoons; per serving—2 teaspoons

LUSCIOUS BANANA CAKE

2 cups cake flour
1 1/2 teaspoons baking powder
1/2 teaspoon baking soda
1 teaspoon salt
1 cup mashed banana
2/3 cup buttermilk
2 egg yolks
3/4 cup plus 1/3 cup sugar
1 teaspoon vanilla
3 egg whites
1/3 cup oil
Whipped Cream Substitute
1 banana, sliced

Preheat oven to 350° F. Mix together flour, baking powder, baking soda, and salt. Set aside. Blend mashed banana and buttermilk. Add egg yolks, 3/4 cup sugar, and vanilla. Blend on low speed until thoroughly mixed. Beat egg whites until stiff, gradually adding remaining 1/3 cup sugar. Place dry ingredients in a mixing bowl; make a well in the center; add the oil and blended banana mixture. Beat together until smooth. Gently fold beaten egg whites into mixture. Pour batter into two 9-inch nonstick or oiled cake pans. Bake 35–40 minutes or until done. Remove from pans and cool. Layer together with Whipped Cream Substitute and banana slices. Serves 10

Fat: Total—2 teaspoons; per serving—1/5 teaspoon
Oil: Total—16 teaspoons; per serving—1 3/5 teaspoons

FROSTED BANANA SQUARES

2 cups all-purpose flour
1 cup sugar
1 teaspoon baking soda
1/2 teaspoon salt
1 cup mashed ripe bananas
2/3 cup mayonnaise
1/4 cup water
1 1/2 teaspoons vanilla
1/2 cup finely chopped nuts

Preheat oven to 350° F. In large bowl combine flour, sugar, baking soda, and salt. Add banana, mayonnaise, water, and vanilla. Beat at medium speed 2 minutes or until smooth. Stir in nuts. Pour into an oiled 9″ × 9″ × 2″ pan. Bake 35–40 minutes or until cake tester inserted in center comes out clean. Cool in pan on wire rack. Frost as desired. Cut into squares. Serves 9

Fat: None
Oil: Total—28 teaspoons; per serving—3 1/9 teaspoons

PINEAPPLE UPSIDE DOWN CAKE

1 tablespoon oil
1 cup packed light brown sugar
1 15 1/2-ounce can pineapple tidbits or slices, drained, saving liquid
3 egg whites
1 cup sugar
3 egg yolks
1 cup cake flour
1 teaspoon baking powder
1/2 cup pineapple juice or syrup

Preheat oven to 350° F. Pour oil in a 10-inch ovenproof skillet. Add brown sugar and spread evenly. Put pineapple tidbits on brown sugar and let bubble on medium heat until sugar is dissolved. (Or pineapple slices can be placed in pan with a cherry in the center of each slice.) Beat egg whites with 1/4 cup sugar until stiff. Beat egg yolks until lemon colored, then gradually add 3/4 cup sugar, beating well after each addition. Add flour that has been mixed with the baking powder alternately with the pineapple juice. Gently fold in the egg whites and pour over the pineapple-brown sugar mixture. Bake 35–40 minutes or until done. Serves 6

Fat: Total—3 teaspoons; per serving—1/2 teaspoon
Oil: Total—3 teaspoons; per serving—1/2 teaspoon

APPLE SPICE CUPCAKES

2 cups cake flour
1/2 teaspoon salt
1/4 teaspoon baking soda
1/2 teaspoon each, cinnamon, cloves, and nutmeg
2 eggs
1/4 cup oil
1 cup sugar
1 teaspoon vanilla
1/2 cup cold double-strength decaffeinated coffee
1 cup chopped raisins
1 cup peeled and chopped apples

Preheat oven to 375° F. Mix flour, salt, baking soda, cinnamon, cloves, and nutmeg. Beat eggs, gradually adding oil, then sugar and vanilla. Beat well. Add dry ingredients alternately with coffee. Stir in fruit. Oil cupcake pans and fill half full. Bake 20 minutes. Yields 1 dozen cupcakes

Fat: Total—2 teaspoons; per cupcake—1/6 teaspoon
Oil: Total—12 teaspoons; per cupcake—1 teaspoon

QUICK CHOCOLATE CUPCAKES

1 1/2 cups all-purpose flour
1 cup sugar
3 tablespoons baking powder
Pinch of salt
1/4 cup skim milk
6 tablespoons chocolate syrup
4 tablespoons oil
1 teaspoon vanilla
1 egg

Preheat oven to 375° F. Mix together flour, sugar, baking powder, and salt. Add skim milk, chocolate syrup, oil, vanilla, and egg; beat well. Oil cupcake pan and fill 2/3 full. Bake 15–20 minutes. Yields 1 dozen cupcakes

Variation: Substitute buttermilk for skim milk; use 1 teaspoon baking soda and 2 teaspoons baking powder.

Fat: Total—1 teaspoon; per cupcake—1/12 teaspoon
Oil: Total—12 teaspoons; per cupcake—1 teaspoon (chocolate syrup per cupcake—1 1/2 teaspoons)

RAISED OVEN DOUGHNUTS

1 1/2 cups skim milk
4 tablespoons granulated sugar
2 teaspoons salt
2 teaspoons nutmeg (optional)
1/4 teaspoon cinnamon (optional)
1/3 cup oil plus 2 teaspoons for brushing
4 3/4 cups all-purpose flour
2 eggs, well beaten
2 envelopes active dry yeast dissolved in 1/4 cup warm water
Confectioners' sugar or Glazing Icing

Scald milk; combine with granulated sugar, salt, spices, and oil in a large mixing bowl. Cool to lukewarm. Add flour, eggs, and dissolved yeast, and beat until well mixed. Cover and let stand in a warm place until dough is double in bulk, about 50–60 minutes. Turn dough onto a well-floured board, turning over 2 or 3 times to shape into a soft ball. (Dough will be soft to handle.) Roll dough out lightly to avoid stretching, about 1/2 inch thick. Cut with a 3-inch doughnut cutter and place rings carefully 2 inches apart on a nonstick baking sheet. (The doughnut rings may also be twisted into figure eight or cruller shapes.) Brush doughnuts lightly with oil and let rise in a warm place until double in bulk, about 20 minutes. Bake in preheated oven at 425° F for 8–10 minutes. After removing from oven, dust with confectioners' sugar or cover with Glazing Icing. Yields 3 dozen doughnuts

Fat: Total—2 teaspoons; per doughnut—negligible
Oil: Total—18 teaspoons; per doughnut—1/2 teaspoon

GINGERBREAD

1/3 cup oil
1/2 cup wheat germ
1 egg
2/3 cup molasses
1/3 cup sugar
3/4 cup nonfat yogurt
1 cup whole wheat flour
3 teaspoons baking powder
1/4 cup nonfat dry milk powder
2 teaspoons ginger
1 teaspoon cinnamon

Preheat oven to 350° F. Combine oil, wheat germ, egg, molasses, sugar, and nonfat yogurt, and stir. Combine wheat flour, baking powder, dry milk powder, ginger, and cinnamon. Combine wet ingredients with dry ingredients, and stir lightly until combined. Do not overmix. Spoon into an 8-inch-square oiled, dusted pan. Bake 45 minutes until knife inserted into bread comes out clean. Serves 8

Fat: 1 teaspoon; per serving—negligible
Oil: 16 teaspoons; per serving—2 teaspoons

CHAPTER 27

Cookies

Cookies made with oil are a challenge because the oil produces a different texture from cookies made with shortening or butter. Altering your favorite recipe may take several trials; however, the following recipes have been kitchen-tested many times. No two people will bake the same cookie recipe alike, so you will have to use your own ingenuity to decide whether you need more or less flour, old-fashioned or quick oats, raisins, and so forth. The most important rule to remember when baking cookies is DO NOT OVERBAKE. Cookies made with oil tend to dry out after a couple of days, so we recommend storing them in the freezing compartment and using them as needed.

BASIC COOKIE RECIPE

2 eggs
1/3 cup oil
1 cup granulated sugar
1/2 cup packed brown sugar
2 teaspoons vanilla
2 cups all-purpose flour
1 teaspoon baking powder
1 teaspoon salt

Preheat oven to 375° F. Beat eggs, gradually adding oil, sugars, and vanilla. Add dry ingredients and blend well. Drop from teaspoon, 2 inches apart, onto nonstick cookie sheet. Bake for 8–10 minutes. Yields 2 dozen

Fat: Total—2 teaspoons; 2 cookies—1/6 teaspoon
Oil: Total—16 teaspoons; 2 cookies—1 1/3 teaspoons

DROP SUGAR COOKIES

2 eggs
2/3 cup oil
2 teaspoons vanilla
3/4 cup sugar
2 1/4 cups all-purpose flour
2 teaspoons baking powder
1/2 teaspoon salt

Preheat oven to 400° F. Beat eggs well, gradually add oil and vanilla. Blend in sugar. Mix together flour, baking powder, and salt. Add to egg mixture. Dough will be soft. Drop by teaspoons, 2 inches apart, on nonstick cookie sheet. Press each cookie flat with bottom of glass dipped in sugar. Bake 8–10 minutes. Yields 2 dozen

Fat: Total—2 teaspoons; 2 cookies—1/6 teaspoon
Oil: Total—32 teaspoons; 2 cookies—2 2/3 teaspoons

CRISP ROLLED COOKIES

2 cups all-purpose flour
1 teaspoon baking powder
1/2 teaspoon salt
1 egg
1 cup sugar
1/4 cup oil
3 tablespoons skim milk
1 teaspoon vanilla

Preheat oven to 375° F. Mix together flour, baking powder, and salt. Beat egg; gradually add sugar, oil, skim milk, and vanilla. Add dry ingredients. Roll dough out to thin sheet and cut into shapes. Sprinkle with sugar and bake on a nonstick cookie sheet for 6–7 minutes. Yields 2 dozen

Fat: Total—1 teaspoon; 2 cookies—1/12 teaspoon
Oil: Total—12 teaspoons; 2 cookies—1 teaspoon

CHEWY OATMEAL COOKIES

2 eggs
2/3 cup oil
1 cup granulated sugar
1 cup packed brown sugar
1 teaspoon vanilla
1/2 teaspoon salt
1 teaspoon baking soda
3 tablespoons boiling water
2 cups all-purpose flour
1 cup old-fashioned rolled oats
1 cup quick rolled oats
1/2 cup raisins
1 cup chopped nuts (optional)

Preheat oven to 350° F. Beat eggs until fluffy. Add oil, sugars, vanilla, and salt. Dissolve baking soda in boiling water and add to mixture. Combine flour and oats, gradually add to oil mixture, and mix until smooth. Add raisins and nuts. Drop from spoon onto nonstick cookie sheet. Bake 10–12 minutes. Remove from pan at once to cooling rack. Yields 6 dozen

Fat: Total—2 teaspoons; 2 cookies—negligible
Oil: Total—32 teaspoons (56 teaspoons if nuts are used); per 2 cookies—1 teaspoon (1 1/2 teaspoons if nuts are used)

CARROT RAISIN OAT COOKIES

1/3 cup packed brown sugar
1/3 cup oil
1/3 cup molasses
1 egg
1/2 teaspoon baking powder
1/2 teaspoon baking soda
1/4 cup nonfat dry milk powder
1 teaspoon salt
1/2 teaspoon cinnamon
1 cup all-purpose flour
1 cup grated raw carrot
3/4 cup raisins
1 1/2 cups quick or old-fashioned rolled oats

Preheat oven to 400° F. In a large bowl beat together sugar, oil, molasses, and egg. Blend in baking powder, baking soda, nonfat dry milk powder, salt, cinnamon, and flour. Mix well. Stir in carrot, raisins, and oats. Mix well. Drop by level measured tablespoonfuls onto a nonstick baking sheet. Bake in preheated oven for 10 minutes. With metal spatula remove cookies from pan and let cool. Yields 3 dozen

Fat: Total—1 teaspoon; per serving—negligible
Oil: Total—24 teaspoons; per 2 cookies—1 1/3 teaspoons

RANGER COOKIES

2 eggs
3/4 cup oil
1 cup packed brown sugar
1 cup granulated sugar
2 teaspoons vanilla
1/2 teaspoon salt
2 cups all-purpose flour
1 teaspoon baking soda
2 cups crisp rice cereal
2 cups quick rolled oats
1/2 cup chopped nutmeats (optional)

Preheat oven to 350° F. Beat eggs until fluffy; add oil, sugars, vanilla, and salt. Combine flour and baking soda, and add to mixture. Stir in crisp rice cereal, oatmeal, and nuts. Do not add more flour and do not refrigerate. Bake immediately. Drop by teaspoonfuls onto nonstick pans and press dough with fork before baking. Bake 10–15 minutes. Yields 8 dozen

Fat: Total—2 teaspoons; per 2 cookies—negligible
Oil: Total—36 teaspoons (48 teaspoons if nuts are used); per 2 cookies—3/4 teaspoon (1 teaspoon if nuts are used)

BRANALL COOKIES

2 eggs
1/2 cup oil
1/2 cup molasses
3/4 cup packed brown sugar
1/4 cup granulated sugar
1 teaspoon baking soda
4 teaspoons hot water
1/2 cup all-purpose flour
1/2 teaspoon salt
2 teaspoons cinnamon
1 teaspoon ground cloves
1/2 teaspoon ground ginger
2 1/2 cups whole wheat flour
1/4 cup wheat germ
1 cup raw bran
1 cup graham flour
1 cup walnuts (optional)

Preheat oven to 350° F. Beat eggs; add oil, molasses, and sugars. Dissolve baking soda in hot water and add to mixture. Sift flour with salt and spices and add to egg mixture; then stir in whole wheat flour, wheat germ, bran, graham flour, and nuts. Form into balls. Place on oiled cookie sheets, and flatten with a wet fork. Bake 12–15 minutes. Yields approximately 6 dozen

Variation: Raisins or dates can be added. Try soaking them in wine (port) or fruit juice 24–48 hours before using, then drain well.

Fat: Total—2 teaspoons; per 2 cookies—negligible
Oil: Total—24 teaspoons (48 teaspoons if nuts are used); per 2 cookies—2/3 teaspoon (1 1/3 teaspoons if nuts are used)

MOLASSES SUGAR COOKIES

2/3 cup oil
1/4 cup molasses
1 egg
1 cup packed brown sugar
1/4 teaspoon salt
2 1/4 cups all-purpose flour
1 teaspoon baking powder
1 teaspoon baking soda
1/2 teaspoon ground cloves
1 teaspoon ginger
1 teaspoon cinnamon
Granulated sugar

Preheat oven to 375° F. Beat together oil, molasses, and egg thoroughly. Add sugar. Mix together dry ingredients and spices, and add to first mixture. Mix well. Chill dough for 1 hour. Form into 1-inch balls. Roll balls in granulated sugar. Place 2 inches apart on nonstick cookie sheet. Sprinkle each cookie with 2 or 3 drops of water. Bake 8–10 minutes. Do not overbake. Yields 4 dozen

Fat: Total—1 teaspoon; per 2 cookies—negligible
Oil: Total—32 teaspoons; per 2 cookies—1 1/3 teaspoons

PEANUT BUTTER COOKIES

1 egg
1/2 cup packed brown sugar
1/2 cup granulated sugar
1/3 cup oil
1/2 teaspoon vanilla
2/3 cup nonprocessed peanut butter
1 1/4 cups all-purpose flour
1/2 teaspoon baking powder
1/2 teaspoon baking soda
1/4 teaspoon salt

Preheat oven to 350° F. Beat egg. Add sugars gradually, then oil, vanilla, and peanut butter. Beat well. Combine flour, baking powder, baking soda, and salt. Stir into peanut butter mixture; stir until well blended. Form into balls about 1 inch in diameter. Place on nonstick cookie sheet about 2 inches apart. Press cookies flat with flour-coated tines of fork. Bake 10–12 minutes. Yields 4 dozen

Fat: Total—1 teaspoon; per 2 cookies—negligible
Oil: Total—32 teaspoons; per 2 cookies—1 1/3 teaspoons

ORANGE COOKIES

1 egg
2/3 cup packed light brown sugar
1/4 cup oil
1/4 cup orange juice
2 teaspoons grated orange peel
1 1/2 cups all-purpose flour
1/2 teaspoon baking soda
1/2 teaspoon baking powder
1/2 teaspoon salt

Preheat oven to 350° F. Beat egg; gradually add sugar and oil, then orange juice and grated orange peel. Combine flour, baking soda, baking powder, and salt. Add to egg mixture. Drop with teaspoon onto nonstick cookie sheet and bake 8 minutes. When cookies are cool, ice with Orange Icing. Yields 2 dozen

Fat: Total—1 teaspoon; per 2 cookies—negligible
Oil: Total—12 teaspoons; per 2 cookies—1 teaspoon

ORANGE ICING

2 tablespoons orange juice
1 tablespoon grated orange peel
1/8 teaspoon salt
1 cup confectioners' sugar

In a small saucepan heat, but do not boil, the orange juice, orange peel, and salt. Stir in enough confectioners' sugar to make consistency for easy spreading. Yields 1 cup

Fat: None
Oil: None

SPICY APPLE COOKIES

2 cups all-purpose flour
1 teaspoon baking powder
1/2 teaspoon baking soda
1/2 teaspoon salt
1/4 teaspoon nutmeg
1/4 teaspoon cinnamon
1/3 cup oil
1 cup packed brown sugar
1 egg
1 tablespoon water
1 cup raisins
1 1/4 cups peeled grated raw apples

Preheat oven to 375° F. Combine flour, baking powder, baking soda, salt, nutmeg, and cinnamon. Add oil, sugar, egg, and water, and beat until smooth. Stir in raisins and apples. Drop with teaspoon onto nonstick cookie sheet. Bake 12–15 minutes. These are soft cookies. Yields 4 dozen

Fat: Total—1 teaspoon; per 2 cookies—negligible
Oil: Total—16 teaspoons; per 2 cookies—2/3 teaspoon

RAGGED ROBINS

2 eggs
1/2 cup sugar
1 teaspoon vanilla
1 cup chopped dates
2 cups cornflakes

Preheat oven to 350° F. Beat eggs until lemon-colored; gradually add sugar and vanilla. Add dates and cornflakes. Shape into balls. Bake on waxed-paper-covered cookie sheet until light brown. Yields 2 dozen

Fat: Total—2 teaspoons; per 2 cookies—1/6 teaspoon
Oil: None

DATE COOKIES

2 cups all-purpose flour
2 teaspoons baking powder
1/2 teaspoon salt
1/2 teaspoon cinnamon
1 egg
1/2 cup oil
1 cup packed brown sugar
1/2 cup skim milk
1/2 teaspoon almond extract
1/2 teaspoon vanilla
1/2 cup chopped dates

Preheat oven to 400° F. Combine flour, baking powder, salt, and cinnamon. Set aside. Beat egg; gradually add oil, then add brown sugar. Add combined dry ingredients, milk, almond extract, and vanilla. Fold in dates. Drop by teaspoonfuls onto nonstick cookie sheet. Bake for 15 minutes until nicely browned. Yields 4 dozen

Fat: Total—1 teaspoon; per 2 cookies—negligible
Oil: Total—24 teaspoons; per 2 cookies—1 teaspoon

CHOCOLATE BROWNIES

2 eggs
3/4 cup granulated sugar
1/2 teaspoon vanilla
1/2 cup chocolate syrup
1/3 cup oil
3/4 cup all-purpose flour
1/2 teaspoon salt
1/2 cup chopped nuts

Preheat oven to 350° F. Beat eggs until foamy. Add sugar and vanilla. Beat until thick. Add chocolate syrup and oil. Beat until smooth, then add flour and salt. Mix thoroughly; add nuts or sprinkle them on top for a crisp crust. Spread in an 8-inch nonstick square pan. Bake for 30 minutes. Cut into squares while warm and remove from pan. Yields 16 brownies

Fat: Total—2 teaspoons; per brownie—1/8 teaspoon
Oil: Total—28 teaspoons; per brownie—1 3/4 teaspoons (chocolate syrup per brownie—1 1/2 teaspoons)

SEAFOAM NUT KISSES

1 egg white
1/4 cup nonfat dry milk powder
1 tablespoon water
3/4 cup packed brown sugar
1/8 teaspoon salt
1 tablespoon all-purpose flour
1 cup chopped nuts or fruits or cereals

Preheat oven to 325° F. With electric mixer at high speed, beat egg white, dry milk powder, and water in small mixing bowl until stiff. Beat in brown sugar a tablespoon at a time to make a thick glossy meringuelike mixture. Scrape sides of bowl often. Fold in salt, flour, nuts, fruits, or cereals. Drop by teaspoonfuls onto waxed-paper-covered cookie sheet. Bake about 15 minutes until light brown. Remove at once and cool on wire rack. Yields 2 dozen

Fat: None
Oil: Total—24 teaspoons (if nuts are used); per 2 cookies—2 teaspoons (if nuts are used)

DATE BARS

2 eggs
1/2 cup packed brown sugar
1/2 teaspoon vanilla
1/2 teaspoon baking powder
1/2 cup all-purpose flour
1/2 teaspoon salt
2 cups chopped dates
1/2 cup chopped nuts

Preheat oven to 325° F. Beat eggs until light and lemon color; gradually add sugar and vanilla. Combine baking powder, flour, and salt, and fold into the egg mixture. Then add the dates and nuts. Spread mixture in an oiled 8-inch square pan. Bake 25–30 minutes or until done. Cool and cut into squares. Yields 16 bars

Fat: Total—2 teaspoons; per bar—1/8 teaspoon
Oil: Total—12 teaspoons (if nuts are used); per bar—3/4 teaspoon (if nuts are used)

PFEFFERNUSSE

4 eggs
1 pound confectioners' sugar
4 cups all-purpose flour
2 teaspoons baking powder
1/2 teaspoon salt
1 tablespoon cinnamon
1 teaspoon nutmeg
1 teaspoon ground cloves
1 cup chopped nuts
1/4 cup chopped citron
1/4 cup chopped lemon peel

Preheat oven to 325° F. Beat eggs until light. Gradually add confectioners' sugar. Combine flour, baking powder, salt, and spices, then add to egg mixture. Stir in the nuts, citron, and lemon peel. Chill dough 30 minutes. Shape into small balls. Place 1 inch apart onto nonstick cookie sheet. Bake until light brown, about 15 minutes. Remove from pan while slightly warm. Cool and store in tightly covered container 5–6 days before using. Yields 5 dozen

Fat: Total—4 teaspoons; per 2 cookies—2/15 teaspoon
Oil: Total—24 teaspoons (if nuts are used); per 2 cookies—4/5 teaspoon (if nuts are used)

LEBKUCHEN

1/2 cup honey
1/2 cup molasses
1 egg
3/4 cup packed brown sugar
1 tablespoon lemon juice
1 tablespoon grated lemon peel
2 3/4 cups all-purpose flour
1/2 teaspoon baking soda
1 teaspoon each, cinnamon, nutmeg, ground cloves, and allspice
1/3 cup chopped citron
1/4 cup chopped nuts
Glazing Icing

Preheat oven to 400° F. Mix honey and molasses (or use all honey) and bring to boil. Cool thoroughly. Stir in the egg, sugar, lemon juice, and lemon peel. Combine dry ingredients and spices, and stir into mixture. Add citron and nuts. Chill dough overnight. Roll small amount at a time, keeping rest chilled. Roll out 1/4 inch thick and cut into oblong pieces 1 1/2″ × 2 1/2″. Place 1 inch apart on nonstick baking sheet. Bake until no imprint remains when touched lightly, approximately 10–12 minutes. While cookies bake, make Glazing Icing. Brush icing over cookies when right out of the oven. Quickly remove from baking sheet. Cool and store to mellow. Yields 6 dozen

Fat: Total—1 teaspoon; per 2 cookies—negligible
Oil: Total—6 teaspoons (if nuts are used); per 2 cookies—1/6 teaspoon (if nuts are used)

DATE-NUT DROPS

1 cup all-purpose flour
1 teaspoon baking powder
1/8 teaspoon salt
3 egg whites
1 cup granulated sugar
1/4 teaspoon grated lemon peel
1/2 teaspoon vanilla
1 cup chopped dates
1 cup chopped nuts

Preheat oven to 350° F. Combine flour, baking powder, and salt. Beat egg whites until foamy; gradually add sugar and beat until stiff. Add lemon peel and vanilla. Gently fold in flour and then dates and nuts. Drop by teaspoonfuls onto nonstick cookie sheet. Bake 8–10 minutes. Yields 4 dozen

Fat: None
Oil: Total—24 teaspoons (if nuts are used); per 2 cookies—1 teaspoon (if nuts are used)

PEANUT DROPS

1/2 cup granulated sugar
1/2 cup light corn syrup
1 cup nonprocessed chunky peanut butter
2 cups cornflakes

Combine sugar and corn syrup and bring to boil, stirring constantly. Continue stirring, reduce heat, and boil slowly for 1 minute. Remove from heat, add peanut butter and cornflakes, and mix well. Drop by teaspoonfuls onto foil. Yields 2 dozen

Fat: None
Oil: Total—24 teaspoons; per 2 cookies—2 teaspoons

CAROB COOKIES

1/2 cup oil
1/3 cup packed brown sugar
1 egg
1 cup all-purpose flour
1 teaspoon baking powder
2 tablespoons carob powder
1/4 teaspoon vanilla

Preheat oven to 350° F. Beat oil and sugar together until light and fluffy. Beat in egg. Add remaining ingredients and mix well. With floured hands, roll mixture into 1-inch balls. Place on oiled baking sheets. Flatten the balls with flour-covered fork. Bake 10 minutes or until golden. Yields 1 1/2 dozen

Fat: Total—1 teaspoon; per 2 cookies—negligible
Oil: Total—24 teaspoons; per 2 cookies—2 2/3 teaspoons

UNBAKED CAROB BALLS

1 cup honey
1 cup nonprocessed peanut butter
1 cup nonfat dry milk
1 cup carob powder
1/2 cup raisins

Combine all ingredients. Mix well and form into balls. Yields 3 dozen

Fat: None
Oil: Total—24 teaspoons; per carob ball—2/3 teaspoon

CHAPTER 28

Desserts

Desserts are not an important part of the Swank low-fat diet. Conventional desserts are similar to meat sauces in that they are satisfying to the palate, but at the same time are rich in calories and especially high in fats. To satisfy those who feel a meal is incomplete without something to top it off, we advocate fresh or canned fruits. For others, we are adding a few desserts that our patients have found tasteful and yet lack both fat and oil.

There are those who feel strongly that sugars should be eliminated from the diet. We do not go that far. We have reduced substantially the amounts of sugar each individual will receive, substituting more complicated carbohydrates such as starches and rice, which are digested more slowly, and proteins such as skim milk and nonfat dry milk powder, cottage cheese, eggs, gelatin, and nuts, all of which delay the absorption of the sugar. With the help of chopped fruits, these desserts become substantially higher in nutritional values.

There are many commercially prepared fruit sorbets and Italian fruit ices available. Even though they appear high in sugar, the average serving is small as it does not take much to be satisfying.

For most of us a satisfactory end to the meal is essential. We believe we have provided many dessert ideas in this section without adding to the problem of keeping the fat intake below 3 teaspoons each day.

BASIC CUSTARD RECIPES

2 or 3 whole eggs or 4–6 egg yolks
1/8 teaspoon salt
4 tablespoons sugar
2 cups skim milk enriched with 1/4 cup nonfat dry milk powder
Flavoring of your choice

SOFT CUSTARD

Blend eggs, salt, and sugar. Scald skim and powdered nonfat dry milk in top of double boiler, and pour slowly over egg mixture.

Return to double boiler and cook over steaming hot (not boiling) water until mixture coats spoon. Remove top of double boiler from hot water immediately to prevent further cooking. Add the flavoring.

FLOATING ISLAND

Make custard with egg yolks only. Use whites to make meringue islands. Drop on warm custard, or cook in simmering water until set, about 5 minutes, and arrange on custard.

SPANISH CREAM

Make custard with egg yolks only. Soften 1 tablespoon unflavored gelatin in 1/4 cup cold water and add to mixture while cooking. Cool slightly and fold in stiffly beaten whites. Chill until firm.

TRIFLE

Line deep bowl with sliced sponge cake. Pour a small amount of sherry over cake if desired. Add cooked custard. Top with sweetened crushed fruit or berries. Chill. Serve with Whipped Cream Substitute.

BAKED CUSTARD

Blend eggs, salt, and sugar. Do not beat eggs because the incorporated air may make a porous custard. Blend skim milk with powdered nonfat dry milk and scald, then slowly pour over egg mixture, stirring constantly. Strain. Add flavoring. Pour into custard cups. Place cups in a pan and fill pan with hot water to 1 inch from the top of the cups. Bake in a slow 325° F oven until a knife inserted in the center of the custard comes out clean. Remove from hot water immediately. If one large pan is used for baking, use 3 whole eggs or 6 egg yolks to make custard. Yields 6 servings

CARAMEL OR MAPLE FLAVORING

Place a tablespoon of caramel or maple syrup in the bottom of each custard cup before adding mixture. The syrup will form a sauce when the custard is turned out.

BREAD PUDDING

Soak 3 slices of bread, cut in cubes, in skim milk. Reduce eggs by half. Add raisins if desired.

Fat: Total—2–6 teaspoons; per serving—1/3–1 teaspoon
Oil: None

FLAN
(Custard with Caramel)

1 1/4 cups sugar
1/4 cup oil
2 cups milk (1 cup nonfat dry milk beaten with water to make 2 cups)
3 eggs
1/4 cup sugar
1 teaspoon vanilla

Preheat oven to 325° F. Mix 1 cup sugar and oil in moderately hot frying pan until sugar is caramel-colored. Pour into custard cups or pie or cake pan. In blender add milk, eggs, remaining 1/4 cup sugar, and vanilla. Blend. Pour mixture over caramel. Place baking dish(es) in a pan of boiling water. Bake for 1 hour or until a knife placed in center comes out clean. Yields 6 servings

Fat: Total—3 teaspoons; per serving—1/2 teaspoon
Oil: Total—12 teaspoons; per serving—2 teaspoons

RICE PUDDING SUPREME

1 cup water, lightly salted
1/2 cup rice
4 cups skim milk
1/2 cup nonfat dry milk powder
3 eggs
1/2 cup sugar
1 cup plump raisins, presoaked in port wine
1/2 teaspoon vanilla
1 tablespoon cinnamon
3 tablespoons sugar

In a large pot bring 1 cup lightly salted water to a boil. Pour rice slowly into the water. Do not stir. Cover tightly and cook exactly 7 minutes. The rice will appear slightly underdone. Add the skim milk and nonfat dry powdered milk. Stir. Bring to a boil, cover, and cook slowly over low heat for 1 hour. Beat eggs, and add the 1/2 cup sugar, raisins, and vanilla. Pour mixture into rice, stirring slowly until the rice begins to thicken. Serve hot, warm, or cold with mixture of cinnamon and sugar sprinkled lightly and evenly over the top. Serves 6

Fat: Total—3 teaspoons; per serving—1/2 teaspoon
Oil: None

RHUBARB CRISP

3 cups 1/2-inch pieces rhubarb (1 1/2 pounds)
3/4 cup granulated sugar
1 egg, well beaten
2 tablespoons all-purpose flour
4 tablespoons oil
1/3 cup packed brown or granulated sugar
2/3 cup all-purpose flour

Preheat oven to 375° F. Mix rhubarb, 3/4 cup sugar, egg, and 2 tablespoons flour together, and spread into a deep dish. Mix oil, 1/3 cup sugar, and 2/3 cup flour together until crumbly; crumble over rhubarb mixture, pressing it down. Bake for 30 minutes or until rhubarb is tender when tested with a fork. Yields 6 servings

Fat: Total—1 teaspoon; per serving—1/6 teaspoon
Oil: Total—12 teaspoons; per serving—2 teaspoons

APPLE CRISP

4–5 tart cooking apples
Cinnamon
Nutmeg
Ground cloves
1/3 cup granulated sugar
1 cup quick rolled oats
1/2 cup all-purpose flour
1 cup packed brown sugar
3 tablespoons oil

Preheat oven to 375° F. Peel apples and slice into a deep baking dish. Sprinkle with spices (if desired) and granulated sugar. Blend together the oats, flour, brown sugar, and oil, then press this mixture on top of the apple slices. Bake for 30 minutes or until apples are tender when tested with a fork. Yields 6 servings

Variation: Crust for Rhubarb Crisp may be substituted.

Fat: None
Oil: Total—9 teaspoons; per serving—1 1/2 teaspoons

BERRY COBBLER

2/3–1 cup granulated sugar
2 tablespoons cornstarch
3/4 cup water
3 cups fresh or frozen berries
1 teaspoon cinnamon or other flavorings
1 cup all-purpose flour
1 1/2 teaspoons baking powder
1/2 teaspoon salt
1/3 cup skim milk
3 tablespoons oil

Preheat oven to 425° F. Mix sugar and cornstarch in saucepan; stir in water. Boil 1 minute, stirring constantly. Add fruit. Pour into an 8-inch baking dish or pie pan, top with cinnamon or desired flavoring. Combine flour, baking powder, and salt. Mix skim milk and oil, and add all at once to flour, stirring with fork until mixture forms a ball. Drop mixture by teaspoonfuls onto fruit. Bake 25–30 minutes until lightly browned. Yields 6 servings

Variation: For canned fruits use 3 cups drained fruit and 3/4 cup of the fruit syrup instead of the fresh fruit and water. Use only 1/2 cup sugar.

Fat: None
Oil: Total—9 teaspoons; per serving—1 1/2 teaspoons

CHOCOLATE TEMPTATION

1 cup all-purpose flour
1/4 teaspoon salt
2 teaspoons baking powder
1/2 cup sugar less one tablespoon
1/2 cup skim milk
4 tablespoons chocolate syrup
1 tablespoon oil
1/2 cup coarsely chopped nuts (optional)

TOPPING

1/4 cup packed brown sugar
3 tablespoons granulated sugar
2 tablespoons chocolate syrup
1 cup boiling water
Whipped Cream Substitute

Preheat oven to 350° F. In a large bowl, mix dry ingredients. Add milk, chocolate syrup, and oil all at once, beating until smooth. Add nuts. Spread batter in a 9-inch square pan. For topping, sprinkle sugars over top of batter. Mix chocolate syrup and water, and pour over entire mixture. (Pour water from measuring cup into tablespoon, letting it overflow onto batter.) Bake immediately for 45 minutes. Serve hot or cold with Whipped Cream Substitute. Yields 6 servings

Fat: None
Oil: Total—3 teaspoons (15 teaspoons if nuts are used); per serving—1/2 teaspoon (2 1/2 teaspoons if nuts are used)
(chocolate syrup per serving—3 teaspoons)

EASY CHEESECAKE

1 3/4 cups graham cracker crumbs
1/4 cup oil
1 3-ounce package lemon-flavored gelatin
1 cup hot water or fruit juice
1 teaspoon salt
2 cups rinsed low-fat or dry-curd cottage cheese
1 cup Whipped Powdered Milk
1 teaspoon vanilla

Combine 1 1/2 cups crumbs with oil. Press 1 1/4 cups of crumb mixture in bottom and on sides of a 12″ × 9″ nonstick pan. Mix gelatin with hot water until completely dissolved. Stir in salt. Chill until mixture begins to thicken. If a smooth consistency is desired, mix the cottage cheese in a blender before adding to gelatin mixture along with the whipped powdered milk and vanilla. Turn into the crumb-lined pan; sprinkle with remaining 1/2 cup crumbs. Chill until firm. Yields 16 servings

Variations: Orange or pineapple juice may be substituted for the water. Garnish with drained orange segments or pineapple slices.

Fat: None
Oil: Total—12 teaspoons; per serving—3/4 teaspoon

CHEESECAKE

5 eggs
2 cups dry-curd or rinsed low-fat cottage cheese
3 tablespoons all-purpose flour
1 teaspoon grated lemon peel
2 teaspoons vanilla
1 cup granulated sugar
1 cup nonfat yogurt

Preheat oven to 325° F. Mix the eggs, cottage cheese, flour, lemon peel, and vanilla in blender until smooth. Pour into bowl and stir in sugar and yogurt. Pour into 9″ × 12″ nonstick pan. Bake for 40 minutes or until center is slightly less than firm. (The cake sets as it cools.) Chill. Garnish with berries or sliced fruit. Yields 15 servings

Fat: Total—5 teaspoons; per serving—1/3 teaspoon
Oil: None

HOLIDAY STEAMED PUDDING

1/4 cup oil
1/2 cup molasses
1 egg
2 cups soft bread crumbs
1/4 cup all-purpose flour
1 teaspoon cinnamon
1/2 teaspoon salt
1/4 teaspoon each, cloves, nutmeg, and allspice
1/2 teaspoon baking soda
1 cup milk
1/2 cup raisins
1/2 cup candied fruits
1/2 cup chopped nuts (optional)

Combine oil, molasses, and egg. Beat well. Add bread crumbs, flour, seasonings, baking soda, and milk. Fold in raisins, candied fruits, and nuts. Turn batter into a 2-quart mold (or 8 individual molds). Cover and steam for 2 hours (1 hour for individual molds). Cool for 10 minutes before removing from molds. Serve hot with sauce, or cool, wrap well, and store. (Brandy can be substituted for all or part of the milk.) Serves 8

Fat: Total—1 teaspoon; per serving—1/8 teaspoon
Oil: Total—12 teaspoons (24 teaspoons if nuts are used); per serving—1 1/2 teaspoons (3 teaspoons if nuts are used)

CAROB CHIFFON DESSERT

1 envelope unflavored gelatin
1/4 cup sugar
1/4 teaspoon salt
1/3 cup carob powder
3 egg yolks
1 1/2 cups skim milk
1/4 cup nonfat dry milk powder
1 teaspoon vanilla
3 egg whites
Mocha Topping

Mix together gelatin, sugar, salt, and carob powder in top of double boiler. Beat egg yolks. Combine skim milk, and nonfat dry milk powder, and add to egg yolks. Mix well and add to gelatin mixture. Cook over boiling water, stirring constantly until gelatin is thoroughly dissolved, about 5 minutes. Remove from heat. Add vanilla. Chill until mixture begins to thicken. Beat egg whites until stiff and fold into gelatin mixture. Turn into individual molds and chill until firm. Unmold and serve with Mocha Topping. Yields 8 servings

Fat: Total—3 teaspoons; per serving—3/8 teaspoon
Oil: None

LEMON FLUFF

1 3-ounce package lemon-flavored gelatin
1 1/2 cups boiling water
1/4 cup lemon juice
3/4 cup sugar
1 14 1/2-ounce can evaporated skim milk, chilled 3–4 hours or longer
*2 cups graham cracker crumbs or crumbled vanilla wafers**

Dissolve gelatin in boiling water. Chill until partially set. Then whip until light and fluffy. Add lemon juice and sugar slowly. Whip chilled milk until it forms soft peaks. Fold gently into gelatin mixture. Press crumbs into an 8″ × 12″ baking dish, reserving 1/4 cup to sprinkle on top. Chill in refrigerator until set or overnight. Serves 12

Fat: None
Oil: None

* Per day 2–3 graham crackers or vanilla wafers are permissible.

BAKED LEMON PUDDING

2 tablespoons oil
1 cup sugar
2 egg yolks
1 juiced lemon and grated peel
3 tablespoons all-purpose flour
1 cup skim milk
2 egg whites, stiffly beaten

Preheat oven to 325° F. Beat oil, sugar, and egg yolks. Add lemon juice and grated peel. Add flour slowly. Add milk and beat gently. Fold in egg whites. Pour into baking dish and set in pan of water. Bake for 30–35 minutes. When finished, pudding has a light sponge cake top with lemon custard base. It can also be baked in individual cups. Serves 8

Fat: Total—2 teaspoons; per serving—1/4 teaspoon
Oil: Total—6 teaspoons; per serving—3/4 teaspoon

FRUIT WHIP

3 egg whites
1/2 cup sugar
2 tablespoons lemon juice
3 tablespoons fruit juice
1 teaspoon grated lemon peel
Dash of salt
1/2 cup chopped and cooked prunes, apricots, etc.

Combine all ingredients except fruit in top of double boiler. Cook, beating constantly with an electric beater, until mixture forms peaks, approximately 7 minutes. Fold in fruit. Chill until ready to serve. Serves 6

Fat: None
Oil: None

RASPBERRY FRUIT ICE ALASKA

4 oranges
3 10-ounce packages frozen raspberries
3 egg whites
1/4 cup sugar
1 teaspoon finely grated orange peel

Juice oranges. Scrape out the pith and set orange peel shells aside. Press raspberries through a fine wire strainer, discarding seeds. Stir in 1/4 cup orange juice. Pour into a freezer tray and partially freeze. Remove and whip until smooth. Carefully spoon raspberry purée into orange shells. Return to freezer and freeze until firm. Beat egg whites to stiff peaks, gradually adding sugar and 2 tablespoons orange juice. Fold in finely grated orange peel. Frost frozen purée in orange shells with meringue. Place shells on baking sheet and broil quickly until meringue is golden brown, approximately 5 minutes. Serves 8

Variation: As an alternate when fresh fruit is available, use 3 cups raspberries or strawberries with 1/2 cup sugar to make the fruit ice.

Fat: None
Oil: None

FRESH RASPBERRY SHERBET

1 envelope unflavored gelatin
3/4 cup sugar
2 cups water
1 quart fresh or frozen raspberries
2 tablespoons lemon juice
2 egg whites
1/8 teaspoon salt

In a saucepan combine gelatin and 1/4 cup of sugar. Stir in water. Heat, stirring, until the sugar and gelatin are completely dissolved. Remove from heat and cool. Press raspberries through a fine wire strainer, discarding seeds. Add raspberry purée and lemon juice to the sugar mixture. Refrigerate until the consistency of unbeaten egg whites. Beat egg whites with salt until frothy. Gradually add remaining 1/2 cup sugar, beating after each addition until glossy. Fold into partially set gelatin. Turn into a 2-quart freezer tray and freeze until firm. Turn into bowl, break up with a spoon, and beat until fluffy. Return to freezer, cover, and store until needed. Yields about 2 quarts

Fat: None
Oil: None

RASPBERRY BAVARIAN

3/4 cup fresh or frozen raspberries
1 3-ounce package raspberry-flavored gelatin
1 cup boiling water
3/4 cup cold water
3 tablespoons lemon juice
3 tablespoons nonfat dry milk
3 tablespoons ice-cold water

Press raspberries through a fine wire strainer, discarding seeds. Dissolve gelatin in the boiling water; add cold water and lemon juice. Refrigerate until mixture begins to thicken, then beat until frothy. Beat nonfat dry milk with ice-cold water until consistency of whipped cream. Fold whipped milk into gelatin. Add strained raspberries. Spoon into six dessert glasses. Chill. Serves 6

Fat: None
Oil: None

CRANBERRY SHERBET

1 can jellied cranberry sauce (16 ounces)
2 tablespoons lemon juice
1/4 cup sweetened pineapple juice
Grated peel of 1 lemon
2 egg whites
2 tablespoons confectioners' sugar

Crush cranberry sauce with fork. Add juices and lemon peel. Pour into freezer tray and freeze until mushy. Beat egg whites until stiff, gradually adding sugar. Fold into frozen mixture. Return to refrigerator and freeze until stiff. Serves 6

Fat: None
Oil: None

LEMON MILK SHERBET

3/4 cup sugar
1/4 teaspoon salt
1 cup water
2–3 cups skim milk
1/2 cup lemon juice
1/2 cup nonfat dry milk powder
3 egg whites
2/3 cup light corn syrup

Combine sugar, salt, and water, and cook for 5 minutes. Cool; add skim milk, lemon juice, and nonfat dry milk powder. Freeze until firm. Turn into a chilled bowl and beat thoroughly. Beat egg whites until stiff, gradually adding 2/3 cup light corn syrup, and continue to beat until very stiff. Fold in frozen mixture and return to freezer. Serves 6

Fat: None
Oil: None

IMITATION SOFT ICE CREAM

3 overripe bananas
3/4 cup skim milk
1/8 teaspoon salt
1 1/2 teaspoons vanilla
1 tablespoon chocolate syrup

Peel and freeze bananas in plastic wrap. In blender add skim milk, salt, vanilla, and chocolate syrup, and blend thoroughly. Add frozen bananas and blend until the consistency of soft ice cream. Serve immediately. Serves 4

Fat: None
Oil: None
(chocolate syrup per serving—3/4 teaspoon)

CHAPTER 29

Icings and Dessert Sauces

Conventional icings, fillings, and dessert sauces, though satisfying to the taste, are often low on the nutritional scale and very high in calories, especially from fats. In these respects they are similar to the usual meat sauces and desserts. To make icings, fillings, and dessert sauces part of the Swank low-fat diet and still retain their desirability, we have eliminated as much fat as possible and substituted oils and other ingredients to maintain their consistency and texture.

Those who feel strongly about refined sugars will note that in many recipes there is a sizable amount of granulated or brown sugar. However, the amounts per serving usually remain well below 1 1/2 teaspoons, and in some recipes there is no refined sugar. Sugar products should be eliminated or reduced if patients have a sensitivity to sugar.

PEANUT BUTTER BROILED ICING

1 tablespoon oil
1/2 cup packed brown sugar
1/3 cup nonprocessed peanut butter
2 tablespoons skim milk
1/3 cup chopped nuts

Mix oil, sugar, and peanut butter. Add milk and nuts, and stir well. Spread on warm cake. Place 4 inches from broiler and broil until top begins to bubble. Yields icing for one 9″ × 12″ loaf

Fat: None
Oil: Total—15 teaspoons

BUTTERSCOTCH ICING

1 cup packed brown sugar
1/2 cup skim milk
1 tablespoon oil
2 cups confectioners' sugar
1 teaspoon vanilla

Heat brown sugar, milk, and oil, stirring until sugar is dissolved. Bring to a boil. Remove from heat. Stir in confectioners' sugar and vanilla. Beat until creamy. Yields icing for two 8-inch layers or one 19″ × 13″ loaf

Fat: None
Oil: Total—3 teaspoons

BROWN SUGAR MARSHMALLOW ICING

12 marshmallows
2 cups packed brown sugar
1/2 cup skim milk
2 tablespoons oil

Cut marshmallows into small cubes. In a covered pan on low heat cook the brown sugar and milk without stirring for 3 minutes. Remove lid and continue cooking to the soft ball stage (238° F). Remove from heat. Add marshmallows and oil, stirring until marshmallows are melted. Cook, and beat to spreading consistency. Thin with milk if necessary. Yields icing for two 8-inch layers

Fat: None
Oil: Total—6 teaspoons

MARSHMALLOW ICING OR FILLING

2 egg whites
1 cup light corn syrup
1/8 teaspoon salt
1 teaspoon vanilla

Combine egg whites, corn syrup, and salt in top of double boiler. Place over rapidly boiling water and cook, beating constantly with electric mixer or rotary beater for 7 minutes or until frosting stands in peaks. Remove from heat and add vanilla, beating well. Yields icing for two 8-inch layers

Fat: None
Oil: None

GLAZING ICING

2 cups confectioners' sugar
3 tablespoons boiling water
1 teaspoon vanilla

In medium-sized bowl combine sugar and boiling water. Beat until a smooth, spreading consistency. Add vanilla. Yields glazing for two 8-inch layers

Fat: None
Oil: None

CHOCOLATE ICING

1 1/2 cups confectioners' sugar
2 tablespoons chocolate syrup
Skim milk

Combine sugar and chocolate syrup. Add enough milk to obtain a spreading consistency. Yields icing for one 9″ × 12″ loaf

Fat: None
Oil: None
(chocolate syrup—6 teaspoons)

THREE-MINUTE ICING OR TOPPING

2 egg whites
1/2 cup sugar
1/8 teaspoon salt
2 tablespoons cold water
1 teaspoon vanilla or almond extract

Mix all ingredients except flavoring extract in top of a double boiler until blended. Place over boiling water. Beat with a wire whisk or electric mixer for 3 minutes or until stiff. Remove top of double boiler from the boiling water and add vanilla or almond extract to frosting. Beat well. Spread on pie, cake, jellied fruit, or molded desserts. This can be used as a substitute for whipped cream or meringue. Yields icing for one 8-inch layer cake or pie

Fat: None
Oil: None

MOCHA TOPPING

1/4 cup ice water
1/4 cup nonfat dry milk powder
1/4 teaspoon vanilla
1 tablespoon sugar
1 teaspoon instant decaffeinated coffee

Beat together ice water and nonfat dry milk powder with a rotary beater or electric mixer until mixture is stiff and stands in peaks. Gradually beat in vanilla, sugar, and decaffeinated instant coffee. Yields 1 cup

Fat: None
Oil: None

BROWN SUGAR TOPPING

1 egg white
3/4 cup packed brown sugar
3/4 cup dark or light corn syrup
2 tablespoons cold water
Flavoring (optional)

Mix all ingredients in top of double boiler. Place over boiling water and beat for 5 minutes or until thick. Yields 1 cup

Fat: None
Oil: None

CAROB CREAM FROSTING

1 tablespoon oil
1/3 cup dark or light corn syrup
1/4 teaspoon salt
1/2 teaspoon vanilla
1/2 cup carob powder
1–2 tablespoons skim milk
3 cups confectioners' sugar

Blend oil, corn syrup, salt, and vanilla. Stir in carob powder. Add milk and confectioners' sugar alternately, beating until smooth and creamy after each addition. Add enough milk to make a good spreading consistency. Yields icing for two 9-inch layers

Fat: None
Oil: Total—3 teaspoons

HONEY FROSTING

1/2 cup honey
1/8 teaspoon salt
1 egg white
1 teaspoon lemon juice

Place honey and salt in a small saucepan, bring to the boiling point, and boil 2 minutes or until the honey forms a soft ball when dropped into cold water (238° F). Pour honey in a thin stream over stiffly beaten egg white, continuing to beat until all the honey is added and the frosting stands in peaks. Blend in lemon juice. Yields frosting for two 8-inch layers

Fat: None
Oil: None

HOT RUM SAUCE

1 cup sugar
1 cup water
2 slices lemon
1 slice orange
1 stick cinnamon
1 whole clove
1 tablespoon cornstarch (optional)
1/4–1/2 cup rum or brandy

In a medium-sized saucepan mix the sugar, water, lemon, orange, and spices; bring to a boil and simmer for 5 minutes. Strain. If a thicker consistency is desired, mix cornstarch with 2 tablespoons of the cooled sauce. Heat the remaining sauce to a boil, stir in the cornstarch, and cook, stirring, until thickened. Add rum or brandy after sauce is removed from heat. Yields 1 1/2 cups

Fat: None
Oil: None

ORANGE SAUCE

Peel of 1/2 lemon, grated
Grated peel and juice of 2 oranges
2 tablespoons granulated sugar
2 tablespoons confectioners' sugar
2 tablespoons Cointreau or brandy

Combine lemon and orange peels and orange juice in a small saucepan with 2 tablespoons of granulated sugar and 2 tablespoons confectioners' sugar. Bring to a boil. Add the Cointreau or brandy. Yields 1 cup

Fat: None
Oil: None

HARD SAUCE FOR PLUM PUDDING

2 tablespoons butter-flavored oil
2–3 tablespoons brandy or rum
1/2 cup confectioners' sugar
1 egg white (optional)

Combine oil and brandy or rum, and mix with electric mixer. Gradually add the confectioners' sugar until thickened. Beat in egg white if a fluffier consistency is desired. Chill before serving. Yields 2/3 cup

Fat: None
Oil: Total—6 teaspoons

CHAPTER 30

Candy

The choice of commercial candies is limited since the use of butter, chocolate, and cocoa butter is prohibited on this diet. Gelatin candies, jelly beans, and hard fruit candies are available commercially and are not restricted. However, we have tried to help your sweet tooth by including a few recipes you might enjoy. If you are tempted with carob candy bars, it is unfortunate to note that they usually contain cocoa butter and sometimes palm oil. Be sure to read the labels carefully to check the contents of a tempting confection to make sure that there is no forbidden food among the ingredients. If you are in doubt about the ingredients, then avoid the temptation.

PEANUT BUTTER FUDGE

2 cups sugar
2 tablespoons light corn syrup
1/4 teaspoon salt
2/3 cup canned evaporated skim milk
1/2 cup nonprocessed peanut butter
1 teaspoon vanilla

Combine sugar, corn syrup, salt, and skim milk. Cook over low heat until sugar is dissolved, stirring occasionally. Increase heat to Medium and bring to a boil. Cook to soft ball stage (238° F), stirring occasionally. Remove from heat, stir in peanut butter and vanilla, and continue to stir until it begins to thicken. Pour into a 9-inch square pan. Cool and cut into squares. Yields 36 pieces

Fat: None
Oil: Total—12 teaspoons; per square—1/3 teaspoon

PEANUT BUTTER SQUARES

1/2 cup sugar
1/2 cup corn syrup
3/4 cup nonprocessed peanut butter
Pinch of salt
1 cup crisp rice cereal
2 cups cornflakes
1 teaspoon vanilla

Stir sugar and corn syrup in pan over low heat. When sugar is dissolved, quickly add peanut butter, salt, cereals, and vanilla. Mix and spread in a 9″ × 15″ pan. When cold, cut into squares. Yields 36 squares

Fat: None
Oil: Total—18 teaspoons; per 1 piece—1/2 teaspoon

CAROB FUDGE

6 tablespoons carob powder
2 cups granulated or packed brown sugar
2/3 cup skim milk
2 tablespoons oil
1/4 teaspoon salt
1 1/2 teaspoons vanilla

In a medium saucepan combine carob powder with sugar; add milk, oil, and salt. Cook to soft ball stage (238° F on a candy thermometer). Add vanilla. Beat until mixture is creamy. Pour into a well-oiled 8″ × 9″ pan. Cut into squares when cool. Yields 36 pieces

Fat: None
Oil: Total—6 teaspoons; per 1 piece—1/6 teaspoon

PEANUT BRITTLE

2 cups sugar
1/2 cup water
1 cup light corn syrup
2 cups raw peanuts
Dash of salt
1 teaspoon baking soda
1 teaspoon vanilla

Combine sugar, water, and corn syrup in large, heavy saucepan; boil until hard ball stage (300° F on a candy thermometer) is reached. Remove from heat; add peanuts and salt. Mixture will be quite thick. Return to heat and boil until mixture and nuts are golden brown. Be very careful not to burn. Remove from heat; add baking soda and vanilla. Pour onto oiled cookie sheet and smooth out until thin. Crack when cooled. Yields 2 pounds

Fat: None
Oil: Total—40 teaspoons

NORWEGIAN "BURNED ALMONDS"

1 cup sugar
1 tablespoon water
1 cup blanched almonds

Combine sugar and water in heavy skillet over medium-high heat. Stir constantly until sugar begins to dissolve. Add almonds and continue to stir until sugar turns golden brown and the almonds are shiny. This will take approximately 15 minutes. Pour onto cookie sheet or aluminum foil and quickly separate almonds. Let cool. Remove from cookie sheet or aluminum foil and store in a tightly covered jar. Yields 1 cup

Fat: None
Oil: Total—20 teaspoons

SPICED NUTS

2 cups confectioners' sugar
1/2 cup cornstarch
2 teaspoons salt
1 teaspoon nutmeg
1/4 cup cinnamon
2 teaspoons ginger
1 tablespoon ground cloves
1 egg white
2 tablespoons cold water
1 3/4 cups whole or half nutmeats

Preheat oven to 250° F. Stir together thoroughly sugar, cornstarch, salt, and spices. Beat egg white lightly and add cold water. Place nuts in a wire strainer and dip into egg mixture until each nut is well coated. Drain. Roll nuts in small amount of the spice mixture. Spread one half of the remaining spice mixture in a shallow pan and add nuts, separating each nut. Cover nuts with remaining spices and bake for 3 hours. Remove from the oven and sift, saving remaining spice mixture for future use. Yields 1 pound

Fat: None
Oil: Total—42 teaspoons

CHERRY DIVINITY

2 cups sugar
2/3 cup water
1/2 cup light corn syrup
2 egg whites, stiffly beaten
1 teaspoon vanilla
Dash of salt
3/4 cup candied cherries, thinly sliced

Bring 1/2 cup sugar and 1/3 cup water to a boil, and boil until a small amount of syrup forms a slightly firm ball in cold water (240° F). While this mixture is boiling, bring remaining sugar, water, and corn syrup to a boil, and boil until a small amount of syrup forms a hard ball in cold water (252° F). Remove first syrup from heat and cool slightly. Pour slowly over egg whites, beating constantly until mixture loses its gloss, 1 1/2 minutes. Add second syrup slowly, beating as before. Fold in vanilla, salt, and cherries, and turn immediately into an 8″ × 8″ oiled pan. Cool until firm. Cut in 1 1/2″ × 1″ pieces. Yields 2 dozen pieces

Fat: None
Oil: None

APPLE CONFECTIONS

2 1/2 cups applesauce
4 envelopes unflavored gelatin
4 cups granulated sugar
1 teaspoon vanilla
1 cup chopped nuts
Confectioners' sugar

Combine 1 cup of the applesauce with the gelatin. Mix remaining applesauce with the granulated sugar. Combine both mixtures. Cook for 15 minutes; remove from heat and add vanilla and nuts. Pour into an 8½″ × 13″ pan and cool. Cut into squares and roll in confectioners' sugar. Yields 48 squares

Fat: None
Oil: Total—24 teaspoons; per 2 candies—1 teaspoon

ORANGE DELIGHT

3 tablespoons unflavored gelatin
½ cup cold water
2 cups sugar
½ cup hot water
6 tablespoons orange juice
1 8-ounce can crushed pineapple, drained (⅔ cup)
Confectioners' sugar

Soften gelatin in cold water. Combine sugar with hot water and stir over moderate heat until sugar has dissolved. Bring to boil and boil for 10 minutes without stirring. Add softened gelatin. Stir until just dissolved, then simmer slowly for an additional 10 minutes. Stir in orange juice. Let cool. Blend in pineapple. Rinse an 8″ × 8″ pan with cold water and pour in mixture. Chill 4–6 hours. Cut into 1-inch squares and turn in confectioners' sugar. Yields 64 squares

Fat: None
Oil: None

PINEAPPLE KISSES

2 egg whites
½ cup granulated sugar
½ teaspoon vanilla or almond extract
1 8-ounce can pineapple chunks
Slivered almonds or chopped walnuts

Preheat oven to 300° F. Beat egg whites until stiff. Add sugar gradually and continue beating. Add flavoring. Rinse off cookie sheet, leaving the surface damp. Cover cookie sheet with a piece of unglazed paper. About 2 inches apart, spread 1-inch rounds of meringue. Top each round with a piece of well-drained pineapple and cover with meringue. Sprinkle with slivered almonds or chopped walnut meats. Bake 45–50 minutes. Yields 1 dozen

Fat: None
Oil: None
Topping: 1/4 cup walnuts—6 teaspoons oil
1/4 cup almonds—5 teaspoons oil

POPCORN BALLS

1 1/4 cups granulated sugar
1 1/4 cups packed brown sugar
1/2 cup light corn syrup
2/3 cup water
1 tablespoon oil
3 1/2 cups popped corn
1 1/4 teaspoons salt

Place granulated and brown sugars, corn syrup, and water in a saucepan. Stir over moderate heat until sugar is dissolved. Add oil and continue cooking, without stirring, to soft ball stage (240° F on a candy thermometer). Put popped corn in a large bowl and sprinkle with salt. Pour the hot syrup over popped corn and mix thoroughly. Shape in small balls, wrap in waxed paper. Yields 6

Fat: None
Oil: Total—3 teaspoons; per popcorn ball—negligible

CHAPTER 31

Menus for One Week

The following menus have been planned to give you an example of how to distribute the fat and oil throughout the day, how to obtain variety, and how to utilize some of the recipes included in this book.

We have attempted to keep the menus simple for those patients who are working or suffering from fatigue. They are meant to give you ideas and can be adjusted to suit your preferences. Desserts have been included so that you can see how to incorporate them into a daily menu. Leftovers have not been utilized, nor have the calorie and protein amounts been indicated.

The number of teaspoons of fat and oil are indicated in separate columns. Amounts are indicated mainly for those foods that have to be measured for their fat and oil content. Beverages are not indicated, with the exception of skim milk.

We have not included low calorie menus in this edition. It has been our experience that very obese patients do not successfully lose weight by using low calorie menus of nine hundred to a thousand calories per day. To reduce the calories to a sufficient level for weight reduction in these patients, it would be necessary to lower the calorie intake to fewer than five hundred calories. Careful supervision is necessary when the calories are reduced to this level. It is for this reason that we have eliminated all low-calorie menus.

After a patient carefully follows the diet for at least six months, we suggest more drastic programs that are carefully monitored if the patient is obese and desires to lose weight.

Those overweight patients who do not lose weight on our regular low-fat diet have almost always failed to lose weight on our low-calorie, low-fat diet of nine hundred to a thousand calories per day.

SAMPLE MENUS

SUNDAY

	Serving Size	Teaspoons of FAT	Teaspoons of OIL
Breakfast			
Pancakes* with syrup	4	1/2	
1 egg, poached	1	1	
Juice			
Coffee or tea (optional)	1 cup		
Cod-liver oil and 1 multiple vitamin			1
Snack			
Skim milk	8 ounces		
Ry-Krisp			
Lunch			
Pasta Salad*	1 serving		4
Saltine crackers	2–3		
Skim milk	8 ounces		
Snack			
1 piece fresh fruit			
Nuts to equal 1 teaspoon oil	10–12 peanuts, almonds, cashews		1
Dinner			
Teriyaki Chicken*			
Stir-Fried Vegetables*	1 serving		1
Rice			
Fruit sorbet			
	TOTAL	1 1/2	7

MONDAY

	Serving Size	Teaspoons of FAT	Teaspoons of OIL
Breakfast			
Breakfast drink—Banana strawberry*			
Whole wheat toast with old-fashioned (nonprocessed) peanut butter	2 teaspoons		1

	Serving Size	Teaspoons of FAT	OIL
Cod-liver oil and 1 multiple vitamin			1
Snack			
Skim milk	8 ounces		
Lunch			
Turkey sandwich (white meat only) with 2 teaspoons mayonnaise			1
1 piece fresh fruit			
1 glass skim milk	8 ounces		
2 Chewy Oatmeal Cookies*	2		1 1/2
Snack			
Nuts to equal 1 teaspoon oil	10–12 peanuts, almonds, cashews		1
Dinner			
Salmon Patties*	2 servings	1/3	2
Assorted vegetable salad with 2 teaspoons dressing	2 teaspoons		1
Baked potato			
Fresh fruit			
	TOTAL	1/3	8 1/2

TUESDAY

	Serving Size	FAT	OIL
Breakfast			
1/2 cup Granola*	1/2 cup		4
Fruit or juice			
Coffee or tea (optional)			
Cod-liver oil and 1 multiple vitamin			1
Snack			
1 piece fresh fruit			
Lunch			
Tuna fish sandwich on whole wheat bread (water-packed tuna) with 2 teaspoons mayonnaise	2 teaspoons		1

	Serving Size	*Teaspoons of* FAT	OIL
1 piece fresh fruit			
Skim milk	8 ounces		
Snack			
Nuts to equal 1 teaspoon oil	10–12 peanuts, almonds, cashews		1
Dinner			
Easy Oven Chicken*	1 serving		1½
Assorted green salad with 2 teaspoons Omar's Special Dressing*	2 teaspoons		1
Angel Food Cake*			
	TOTAL	0	9½

WEDNESDAY

Breakfast			
Whole wheat toast with nonprocessed peanut butter	2 teaspoons		1
Cold cereal and skim milk			
1 glass juice			
Tea or coffee (optional)			
Cod-liver oil and 1 multiple vitamin			1
Snack			
Skim milk with 1 tablespoon chocolate syrup	8 ounces		
Lunch			
Peanut butter and jelly sandwich	4 teaspoons		2
1 piece fresh fruit			
Skim milk	8 ounces		
Snack			
Nuts to equal 1 teaspoon oil	10–12 peanuts, almonds, cashews		1

	Serving Size	Teaspoons of FAT	Teaspoons of OIL
Dinner			
Fish-and-chips			
White fish—deep-fried using Beer Batter*			app. 2
Oven-Fried Potatoes*	1 serving		1½
Assorted fresh vegetable salad with lemon juice dressing			
Fresh fruit			
TOTAL		0	8½

THURSDAY

	Serving Size	Teaspoons of FAT	Teaspoons of OIL
Breakfast			
1 poached egg	1	1	
Whole wheat toast and jam			
Fresh fruit			
Coffee or tea (optional)	1 cup		
Cod-liver oil and 1 multiple vitamin			1
Snack			
Skim milk	8 ounces		
Lunch			
1 bowl Vegetable Soup* (or commercial dehydrated)			
Whole wheat roll (commercial)			
Fresh fruit			
1 Chocolate Brownie*	1		1¾
Snack			
Nuts to equal 1 teaspoon oil	10–12 peanuts, almonds, cashews		1
Dinner			
Teriyaki Shrimp*			
Steamed vegetables			
Baked potato or rice			
Fresh Apple Cake*	1 serving		1
TOTAL		1	4¾

	Serving Size	Teaspoons of FAT	OIL
FRIDAY			
Breakfast			
1 bagel with Yogurt Cream Cheese*			
Fresh fruit			
Skim milk	8 ounces		
Cod-liver oil and 1 multiple vitamin			1
Snack			
Skim milk	8 ounces		
Lunch			
Fresh vegetable salad with 4 teaspoons French Dressing*	4 teaspoons		2
Whole wheat roll or 2 saltine crackers			
1 glass skim milk	8 ounces		
2 Sugar Cookies*	2		2 2/3
Snack			
Fresh fruit			
Dinner			
Spaghetti with Meatless Spaghetti Sauce*	1 serving		1
Assorted vegetable salad with 2 teaspoons Russian Dressing*	3 teaspoons		1
French bread			
Fresh Raspberry Sherbet*			
	TOTAL	0	7 2/3

	Serving Size	Teaspoons of FAT	OIL
SATURDAY			
Breakfast			
Waffles*	1	1/6	1
Fresh fruit			
Skim milk	8 ounces		
Coffee or tea (optional)			
Cod-liver oil and 1 multiple vitamin			1

	Serving Size	Teaspoons of FAT	OIL
Snack			
1 piece Pumpkin Bread*			1 1/2
Skim milk	8 ounces		
Lunch			
Chicken salad in Pita Bread			
Fresh fruit			
Skim milk	8 ounces		
Snack			
Nuts to equal 1 teaspoon oil	10–12 peanuts, almonds, cashews		1
Dinner			
Tuna Pot Pie*	1 serving		1
Assorted green salad with 2 teaspoons Omar's Special Dressing*	2 teaspoons		1
Roll			
Apple Crisp*			1 1/2
	TOTAL	1/6	8

BIBLIOGRAPHY

1. Jack C. Drummond. *The Englishman's Food: A History of Five Centuries of English Diet.* London: Jonathon Cape, 1939.
2. U.S. Department of Agriculture. *Consumption of Food in the United States—1909–1948.* Washington, D.C.: U.S. Department of Agriculture, 1949.
3. Food and Agriculture Organization of the United Nations. *The State of Food and Agriculture in 1948.* Washington, D.C.: Food and Agriculture Organization of the United Nations, 1948.
4. ———. *The State of Food and Agriculture.* Rome: Food and Agriculture Organization of the United Nations, 1964.
5. Remarks by Dr. David L. Call, professor of Food Economics and director of Cooperative Extension at Cornell University, at the Newspaper Editors Conference, October 7, 1975.
6. Alan E. Banik. *Hunza Land.* Long Beach, Calif.: Whitehorn Publishing Company, 1960. Alan E. Banik, and Renee Taylor.
7. William Durant. *History of Civilization.* Vol. 3, *Caesar and Christ.* New York: Simon & Schuster, 1944.
8. Armin Ackermann. "Die Multiple Sklerose in der Schweiz." *Schweiz Medical Wochenschr* 61 (1931):1245.
9. Roy L. Swank. "Multiple Sclerosis: A Correlation of Its Incidence with Dietary Fat." *American Journal of the Medical Sciences* 220 (1950):421–30.
10. Roy L. Swank et al. "Multiple Sclerosis in Rural Norway: Its Geographic and Occupational Incidence in Relation to Nutrition." *New England Journal of Medicine* 246 (1952):721–28.
11. Milton Alter. "Multiple Sclerosis in Mexico." *Archives of Neurology* 23 (1970):451–59.
12. Uri Leibowitz, Esther Kahana, and Milton Alter. "The Changing Frequency of Multiple Sclerosis in Israel." *Archives of Neurology* 29 (1973):107–10.
13. Uri Leibowitz. *Multiple Sclerosis: Clues to its Cause.* Amsterdam: North Holland Publishing Company, 1973.

14. Roy L. Swank. *A Biochemical Basis of Multiple Sclerosis.* Springfield, Ill.: Charles C. Thomas, 1961.
15. Milton Alter, Muhammond Yamoor, and Mary Harshe. "Multiple Sclerosis and Nutrition." *Archives of Neurology* 31 (1974):267–72.
16. James H. D. Millar et al. "Doubleblind Trial of Linoleate Supplement of Diet in Multiple Sclerosis." *British Medical Journal* 1 (1973):765–68.
17. Shigeo Okiaka et al. "Multiple Sclerosis and Allied Diseases in Japan." *Neurology* 8 (1958):756–63.
18. Robert H. Dworkin et al. "Linoleic Acid and Multiple Sclerosis: A Reanalysis of Three Double-Blind Trials." *Neurology* 34 (1984):1441–45.
19. Eustace L. Benjaman. "Report of Two Hundred Necropsies on Natives in Okinawa." *United States Navy Medical Bulletin* 46 (1946):495–500.
20. William F. Enos, James C. Beyer, and Robert H. Holmes. "Pathogenesis of Coronary Disease in American Soldiers Killed in Korea." *Journal of the American Medical Association* 158 (1955):912–14.
21. Haqvin Malmros. "The Relationship of Nutrition to Health. A Statistical Study of the Effect of Wartime on Arteriosclerosis, Cardiosclerosis, Tuberculosis, and Diabetes." *Acta Medica Scandinavica* 246 (1950):137–53.
22. Axel Strom, and Adelsten Jensen. "Mortality from Circulatory Disease in Norway." *Lancet* 1 (1951):126–28.
23. Ancel Keys. "Atherosclerosis: A Problem in Newer Public Health." *Journal of Mount Sinai Hospital* 20 (1953):119–39.
24. Ancel Keys, and Joseph T. Anderson. "The Relationship of Diet to the Development of Atherosclerosis." *Publication 338 of the National Academy of Science, National Research Council, Washington, D.C.,* 1955.
25. Robert D. Briggs et al. "Myocardial Infarction in Patients Treated with Sippy and Other High-Milk Diets." *Circulation* 21 (1960):538–42.
26. George Christakis et al. "Effect of the Anti-Coronary Club Program on Coronary Heart Disease Risk Factor Status." *Journal of the American Medical Association* 198 (1966):597–607.
27. Israel S. Wechsler. "Statistics of Multiple Sclerosis." *American Medical Association Archives of Neurology and Psychiatry* 8 (1922):59–63.
28. George Schaltenbrand. "Discussion on the Demyelinating Disease." *Proceedings of the First International Congress of Neuropathy* Rome, 1952.
29. Charles C. Limburg. "Geographic Distribution of Multiple Sclerosis and Its Estimated Prevalence in the United States." *Proceedings of the Association for Research of Nervous and Mental Disease* 28 (1950):15.

30. Thomas C. Guthrie. "Visual and Motor Changes in Patients with Multiple Sclerosis." *American Medical Association Archives of Neurology and Psychiatry* 65 (1951):437–51.
31. Wesley Watson. "Effect of Lowering Body Temperature on the Symptoms and Signs of Multiple Sclerosis." *New England Journal of Medicine* 261 (1959):1253–59.
32. Carl E. Hopkins, and Roy L. Swank. "Multiple Sclerosis and Local Weather." *American Medical Association Archives of Neurology and Psychiatry* 74 (1955):203–07.
33. F. Curtius et al. "Multiple Sklerose und Erbanlange." *Zeitschrift für die Geselschaft Neurology und Psychiatry* 160 (1937):226–27.
34. Douglas McAlpine et al. "Familial Incidence of Disseminated Sclerosis and Its Significance." *Brain* 74 (1951):191–232.
35. Roland P. Mackay. "Familial Occurrence of Multiple Sclerosis and Its Implications." *Annals of Internal Medicine* 33 (1950):298–320.
36. James H. D. Millar et al. "Familial Incidence of Disseminated Sclerosis in Northern Ireland." *Ulster Medical Journal* 2 (1954):23–29.
37. Adele D. Sadovnick, and Patrick MacLeod. "The Familial Nature of Multiple Sclerosis: Empiric Recurrence Risks for First, Second and Third Degree Relatives of Patients." *Neurology* 31 (1981):1039–41.
38. Ludwig V. Chiavacci, Hans Hoff, and Necmittin Polvan. "Frequency of Multiple Sclerosis in Greater New York." *American Medical Association Archives of Neurology and Psychiatry* 64 (1950):546–53.
39. Preliminary Report of the Study of the Prevalence of Multiple Sclerosis in Los Angeles, King and Pierce Counties. *Neurological Diseases Environmental Studies.* Director Roger Detel, M.D., 1976.
40. Roy L. Swank, and Robert B. Bourdillon. "Multiple Sclerosis: Assessment of Treatment with a Modified Low-Fat Diet." *Journal of Nervous and Mental Disease* 131 (1960):468–88.
41. Walter B. Matthews et al. *McAlpine's Multiple Sclerosis.* Edinburgh, London, Melbourne, and New York: Churchill Livingston, 1985.
42. Michael L. Daley, Roy L. Swank, and Catherine M. Ellison. "Flicker Fusion Thresholds in Multiple Sclerosis: A Functional Measure of Neurological Damage." *Archives of Neurology* 36 (1979):292–95.
43. Michael L. Daley, and Roy L. Swank. "Qualitative Posturography: Use in Multiple Sclerosis." *IEEE Transaction on Biomedical Engineering* 9 (1981):668–71.
44. Ephraim Field, and Greta Joyce. "Simplified Laboratory Test for Multiple Sclerosis." *Lancet* 2 (1985):27–28.
45. Cherry H. Tamblyn. "Red Cell Electrophoretic Mobility Test for Early Diagnosis of Multiple Sclerosis." *Neurological Research* 2 (1980):69–83.
46. Marta Elian, and Geoffrey Dean. "To Tell or Not to Tell the Diagnosis of Multiple Sclerosis." *Lancet* 2 (1985):27–28.
47. Isabelle Korn-Lubetzki et al. "Activity of Multiple Sclerosis During

Pregnancy and Puerperium." *Annals of Neurology* 16 (1984):229–31.

48. Sigrid Poser, and Wolfgang Poser. "Multiple Sclerosis and Gestation." *Neurology* 33 (1983):1422–27.
49. Leo Alexander et al. "Blood and Plasma Transfusions in Multiple Sclerosis." *Transactions of the Association of Neurological Diseases, Multiple Sclerosis and the Demyelinating Diseases* (1950):1978.
50. M. Demole. "Alimentation Militare, 1942." *Schweiz Medical Wochenschr* 78 (1943):827.
51. Roy L. Swank. "Multiple Sclerosis: Twenty Years on a Low-Fat Diet." *Archives of Neurology* 23 (1970):460–74; also *Archives of Neurology and Psychiatry* 69 (1953):91–103.
52. John F. Kurtzke. "Rating Neurologic Impairment in Multiple Sclerosis: An Expanded Disability Status Scale." *Neurology* 33 (1983):1444.
53. Paul Thygesen. *The Course of Disseminated Sclerosis.* Copenhagen: Rosenkilde and Bagger, 1953.
54. Leo Alexander, Austin W. Berkeley, and Alene M. Alexander. "Prognosis and Treatment of Multiple Sclerosis—Quantitative Nosometric Study." *Journal of the American Medical Association* 166 (1958):1943–48.
55. R. S. Allison. "Survival in Disseminated Sclerosis: A Clinical Study of a Series of Cases First Seen Twenty Years Ago." *Brain* 73 (1950):103–20.
56. Richard Brickner, and Norman Q. Brill. "Dietetic and Related Studies on Multiple Sclerosis." *American Medical Association Archives of Neurology and Psychiatry* 46 (1946):16–35.
57. Roland P. Mackay, and Asao Hirando. "Forms of Benign Multiple Sclerosis." *Archives of Neurology* 17 (1967):588–600.
58. Tibor Lehoczky et al. "Forme bénigne' de la sclérose en plaque." *Presse Medicale* 71 (1963):2294–96.
59. Alexander MacLean, and Joseph Beckson. "Mortality and Disability in Multiple Sclerosis." *Journal of the American Medical Association* 146 (1951):1367–69.
60. Ragnar Miller. "Studies of Disseminated Sclerosis." *Acta Medica Scandinavica* 222 (1949):1–214.
61. Veterans Administration Multiple Sclerosis Study Group. "Five-Year Follow-Up on Multiple Sclerosis." *Archives of Neurology* 11 (1964):583–92.
62. James W. Dawson. "The Histology of Disseminated Sclerosis." *Review of Neurology and Psychiatry* 15 (1917):47–66.
63. Giorgio Macchi. "Pathology of Blood Vessels in Multiple Sclerosis." *Journal of Neuropathology and Experimental Neurology* 13 (1954):378–84.
64. Tracy J. Putnam. "Evidence of Vascular Occlusion in Multiple Sclero-

sis and Encephalomyelitis." *Archives of Neurology and Psychiatry* 37 (1937):1298–1321.

65. Robert S. Dow, and George Berglund. "Vascular Pattern of Lesions of Multiple Sclerosis." *Archives of Neurology and Psychiatry* 47 (1942):1–18.
66. Tore Broman. "A Supravital Analysis of Disorders in the Cerebral Vascular Permeability in Man." *Acta Medica Scandinavica* 118 (1944):1986.
67. ———. "Supravital Analysis of Disorders in the Cerebral Vascular Permeability. II. Two Cases of Multiple Sclerosis." *Acta Psychiatrica et Neurologica* 46 (1947):58–71.
68. Armin Haeren et al. "A Study of the Blood Cerebrospinal Fluid-Brain Barrier in Multiple Sclerosis." *Neurology* 14 (1964):345–54.
69. David O. Davis, and Barry D. Pressman. "Computerized Tomography of the Brain." *Radiologic Clinics of North America* 12 (1974):297–313.
70. Leon Weisberg. "Contrast Enhancement Visualized by Computerized Tomography in Acute Multiple Sclerosis." *Computer Tomography* 5 (1981):292–300.
71. Louis Bakay. *The Blood Brain Barrier.* Springfield, Ill.: Charles C. Thomas, 1956.
72. ———. "Relationship Between Cerebral Vascularity and P32 Uptake." *American Medical Association Archives of Neurology and Psychiatry* 78 (1957):29–36.
73. Thaddeus Samorajski, and Robert A. Moody. "Changes in Blood-Brain Barrier After Exposure of the Brain." *American Medical Association Archives of Neurology and Psychiatry* 78 (1957):369–76.
74. Tore Broman. *The Permeability of the Cerebrospinal Vessels in Normal and Pathological Conditions.* Copenhagen: Ejnor Munlisgaard, 1949.
75. Roy L. Swank, and Raymond F. Hain. "The Effects of Different-Sized Emboli on the Vascular System and Parenchyma of the Brain." *Journal of Neuropathology and Experimental Neurology* 11 (1952):280–99.
76. Miles Bouton. "Cerebral Air Embolism and Vital Staining." *Archives of Neurology and Psychiatry* 43 (1940):1151–62.
77. James Lee. "Effects of Air Embolism on Permeability of Cerebral Blood Vessels." *Neurology* 9 (1959):619–25.
78. Revis C. Lewis, and Roy L. Swank. "Effect of Cerebral Microembolism on the Perivascular Neuroglia." *Journal of Neuropathology and Experimental Neurology* 12 (1953):57–63.
79. Jan Cammermeyer, and Roy L. Swank. "Acute Cerebral Changes in Experimental Canine Fat Embolism." *Experimental Neurology* 1 (1959):214–32.
80. Roy L. Swank, and Walter Marchand. "Combat Neuroses: Develop-

ment of Combat Exhaustion." *Archives of Neurology and Psychiatry* 55 (1946):236; and Roy L. Swank. "Combat Exhaustion: A Description and Statistical Analysis of Causes, Symptoms, and Signs." *Journal of Nervous and Mental Disease* 109 (1949):475–508.

81. Roy L. Swank, John G. Roth, and David C. Woody. "Cerebral Blood Flow and Red Cell Delivery in Normal Subjects and in Multiple Sclerosis." *Neurological Research* 5 (1983):37–59.
82. G. Gomirat. "Alternazioni dei capillari in malati di sclerose multipla e loro significato." *Rivista di patholgi e nervi* 53 (1939):148–66.
83. Nugret Mutlu. "Capillarioscopic Studies in Cases of Multiple Sclerosis and Other Neuropsychiatric Disorders." *American Medical Association Archives of Neurology and Psychiatry* 66 (1951):363–67.
84. Wilbur Rucker. "Sheathing of Retina Veins in Multiple Sclerosis." *Proceedings of the Association for Research of Nervous and Mental Disorders* 28 (1950):396.
85. Magnus Haarr. "Periphlebitis Tetinae in Association with Multiple Sclerosis." *Acta Psychiatrica et Neurologica—Scandinavica* 28 (1953):175–90.
86. Ray C. Franklin, and Richard Brickner. "Vasospasm Associated with Multiple Sclerosis." *American Medical Association Archives of Neurology and Psychiatry* 58 (1947):125–62.
87. Gerald Grain, and William Jahsman. "Significance of Peripheral Vascular Changes in Multiple Sclerosis." *Proceedings of the Association Research of Nervous and Mental Disorders* 28 (1950):216.
88. Maurice H. Shulman et al. "Capillary Resistance Studies in Multiple Sclerosis." *Journal of Neuropathology and Experimental Neurology* 9 (1950):420–29.
89. Roy L. Swank. "Subcutaneous Hemorrhages in Multiple Sclerosis." *Neurology* 8 (1958):497–98.
90. Melvin Knisely et al. "Sludged Blood." *Science* 106 (1947):431–39.
91. Leon Roizin et al. "Preliminary Studies of Sludged Blood in Multiple Sclerosis." *Neurology* 3 (1953):250–60.
92. Torben Fogg. "On the Pathogenesis of Multiple Sclerosis." *Acta Psychiatrica et Neurologica* 74 (1951):22–31.
93. Shaul Feldman, Gabriel Izak, and David Nelken. "Blood Coagulation Studies and Serotonin Determination in Serum and Cerebrospinal Fluid in Multiple Sclerosis." *Acta Psychiatrica et Neurologica—Scandinavica* 32 (1957):37–49.
94. Morton Nathanson, and Phillip Savitsky. "Platelet Adhesive Index Studies in Multiple Sclerosis and Other Neurologic Disorders." *Bulletin of the New York Academy of Medicine* 28 (1952):462–69.
95. Ephraim J. Field and E. A. Caspary. "Behavior of Blood Platelets in Multiple Sclerosis." *Lancet* 1 (1964):876–79.
96. Helen Wright et al. "Platelet Adhesiveness in Multiple Sclerosis." *Lancet* 2 (1965):1109–10.

97. Roy L. Swank. "Changes in the Blood Produced by a Fat Meal and by Intravenous Heparin." *American Journal of Physiology* 164 (1951):798–811.
98. Chester Cullen, and Roy L. Swank. "Intravascular Aggregation and Adhesiveness of the Blood Plasma Associated with Alimentary Lipemia and Injections of Large Molecular Substances: Effect on Blood-Brain Barrier." *Circulation* 9 (1954):335–46.
99. Roy L. Swank. "Effect of High Fat Feeding on Viscosity of the Blood." *Science* 120 (1954):427–28.
100. ———. "Effects of Fat on Blood Viscosity in Dogs." *Circulation Research* 4 (1956):579–85.
101. ———. "Changes in Blood of Dogs and Rabbits by High Fat Intake." *American Journal of Physiology* 196 (1959):473–77.
102. Roy L. Swank, and Haruomi Nakamura. "Oxygen Availability in Brain Tissues After Lipid Meals." *American Journal of Physiology* 198 (1960):217–20.
103. Roy L. Swank, and Rolf Engel. "Production of Convulsion in Hamsters by High Butterfat Intake." *Nature* 181 (1958):1214–17.
104. Roy L. Swank, and Haruomi Nakamura. "Convulsions in Hamsters After Cream Meals: Electroencephalograms and Available Cerebral Oxygen." *Archives of Neurology* 3 (1960):594–600.
105. Roy L. Swank, and Lavelle Jackson. "Electrolyte Changes in Blood, Urine and Tissues After Lipid and Other Test Meals." *American Journal of Physiology* 204 (1963):1071–76.
106. John Meyer, and Arthur Waltz. "Effects of Changes in Composition of Plasma on Pial Blood Flow." *Neurology* 9 (1959):728–40.
107. Hanlod Harders. "Neue Beobachtungen Zum Diätfehler." *Deutsche Gesellschaft für innere Medizin* 62 (1956):499.
108. Arthur U. Williams, Curtis Higginbotham, and Melvin H. Knisely. "Increased Blood Cell Agglutination Following Ingestion of Fat: A Factor Contributing to Cardiac Ischemia, Coronary Insufficiency and Anginal Pain." *Angiology* 8 (1957):29–39.
109. Eli Davis, and Jacob Landau. *Capillary Microscopy.* Springfield, Ill.: Charles C. Thomas, 1966.
110. Reid S. Connell, Roy L. Swank, and Michael C. Webb. "Pulmonary Microembolism After Blood Transfusion: An Electron Microscopic Study." *Annals of Surgery* 171 (1973):40–50.
111. ———. "The Development of Pulmonary Ultrastructural Lesions During Hemorrhagic Shock." *Journal of Trauma* 15 (1975):116–29.
112. Roy L. Swank, Wolfgang Hissen, and Jack H. Fellman. "5-Hydroxytryptamine (Serotonin) in Acute Hypotensive Shock." *American Journal of Physiology* 207 (1964):215–22.
113. Fredrick J. Seil, Arnold L. Leiman, and James M. Kelly III. "Neuroelectric Blocking Factors in Multiple Sclerosis and Normal Sera." *Archives of Neurology* 33 (1976):418–22.

114. Arthur Weil. "Study of Etiology of Multiple Sclerosis." *Journal of the American Medical Association* 97 (1931):1587–91.
115. Arthur Weil, Joseph Luhan, and Ben Balser. "Demonstration of Myelolytic Substances in Urine and Spinal Fluid in Nervous Diseases." *Transactions of the American Neurological Association* 61 (1935):142–46.
116. Fredrich Wolfgram, and Augustus S. Rose. "The In Vitro Action of Some Organic Acids on Myelin." *Journal of Neuropathology and Experimental Neurology* 17 (1958):399–407.
117. Murray B. Bornstein. "The Immunopathogenesis of Multiple Sclerosis." *Mount Sinai Journal of Medicine* 41 (1974):46–55.
118. Murray B. Bornstein, and Stanley M. Crain. "Functional Studies of Cultured Brain Tissues as Related to Demyelinative Disorders." *Science* 148 (1965):1242–46.
119. Guy Carels, and Jean A. Cerf. "Dépression réversible de l'activité réflexe de la moelle isolée de Grenouille par le sérum de sujets atteints de sclérose en plaques." *Revue Neurologique* 116 (1966):242.
120. Roy L. Swank et al. "Plasma in Multiple Sclerosis: A Possible Abnormality." *Plasma Therapy Transfusion Technology* 4 (1983):301–11.
121. Roy L. Swank et al. "Paper Chromatography of Blood Plasma in Multiple Sclerosis." *Proceedings of the Society for Experimental Biology and Medicine* 76 (1951):183–89.
122. Roy L. Swank. "Blood Plasma in Multiple Sclerosis. Periodic Abnormalities in Paper Chromatograms." *American Medical Association Archives of Neurology and Psychiatry* 69 (1953):281–92.
123. ———. "Effects of Fat Meal and Heparin on Blood Plasma Composition as Shown by Paper Chromatography." *Proceedings of the Society for Experimental Biology and Medicine* 75 (1950):850–54.
124. Ephraim J. Field, and Greta Joyce. "Simplified Laboratory Test for Multiple Sclerosis." *Lancet* 2 (1976):367–68.
125. Cherry H. Tamblyn et al. "Red Cell Electrophoretic Mobility Test for Early Diagnosis of Multiple Sclerosis." *Neurological Research* 2 (1980):69–83.
126. Geoffrey V. F. Seaman, Roy L. Swank, and Charles F. Zukoski. "Red Cell Membrane Differences in Multiple Sclerosis Are Acquired from the Plasma." *Lancet* 1 (1979):1139.
127. Geoffrey V. F. Seaman, Roy L. Swank, and Cherry H. Tamblyn. "Polystyrene Latex Particles as Indicators of Abnormal Plane Properties in Multiple Sclerosis." *Neurology* 34 (1984):547–49.
128. Adele D. Sadovnick, and Patrick M. J. MacLeod. "The Familial Nature of Multiple Sclerosis: Empiric Recurrence Risks for First, Second, and Third-Degree Relatives of Patients." *Neurology* 31 (1981):1039–41.
129. Hugh M. Sinclair. "Deficiency of Essential Fatty Acids and Atherosclerosis, etcetera." *Lancet* 1 (1956):381–83.

130. Robert H. S. Thompson. "A Biochemical Approach to the Problem of Multiple Sclerosis." *Proceedings of the Royal Society of Medicine* 59 (1966):269–76.
131. S. Geil et al. "The Fatty Acid Composition of Phospholipid from Platelets and Red Cells in Multiple Sclerosis." *Journal of Neurology, Neurosurgery and Psychiatry* 33 (1970):506-10.
132. J. Belin et al. "Linoleate Metabolism in Multiple Sclerosis." *Journal of Neurology, Neurosurgery and Psychiatry* 34 (1971):25–29.
133. Valerie C. Wilmot, and Roy L. Swank. "The Influence of Low-Fat Diet on Blood Lipid Levels in Health and in Multiple Sclerosis." *American Journal of the Medical Sciences* 223 (1952):25–34.
134. Roy L. Swank. "Blood Viscosity in Cerebrovascular Disease: Effects of Low-Fat Diet and Heparin." *Neurology* 9 (1959):553–60.
135. ———. "Alteration of Blood on Storage: Measurement of Adhesiveness of 'Aging' Platelets and Leukocytes and Their Removal by Filtration." *New England Journal of Medicine* 256 (1961):728–33.
136. ———. "Adhesiveness of Platelets and Leukocytes During Acute Exsanguination." *American Journal of Physiology* 202 (1962):261–64.

INDEX

Italicized page numbers refer to figures.

RECIPE INDEX